Annotated Instructor's Edition

Unfolding Case Studies

Experiencing the Realities of Clinical Nursing Practice

KELLIE J. GLENDON, MSN, RNC
Associate Professor
School of Nursing
Miami University
Hamilton, Ohio

DEBORAH L. ULRICH, PHD, RN
Professor
School of Nursing
Miami University
Oxford, Ohio

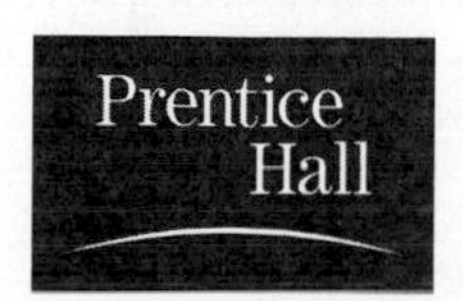

Upper Saddle River, New Jersey 07478

Publisher: *Julie Alexander*
Executive Editor: *Maura Connor*
Acquisitions Editor: *Nancy Anselment*
Director of Production and Manufacturing: *Bruce Johnson*
Managing Production Editor: *Patrick Walsh*
Manufacturing Manager: *Ilene Sanford*
Production Liaison: *Julie Boddorf*
Production Editor: *Karen Fortgang*
Creative Director: *Marianne Frasco*
Cover Design Coordinator: *Maria Guglielmo*
Cover Designer: *John Smith*
Interior Designer: *Julie Boddorf*
Director of Marketing: *Leslie Cavaliere*
Marketing Coordinator: *Cindy Frederick*
Editorial Assistant: *Beth Romph*
Composition: *Peirce Graphic Services, Inc.*
Printing and Binding: *The Banta Company*

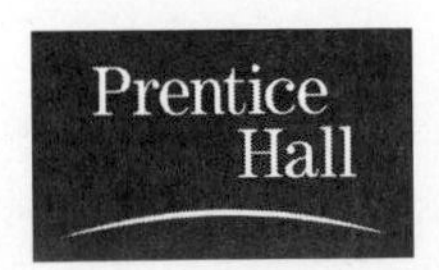

10 9 8 7 6 5 4 3 2
ISBN 0-13-090380-9

This book is dedicated to our future students—tomorrow's professional nurses. Our hope is that they will enter their professional practice with a greater awareness of the realities of clinical decision making and feel that their education has allowed them to excel and grow in their ability to communicate and use critical thinking as they care for their clients.

Contents

Preface

To the Faculty

It is no news to you that the process of teaching and learning has changed dramatically in the last decade. No longer can we give students volumes of information in a lecture format and then expect them to regurgitate it back to us on a test. The new teaching and learning paradigm challenges us to focus on learning and help students learn more effectively. Memorizing facts is often necessary, but it is only the beginning of effective learning. We, as faculty, need to help students learn to think critically, problem solve, and communicate with others if our students are going to be effective in their role as professional nurses. We have all read about new interactive strategies and have probably tried many of them, but we often revert back to our comfort zone of lecture. After all, it was the way we were all taught and we turned out fine. But, the complexity of clinical practice has multiplied, as has the level of critical thinking and problem solving needed by the nurse to practice safely and effectively. Interactive strategies such as our "Unfolding Cases Model" (Glendon and Ulrich, 1997) help students practice how to nurse in this new era of clinical complexity.

Our "Unfolding Cases Model" (Glendon and Ulrich, 1997) is designed to actively involve students as they practice solving problems they may encounter in their professional nursing career. This model is a variation and an extension of the frequently used case study strategy. It presents a case that typifies a common disorder or disease and then follows the client as the situation he or she experiences "unfolds" across time, settings, and/or disease progression. The unfolding case usually has three paragraphs, although some cases may contain more. The first paragraph sets the scene and introduces the characters and the situation they face. Using cooperative learning strategies (see Table 1), groups of students process the focused questions following each paragraph and then share their solutions with the entire class. Paragraph two is then revealed. It usually describes a change in time, a new focus, or new assessment data. Again student groups process the focused questions and share their findings with the class. Further paragraphs are sequentially revealed and processed. Class discussion follows. The final step in the model is an individual reflective writing exercise that encourages students to reflect on the experience, think about different perspectives, or plan future learning needs (see Table 2). This interactive strategy allows students to process information and problem solve both as individuals and as a member of a peer group. Communication skills are practiced and students see and react to others who might have differing perspectives from their own. Being exposed to multiple viewpoints extends the learning for individual students and helps them grow as professionals. The individual reflective writing prompt at the end of the case encourages students to reflect on their own values and beliefs in order to make the learning significant and applicable to their personal growth as individuals and professional nurses.

It is our hope that this workbook will help you to help your students learn more effectively without necessitating a complete change of your lecture material, learning objectives, and ideas of what nurses need to know. It is merely a new vehicle for you to structure your teaching around. Since each student will have her or his own workbook, you need to only assign a case prior to class. Since the cases cover common disorders/problems, it is often possible to structure an entire class around a single case. Let students use the case as a structure for picking out the important concepts from the assigned reading. Ask them to jot down possible solutions/answers to the focused questions. If they have prepared prior to class, not only will they be ready to ask pertinent questions, but they will also be able to process the case as a group more effectively. You might require them to show you their partially completed case prior to class as a way to check their preparedness, or you might even collect them intermittently. This periodic checking will increase students' compliance in preparing and reading prior to class, which is necessary if they are to analyze, think critically, and problem solve as they process the case in class with their peers.

In class, you may begin with a short 10- to 15-minute lecture on the topic of the case, give a short quiz using NCLEX type questions to assure prior individual preparation for class, or just ask students to get into groups of 4–6 to process the case. You might assign permanent groups for the entire quarter or semester, or you might have temporary groups that stay together for only one class. You then direct student groups to process the case one paragraph at a time using a cooperative strategy of your choice (see Table 1). After giving the groups time to process, call on one individual in each group to report their group's answers. You might list these on an overhead or the board. Have each group give one solution at a time until all have been listed. If students miss important points or give wrong solutions, you can clarify, correct misunderstandings, or add other information. A total class discussion evolves, which is usually of a higher quality than it would have been without the group processing. You will find that your students have covered the information on which you normally lecture and they have been active in the process. This will increase the effectiveness of the learning and make it more meaningful to them.

After processing all of the case, you might summarize important points, ask for questions, pose a slightly different problem and ask them if this would change their interventions, or use several NCLEX type questions to assure them that they have indeed learned what is important in this condition or disorder. This will ease their minds and help them see the value of the interactive strategy. The reflective writing prompt at the end of each case might be completed in class, as homework, or as a part of a reflective journal that individual students turn in periodically or at the end of the semester. That is up to you.

The instructor's manual is identical to the student workbook except it includes possible answers/solutions. It is not meant to propose that these answers are the only correct responses, but the manual presents some basic ideas that students should come up with. The answers are brief and are only to help you guide the students as they process the case. Your experiences and expertise should be used here to augment, broaden, and deepen the learning in the class discussion and help bring the situation to life. With critical thinking and the use of cooperative learning strategies, you will find that students come up with a multitude of wonderful solutions that may not be included in the so-called "answer book." Our hope is that you will find other varied and creative solutions to the cases. As always, information continually changes as new research evolves. Therefore, you will need to update answers or solutions to these cases continually.

Each case can be used in a variety of ways with students, although we feel the most effective way is to use it first as a structure for reading the assigned readings from their texts prior to class and then as a strategy in class to cover pertinent information as an alternative to lecture. You might want to use a case as a clinical decision-making test. Students could either process it individually or as groups and it could be graded. A case might be an ideal choice as a "make-up" clinical or as a post-conference discussion. Use it as you see fit.

Our hope is that this collection of cases will help you to help your students be better prepared and more confident as they begin their practice as professional nurses.

Sincerely,

Kellie Glendon and Debbie Ulrich

Glendon, K. and Ulrich, D. (1997). Unfolding cases: An experiential learning model. *Nurse Educator*, 22, 15–18.

Table 1. Cooperative Learning Strategies

Think-Pair-Share (Lyman, 1987)
- The faculty poses a problem or question to the students
- Students are given think time for one minute or more, depending on the difficulty level of the problem, to individually process the problem or question
- Students share their ideas or solutions with a peer in the next few minutes
- Each pair or selected pairs may report a possible solution to the entire class
- A total class discussion follows

Roundtable (Kagan, 1992)
- Students in groups of 4 to 6 sit in a circular fashion
- The faculty propose a problem or question to brainstorm
- Each student verbalizes a possible response to the problem or question in turn as a volunteer records every student's idea or as a pad is passed from one student to the next as they record their own responses
- A member of the group is called upon by the faculty to report the group's ideas
- A total class discussion follows

Pass the Problem (Kagan, 1992)
- The faculty poses a different problem to each group. The roundtable technique begins this strategy as students, in groups, process the problem proposed to their group and write down their ideas in turn
- Once a list of ideas is formulated, the group passes its list to another group
- The new group processes the new problem and may be asked by faculty to clarify it, prioritize the list, or add more solutions to the existing list. This last step is used to encourage critical thinking about the problem.
- The faculty could call on groups to report their ideas or pass the problem again so that more groups gain exposure to the problems posed by the faculty
- A total class discussion follows

Kagan, S. (1992). *Cooperative learning.* San Juan Capistrano, CA: Resources for Teachers
Lyman, F. (1987). Think-pair-share: An expanding teaching technique. *MAA-CIE Cooperative News* 1, 1–2.

Table 2. Reflective Writing

- This strategy is used to complete the entire unfolding case exercise. Each student individually completes the assignment
- This (1) encourages students to reflect on the learning that has occurred, (2) gives them something further to think about, (3) asks them to think about their strengths and areas in need of improvement, (4) asks them to consider what their beliefs and values are, or (5) asks specifically what the role of the nurse is when faced with various situations
- Some of the questions posed by faculty might include: Write a response to the following writing prompt: (1) How have your beliefs changed? (2) How do you feel about it? (3) What will you do now, based on what you know about nursing practice? (4) What is the role of the nurse in this situation?
- May be used as a vehicle for class discussion, part of an ongoing reflective journal kept by all students, or as a personal student diary for self-expression and evaluation

Glendon, K. & Ulrich, D. (1997). Unfolding cases: An experiential learning model. *Nurse Educator,* 22, 15–18.

List of Contributors

Book Contributors

Editors:

Kellie Glendon, MSN, RNC
Associate Professor of Nursing
Miami University
Hamilton, Ohio
Chapter 1 (Cases 1–11); Chapter 2 (Cases 1–6, 8–10), Chapter 4 (Case 12), Chapter 5 (Cases 8–10)

Deborah L. Ulrich, PhD, RN
Professor of Nursing
Miami University
Oxford, Ohio
Chapter 1 (Cases 1–11); Chapter 2 (Cases 1–6, 8–10), Chapter 4 (Case 12), Chapter 5 (Cases 8–10)

Other Contributors

Carol Wolfensperger Bashford, MS, RN, CS
Assistant Professor of Nursing
Miami University
Hamilton, Ohio
Chapter 4 (Cases 10, 13); Chapter 5 (Case 2)

Carolyn M. Burger, MSN, RNC, OCN
Assistant Professor of Nursing
Miami University
Middletown, Ohio
Chapter 4 (Cases 7–9)

Anne R. Carson, MSN, RN, CPNP
Associate Professor of Nursing
Miami University
Middletown, Ohio
Chapter 1 (Case 12); Chapter 2 (Case 7)

Donna Miles Curry, PhD, RN
Associate Professor of Nursing
Wright State University-Miami Valley College of Nursing
Dayton, Ohio
Chapter 5 (Case 6)

Marie Witter Garrison, MSN, RN, CEN
Visiting Assistant Professor of Nursing
Miami University
Hamilton, Ohio
Chapter 4 (Case 14)

Diane Eigsti Gerber, MSN, RN
Consultant-Communicable and Environmental Disease Services
Tennessee State Department of Health
Chapter 5 (Case 7)

Joan Fopma-Loy, DNS, RN, CS
Professor of Nursing
Miami University
Oxford, Ohio
Chapter 3 (Case 11); Chapter 5 (Cases 1, 4)

Katherine Voorhees Hieber, MS, RN, CS
Associate Professor of Nursing
Miami University
Middletown, Ohio
Chapter 4 (Cases 4–6)

Barbara L. Knepshield, PhD, RN
Gerentology Clinical Specialist
Veterans Hospital
Dayton, Ohio
Chapter 4 (Case 18)

Carolyn H. Mason, MS, RN
Visiting Assistant Professor of Nursing
Miami University
Middletown, Ohio
Chapter 5 (Cases 3, 11)

Eugenia M. Mills, PhD, RN
Associate Professor of Nursing
Miami University
Hamilton, Ohio
Chapter 4 (Case 3)

John T. Pack, MSN, RNC
Visiting Assistant Professor of Nursing
Miami University
Hamilton, Ohio
Chapter 4 (Case 2)

Marjorie Thiel Ryan, MSN, RN, CS
Associate Professor of Nursing
Miami University of Ohio
Chapter 3 (Cases 1, 3)

Diana L. Stanforth, MSN, RN, CCRN
Lecturer/Nursing
Indiana University East
Richmond, Indiana
Chapter 4 (Case 11)

Jeraldine Taylor, MS, RN
Associate Professor of Nursing (retired)
Miami University
Middletown, Ohio
Chapter 3 (Cases 2, 6–10)

Janet Teets, MSN, RN
Associate Professor of Nursing
Miami University
Hamilton, Ohio
Chapter 3 (Cases 4–5)

Jean Vanderbeek, MS, RN, CS
Associate Professor of Nursing
Miami University
Middletown, Ohio
Chapter 4 (Cases 15–16)

Paulette Worcester, DNS, RN, CFNP
Assistant Professor of Nursing
Miami University
Hamilton, Ohio
Chapter 4 (Case 1); Chapter 5 (Case 5)

Tao Yin, MSN, RN
Assistant Professor of Nursing
Miami University
Hamilton, Ohio
Chapter 4 (Case 17)

Acknowledgments

We wish to thank the nursing faculty who contributed their time and talent to the development of this book. All of them highly respected, extremely busy, and remarkably generous in developing unfolding cases in their area of expertise.

We wish to thank the hundreds of nurse educators who have attended our presentations on "unfolding cases" and have encouraged us to develop this book to use with students throughout their nursing education.

About the Authors

Kellie J. Glendon, MSN, RNC, is an experienced nurse educator, author, and national speaker on innovative teaching in nursing curricula. Kellie is an Associate Professor of Nursing at Miami University and has been teaching students in the Associate Degree Program for the past 13 years. She was awarded the Excellence in Teaching Award by the Greater Cincinnati Consortium of Colleges and Universities in 1998. Kellie continues to promote creative strategies to enhance critical thinking in nursing students.

Deborah L. Ulrich, PhD, RN, is an experienced nurse educator who has influenced nurse educators through journal articles, national presentations, and a recent book on interactive group learning. Her strategies have challenged educators to experiment with new ways of teaching and learning. Debbie has been a nurse educator for the past 30 years in diverse educational settings.

chapter **1**

Annotated Obstetrical Cases

CASE #1 JEAN MULBERRY

Learning Objectives

1. Interpret client data using discipline specific language.
2. Identify and analyze assessment data characteristic of the antepartum period.
3. Identify nursing interventions for common discomforts of pregnancy.
4. Identify strategies for assessing nutritional state.
5. Analyze Jean's nutritional state and offer educational interventions.
6. Identify educational interventions related to warning signs of pregnancy.

Jean Mulberry is a 26-year-old married female seeing the doctor to confirm a positive home pregnancy test. Jean works full time as an accountant. She had an abortion 10 years ago. She expresses ambivalence about the pregnancy, stating, "I'm really scared. We had agreed to wait another year until we had a down payment for a house." She complains of tender breasts and intermittent nausea. Her last menstrual period was June 10.

Focus Questions

1. What is Jean's gravida, para, TPAL, and due date?

   Jean is gravida 2, para 0 or G2, T0, P0, A1, L0. Using Nagele's rule, which says add 7 days to the first day of last menstrual period, (10 + 7 = 17), then subtract 3 months, Jean's EDC or EDB is March 17.

2. What assessment data does the nurse need to obtain from Jean now and throughout the antepartum period that would identify risks to the pregnancy?

   Risk factors fall into several categories: biophysical, psychosocial, sociodemographic, and environmental (Wong & Perry, 1998). Students might assess any of the following:

   - ***Biophysical*—genetic disorders, nutritional problems such as anorexia, obesity, or pica, current medical problems, previous pregnancy losses; assess blood for infections such as VDRL, HbsAg, HIV or blood type and Rh for incompatibilities; test urine for glucose and protein or leukocytes; screen for TB, rubella titer, or sickle cell.**
   - ***Psychosocial*—mental problems, abuse, cultural norms not safe for pregnancy, use of drugs, alcohol, caffeine, or smoking.**

- ***Sociodemographic*—poverty, poor health, lack of prenatal care, age such as under 15 or over 35, first pregnancy risks for PIH or dystocia, marital status—unmarried at above risk; residence (rural areas increased risk for maternal mortality); ethnicity—African American increased risk**
- ***Environmental*—exposure to radiation, chemicals, pesticides, drugs, pollution, smoke, stress.**

3. Illustrate the normal changes of pregnancy using a body diagram. Include the drawing with this case.

   Students may label on the drawing any of the following related to physical changes (Wong & Perry, 1998).

   - ***Vital signs*—BP lower in second trimester; weight gain of 1 lb. per month in first trimester and then 1 lb. per week in last two trimesters**
   - ***General appearance, mental status*—ambivalence related diagnosis, body changes, pregnancy fears**
   - ***Head and scalp*—chloasma**
   - ***Nose*—nasal congestion**
   - ***Mouth*—hypertrophy of gums; hyperptyalism**
   - ***Respirations*—shortness of breath with later pregnancy; lightening at end**
   - ***Cardiac*—heart rate increases of 10 bpm.; increased blood volume; pseudoanemia; varicosities in lower extremities; palpitations; supine hypotensive syndrome**
   - ***Breasts*—enlarge, areola darkens, Montgomery glands enlarge, vascularity increases, colostrum is produced**
   - ***Abdomen*—stretch marks; diastasis of midline muscles; linea nigra**
   - ***Uterus*—increase in size and weight; presence of Hegars, Chadwicks, and Goodell's signs**
   - ***Gastrointestinal*—heartburn, constipation, morning sickness**
   - ***Endocrine*—hormones decrease insulin effectiveness**
   - ***Renal*—increased output**
   - ***Skeletal*—lordosis**

4. Is there assessment data in this case to indicate a risk to this pregnancy? If so, what?

   Yes, previous abortion could indicate a risk. Assess her anxiety related to being scared—ask questions related to abuse to screen for family abuse such as, "Have you ever been kicked, slapped, etc." (Furniss, Torchen, & Blakewell-Sachs, 1999)—or it may only be normal ambivalence.

5. Are her physiological and psychological symptoms expected at this time? If not, what do they mean in relation to Jean's pregnancy?

   Yes, tender breasts, nausea, and ambivalence are common in first trimester.

6. List other expected changes she may experience in the antepartum period and recommend interventions she could try (Wong & Perry, 1998), such as:

• Nausea and vomiting	**eat small frequent meals; crackers on arising; fluids such as tea or coffee within hour of arising**
• Urinary frequency	**Kegel exercise; limit fluid prior to bedtime**
• Back pain	**good body mechanics; correct posture; pelvic tilt**
• Constipation	**fluids, fiber, regular eating schedule; exercise**

In assessing Jean's nutrition, the nurse finds that she is having 1–2 glasses of wine each night with dinner. Also, she states, "Milk makes me sick—I cannot stand the sight or smell of it."

Focus Questions

1. How should the nurse go about assessing Jean's nutritional status?

   Assess nutrition by using a 3-day review of diet.

2. Should Jean modify her diet to support her pregnancy? If so, how?

   Yes, she should add 300 calories especially in the second and third trimester and increase milk group servings to 3 or more.

3. What suggestions might the nurse give to Jean in relation to her problem with milk?

   Substitute sardines or salmon, beans and legumes, greens, figs, tofu, cheese, and yogurt for milk.

4. What nutritional supplements are indicated?

   Prenatal vitamins and folic acid reduce neural tube defects and iron prevents anemia.

5. How would the nurse best counsel Jean in relation to her wine consumption? Why?

   No amount of alcohol is safe. Counsel her to avoid alcohol. Clients who drink may have a baby with fetal alcohol syndrome (microcephaly, epicanthal folds, short nose, thin upper lip, small chin, or impaired growth and learning disabilities).

As Jean is leaving the office to make her next appointment she says, "You mean I do not need to see anyone for a whole month? What if something goes wrong, how will I know?"

Focus Question

1. How should the nurse respond to Jean's questions, and what specific things should he or she tell Jean at this first visit?

   First, emphasize the importance of regular prenatal care (Davis, Okuboye, & Ferguson, 2000). Counsel her to call the health care provider if she experiences severe vomiting, chills, fever, burning on urination, diarrhea, abdominal cramping, any vaginal bleeding or leakage of fluid, absence of fetal movement, visual disturbances, swelling of the face or hands, headache, convulsion, and epigastric pain. (Wong & Perry, 1998).

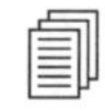

Reflective Writing

Nurses are expected to be caring. What does this mean? Identify some caring behaviors the nurse might exhibit in this situation with a newly pregnant client.

This case has presented normal aspects of pregnancy with ambivalence characteristic of early pregnancy. Characteristics of a caring nurse are: taking the time to really listen to the client's concerns, avoid checking time on watch, sit down instead of going in and out of room, use of therapeutic communication, touch, and answering client's concerns first.

References

Davis, L, Okuboye, S, & Ferguson, S. (2000). Healthy people 2010: Examining a decade of maternal & infant health. *AWHONN Lifelines*, 4(3), 26–33.

Furniss, K., Torchen, C., & Blakewell-Sachs, S. (1999). Learning to ask. *JOGNN*, 28(4), 353.

Wong, D. & Perry, S. (1998). *Maternal child nursing care.* St.Louis: Mosby.

CASE #2 MARIA BOWMAN

Learning Objectives

1. Discuss the implications, abnormal and normal results, nursing interventions related to serum AFP, triple marker test, and amniocentesis.
2. Analyze how cultural background might affect the nurse-client relationship.
3. Identify specific components and significance of the biophysical profile, nonstress test, and L/S ratio.
4. List pros and cons of caring for clients who have procedures that conflict with your own values and beliefs.

Maria Bowman is a quiet, shy, 35-year-old woman from Puerto Rico, gravida one para zero (G1P0), who arrives at the clinic with her husband, Tom, an American naval officer. Tom tells the nurse that in Puerto Rico an Alpha-fetoprotein blood test was done, and they were told that it was abnormal.

Focus Questions

1. What are the implications of this test?

   Serum AFP is a screening tool for neural tube defects (80% accuracy). High levels may be indicative of neural tube defects. Lower levels may indicate Down Syndrome. Down Syndrome is also associated with increased maternal age. Follow-up tests will be performed as this test is only used for screening (Wong & Perry, 1998).

2. When is this test normally done?

   15 to 21 weeks (17 weeks is ideal).

3. Since this test was abnormal, what additional tests might the nurse anticipate being ordered?

   The triple marker test is now also done at 16 to 18 weeks to calculate risk of Down Syndrome (60%) reliability. These are screening tests only; a diagnosis is made through amniocentesis, chromosome studies, and ultrasound (Wong & Perry, 1998).

4. How might Maria's cultural background affect the nurse-client relationship and what might the nurse do to become more culturally competent?

   Nurses must seek to be culturally competent in their interactions with clients of a different culture. Campinha-Bacote (1997) described four ways to become more culturally competent. First the nurse must look at him- or herself, how *culturally sensitive* is the nurse to Maria's cultural beliefs, even if her beliefs are different from the nurse's? The nurse must strive to understand Maria's beliefs and work toward being less ethnocentric. In Maria's culture, there is a reliance on folk healers, use of herbs and rituals, paternalism, strong sense of privacy in families, relaxed sense of time, suspicion of hospitals, and belief that illness is caused by evil spirits. The nurse should gain *cultural knowledge* by reading about different cultures. The strength of cultural beliefs will depend on whether or not Maria has taken on any aspects of Tom's culture or if she responds on the basis of her own cultural background. The nurse would need to assess this carefully and not make assumptions. The nurse must gain *cultural skill.* This means the nurse learns ways of assessing the client's cultural practices and seeks ways of incorporating these practices into the plan of care. The nurse who attempts to

do this will gain trust with the client. The nurse needs to establish if any language barriers exist and begin assessing Maria's knowledge of the test and her feelings. Asking the client about her fears related to the procedure would be important. Finding out what Maria believes would help her during the procedure and could be helpful in this case. Perhaps Maria would like to have a religious item with her to assist her in getting through the procedure. Finally the nurse needs to have *cultural encounters* with clients of different cultures. More than a couple of encounters are necessary in becoming culturally competent. Becoming culturally competent is essential in developing therapeutic relationships.

Maria is scheduled for an amniocentesis. When asked by the nurse if she has questions about the test, Maria says, "I'm afraid the baby will be stuck with the needle and how will I stop the fluid from leaking out?" Her husband tells her firmly, "You're going to have this test." She looks down, remains quiet, and follows the nurse to the exam room. The nurse realizes Maria lacks knowledge.

Focus Questions

1. Considering the assessment data, what should the nurse do first?

   First, the nurse should answer Maria's question. Respecting her concerns will help her trust the nurse. The nurse must also educate her on the test procedure.

2. What specific information should the nurse give Maria and Tom about indications of a test like this and the procedure itself?

   The amniocentesis is performed to determine if any genetic conditions exist; it is performed in late pregnancy to assess fetal maturity (Wong & Perry, 1998). A local anesthetic can be used to numb the skin; a needle is inserted to take fluid out while an ultrasound is performed to locate the baby so as not to puncture it. An adhesive bandage covers the needle opening and the leakage will stop by itself and is usually very minimal.

3. What physical interventions would the nurse perform prior to the test?

   Maternal vital signs and FHR are done prior to and after the procedure. Ask the patient to empty bladder so it will not be punctured.

4. What specific instructions should the nurse give Maria after the test and why?

   Instruct Maria in the signs and symptoms of labor as there is a less than 1% chance that labor could ensue (Wong & Perry, 1998).

Diagnosed at 24 weeks as a gestational diabetic, Maria, now at 36 weeks, comes to the hospital and worriedly states, "My baby is not moving. Is he okay?" A biophysical profile (BPP) score of 10 was obtained.

Focus Questions

1. How would the nurse explain the biophysical profile (BPP) test to Maria and what should Maria expect?

   Maria's findings indicate there is a normal fetus. The nurse needs to know some basic knowledge about the results of the test and why testing is done more frequently in the diabetic client. When the test is performed, the nurse might describe to Maria what is

being looked at. The baby is observed through an ultrasound moving its hands, feet, and body. The test is assessing fetal well-being through the fetus's ability to extend, flex the body, and make breathing movements. The heart rate of the baby is also observed. The baby's heart rate should increase as it moves or kicks. Another measure of fetal wellness is the amount of amniotic fluid available. Polyhydramnios or excess fluid occurs 10 times more often in diabetic pregnancies than nondiabetic pregnancies and is associated with premature rupture of membranes, preterm labor, and postpartum hemorrhage (Wong & Perry, 1998). Amniotic fluid indexes (AFI) of 5 cm. or less is an indication of oligohydramnios; 5.1–8.0 cm. is borderline (Calhoun, 1999). The test results that include the finding of oligohydramnios may indicate a delivery is necessary in babies with scores even as high as 8 out of 10. Oligohydramnios is associated with congenital anomalies, IUGR, and fetal distress in labor (Wong & Perry, 1998). While nurses are not involved in initially discussing results with the client, they are involved in describing what is being looked at and what the patient can expect to see, hear, and feel during this procedure. Simple explanations can help relieve a patient's anxiety about the test. In the past the ultrasound required that women have a full bladder. Today, with more advanced technology, the ultrasound is performed without the requirement of a full bladder and with the patient resting comfortably with pillows. Gel is applied to the abdomen and a scanner is passed over the abdomen. The woman should not feel discomfort and can watch the fetus moving on the screen. There is currently no evidence that there are any risks to the fetus, although the hypothetical risk of biological damage could be reported in the future.

2. How should the nurse respond to the question of lack of fetal movement?

   It was good that Maria realized that lack of fetal movement may indicate a problem, especially with her history of diabetes. Diabetes increases the risk of fetal demise and congenital anomalies. The nurse should instruct Maria to assess fetal movement, for example, by using a screening tool where she consciously observes fetal movement and counts for 1 hour every day. If the baby moves less than 10 times in 1 hour, she should eat something nutritious and repeat counting. If the baby moves less than 10 times in the second hour she should report it to the doctor. This tool is the Piacquadio Protocol (Calhoun, 1999).

3. Since Maria's nonstress test was reactive, what would the strip look like?

   There would be 2 or more accelerations of FHR of 15 beats per minute (BPM) lasting 15 seconds or more associated with each fetal movement in a 20-minute test period (Wong & Perry, 1998).

4. How frequently will testing occur in Maria's case?

   Due to her diabetes, the test is performed two times a week as long as it is reactive; if nonreactive, repeat in 24 hours (Wong & Perry, 1998). The biophysical profile (BPP) may also be indicated.

5. If an amniocentesis were ordered, what would be the significance of the lecithin/sphingomyelin (L/S) ratio? If the result was 2:1? If the result was 3:1?

   The L/S ratio is the comparison of lecithin/sphingomyelin, the surfactant necessary for extrauterine breathing. A 2:1 ratio indicates lung maturity in a nondiabetic pregnancy (Wong & Perry, 1998). So in Maria's case, a 2:1 ratio would indicate a lack of lung maturity. A 3:1 ratio in a diabetic client would indicate lung maturity.

Reflective Writing

Today at the clinic you are caring for another mother who has had an amniocentesis and it is determined that her baby has Down Syndrome. At 18 weeks she decides to abort the baby. You have been assigned to be her nurse for the abortive procedure, but your beliefs are that the baby has a right to live. Will you care for her? What are the pros and cons of your action?

Students may choose to care for her or not. Some of the pros and cons of either action could be:

- *Pros of not taking care of her*

You begin to question your suitability for this setting that does abortions.

You refuse to care for her, and you feel better yourself for not going against your own beliefs.

- *Cons of not taking care of her*

Someone besides you has to care for the client.

In some situations there may be no one to care for the client and your refusal to care for her could affect your job performance evaluations.

- *Pros of taking care of her*

You feel you are fulfilling the role of the nurse as caring for everyone without being judgmental.

- *Cons of taking care of her*

You feel guilty for taking part in caring for her.

You subconsciously could make the client feel guilty by showing your biases and ultimately give poor care.

References

Calhoun, S. (1999). Focus on fluids, examining maternal hydration and amniotic fluid volume, *AWHONN Lifelines*, 3(6), 21–24.

Campinha-Bacote, J. (1997). Cultural competence: A critical factor in child health policy. *Journal of Pediatric Nursing*, 12(4), 260–261.

Wong, D. & Perry, S. (1998). *Maternal child nursing care.* St. Louis: Mosby.

CASE #3 SUZANNE NETHERS

Learning Objectives

1. Interpret the data given and determine which phase of the first stage of labor the client is experiencing.
2. Discuss the appropriate psychological and physiological characteristics of all phases of the first stage of labor.
3. Analyze available data and determine actual or potential nursing diagnoses and/or collaborative problems appropriate to the first stage of labor.
4. Identify appropriate nursing interventions relative to each phase of the first stage of labor.

0800 Suzanne Nethers is an excited and talkative 24-year-old (G1P0) kindergarten teacher married to Jeff, a 26-year-old computer analyst. She is admitted to the labor and delivery suite with signs of bloody show and contractions occurring every 16 minutes and lasting 20–30 seconds.

Jeff reports to the nurse that she is doing really well with her breathing and that they are excited about having a natural childbirth. During the assessment the nurse finds the current pregnancy, family, and medical history are normal; BP 128/64, P. 90, R.24. FHT are 140, strong and regular. Membranes are intact. A vaginal check reveals Suzanne to be 2 cm. dilated, 50% effaced, and at 0 station.

Focus Questions

1. In what stage and phase of labor is Suzanne?

   Stage 1, latent phase

2. What would the nurse need to assess?

   The nurse should assess: cervical dilation, effacement, and station; contraction frequency, duration, and intensity; bloody show, noting color and amount; maternal behavior; intactness of the membranes; duration of labor; maternal VS; maternal voiding; FHT; presentation.

3. What data would prompt the nurse to call the physician or nurse midwife (list warning signs)?

   The nurse should report: IUP over 75; duration of contraction over 90 seconds; contractions occurring less than 2 minutes apart; any fetal bradycardia, tachycardia, or decreased variability or irregular FHT; fluid in the vagina that is excessively bloody or meconium stained; arrest in progress of cervical dilation/effacement or descent of the fetus; maternal temperature over 100.4°; foul smelling vaginal discharge; tachycardia; hypertension; persistent bright or dark red vaginal bleeding; cord prolapse (Wong & Perry, 1998).

4. What nursing diagnoses or collaborative problems and interventions are appropriate at this stage of labor?

Nursing Diagnosis	Interventions	Collaborative
Anxiety r/t labor	**Focal point; teach breathing Involve in care decisions Discuss progress**	**Fetal distress**
Knowledge deficit r/t labor	**Educate on relaxation techniques and breathing techniques to help ease pain**	**Infection**
Risk for fluid volume deficit r/t to altered intake	**Monitor intake and output, VS, and electrolytes; assess skin turgor and mucous membranes for dryness; give IV fluids as ordered. Assess for emesis.**	**Hemorrhage**
Risk for altered elimination r/t sensory loss	**Offer bedpan q 2 hours; have client void or catheterize if necessary**	

Collaborative interventions are directed at monitoring for the problem and if detected to notifying the physician.

1400 Suzanne's contractions are 4 minutes apart, last 45–60 seconds, and are of moderate intensity. Vaginal assessment is 6 cm. dilated, +2 station, 100% effaced. Suzanne is more serious and focused on each contraction, feels helpless and apprehensive, and wants to "get this over with." She asks, "Can I have something to take the edge off this pain?" Jeff is supportive and attentive. She has been ambulating with Jeff in the hallway but now wants to lie down. As she gets into bed, her membranes spontaneously rupture and a tinge of green is noted in the fluid color. There is increasing bloody show.

Focus Questions

1. What stage and phase of labor is she in?

   Stage 1 active phase

2. What nursing diagnoses and interventions are appropriate now?

Pain r/t increasing intensity and frequency of contractions as evidenced by (aeb) client request	**Explain analgesics and anesthesia available; medicate per physician order**
Risk for infection r/t ROM	**Check temperature every hour; check odor and consistency of amniotic fluid; use hygiene and hand washing**

3. What collaborative problems are possible considering this data?

   Fetal distress is possible due to meconium in the amniotic fluid. The nurse should assess FHT and variability, as well as for periodic changes such as variable deceleration or late deceleration. Scalp ph may be done if distress is evident. Assess for cord prolapse as a possible collaborative problem with ROM.

1900 Suzanne's contractions are 2–3 minutes apart, last 70–80 seconds, and are of very strong intensity. She shows frustration, loss of control, has nausea, and vomits small amounts. She tells her husband, "Get away, do not touch me!" As the nurse enters the room, she asks for a bedpan and says she feels like she has to have a bowel movement. She screams, "I have to push!"

Focus Questions

1. What stage and phase of labor is Suzanne currently experiencing?

   Stage 1, transitional phase

2. What interventions are indicated in this stage and phase of labor?

   The nurse should do a vaginal check to assess for complete dilation and effacement because she could be entering the second stage. FHT and maternal VS should be monitored. Support/comfort and teaching the pushing technique is indicated.

3. During the vaginal assessment the nurse finds Suzanne is only 9 cm., yet she continually wants to push. What should the nurse do and why? What if Suzanne were 10 cm.? What if she was 10 cm. and did not have the urge to have a bowel movement or push?

   If Suzanne were 9 cm., she should not push but pant/blow because pushing will tear her cervix and influence future labor. If Suzanne is 10 cm. and she has the urge to have a bowel movement or push, it would be appropriate to encourage her to push, as these findings are indicative of the Ferguson's reflex. New literature is questioning the practice of encouraging the mother to push when completely without the conscious urge to bear down or push. It is suggested that it would be best to encourage the mother to wait for the spontaneous urges to bear down rather than rely on cervical dilation as the sole indicator for the onset of pushing (Mayberry, Wood, Strange, Lee, Heisler, & Neilsen-Smith, 1999).

4. According to practice standards, what documentation would be necessary for the nurse to include in the charting?

   Documentation should include progress of labor-dilation, effacement, station, VS, FHT, description of fetal heart tracing (Harvey, 1997), voiding, contraction pattern, any medications, condition of any tubes (internal or external monitors, IV therapy), status of membranes; narrative note on any changes, maternal behavior, and responses.

Reflective Writing

You are a new nurse on a labor and delivery unit. You observe that L & D nurses have a lot of "old practices" such as confining patients in a supine position for pushing. All of these nurses have been in practice longer than you have been alive. How could you influence a change in practice on this unit?

Students are asked to think about how to effect change as well as how to appropriately communicate their concerns to their peers when they are making the transition from student to professional. The best way to respond to this is to be positive about and talk about new ideas. One way to effect change would be for the new graduates to volunteer to be on education committees at their hospitals. By attending and reporting on new ideas in practice, each new nurse could help make needed changes. By being a role model for using these new practices, the nurse could help change to occur. Enthusiasm sells the idea, so the nurse should try to avoid negativity. Also he or she should get another peer involved and collaborate on writing or preparing for educational programs. The new nurse can advocate for reeducation programs to the Director of Nursing. Discussion about how easy it would be to do what always has been done should take place, and how harmful ignoring new research practices could be.

References

Harvey, C. (1997). A look at new terms, electronic fetal monitoring update. *AWHONN Lifelines*, 1(3), 42–44.

Mayberry, L., Wood, S., Strange, L., Lee, L., Heisler, D., & Neilsen-Smith, K. (1999). Managing second-stage labor, exploring the variables during the second stage. *AWHONN Lifelines* 3 (6), 28–33.

Wong, D. & Perry, S. (1998). *Maternal child nursing care.* St. Louis: Mosby.

CASE #4 LAURA SHINGLE

Learning Objectives

1. Identify normal and abnormal assessment data for the second stage of labor.
2. Discuss nursing interventions appropriate for an emergency precipitous delivery.
3. Identify signs indicating the third stage of labor.
4. Discuss potential complications of precipitous delivery for infant and mother.
5. Differentiate between normal and abnormal assessment data of baby's immediate post-delivery, as well as nursing interventions.

1230 Laura Shingle, a 34-year-old G3P2, presents in ER with contractions q 2–3 minutes lasting 70–90 seconds with strong intensity. She states her water broke in the car, and she now feels the urge to push. Upon initial exam, she is completely dilated, +3 station, vertex presentation. She states she has been in labor since 1030. The physician is here for the delivery room.

Focus Questions

1. What stage of labor is Laura experiencing? At what point does this stage begin and when does it end? Are these data normal or abnormal?

   Second stage goes from complete dilation and effacement to delivery of the baby.

   The majority of the data is normal. Duration of labor is abnormal; only 2 hours and she is delivering.

2. What are the nursing interventions that should occur immediately before and during the delivery?

   The nurse should direct the support person to scrub and gown; assist the client into different positions to help the descent of the fetus (lateral position may provide a more controlled delivery); assist the client with relaxation between pushing/contractions; assist the client with proper breathing such as pant blows; assess FHT and maternal VS; assess bladder for distention—this could impede progress; encourage the client to breathe with contractions and pushing and avoid breath holding or the valsalva maneuver; anticipate maternal and fetal injury r/t rapid delivery; call pediatricians if any sign of fetal distress; cleanse the perineum in preparation for delivery; assist physician with procedures, get bulb suction ready to suction mouth; note the time on the delivery of the baby.

3. What procedures should the nurse anticipate the physician would do to minimize fetal and maternal injury? Describe.

   The Ritgen maneuver may be done to ease delivery of the head and avoid rapid expulsion of the head thereby minimizing damage to maternal tissues. An episiotomy may be done to enlarge the opening. A nuchal cord may be clamped and cut in order to remove from around the neck.

1245 Laura delivers a 9-lb. baby girl. After cord clamping, the baby is taken to the warmer. The physician waits for the placental delivery.

Focus Questions

1. What stage of labor is Laura in now and how long should this stage last?

   Laura is in Stage 3, delivery of the placenta. This lasts less than 30 minutes.

2. What might happen if it takes too long? Why?

   Laura could hemorrhage due to retained placenta.

3. Why is pulling on the cord contraindicated?

   Pulling on the cord causes placental fragmentation; it could pull the cord off; it could invert the uterus.

4. How much bleeding is to be expected? How much is abnormal?

   For a delivery 350 cc. is normal although any bleeding less than 500 cc. is normal. More than 500 cc. is considered a hemorrhage.

5. What are the usual signs prior to separation of the placenta?

   The signs are rise in the fundus, globular shape of the uterus, and gush of blood.

6. What specific things does the nurse look for when assessing the placenta? Why?

   Assess the placenta for intactness. Retained placenta will result in continual hemorrhage until it is removed.

Laura's baby has Apgar scores of 7 and 9. Erythromycin ointment is placed immediately in both eyes. Aquamephyton is given IM into the right vastas lateralis. A left-sided cephalohematoma is noted. Milia and erythema toxicum are present on the face, arms, and chest. Acrocyanosis is present. Temperature is 97°, P.120, R.36. There are Mongolian spots on the buttocks.

Focus Questions

1. List criteria and possible points for the Apgar score.

   There is a total of ten possible points. A maximum of 2 points in each of five areas are evaluated. They are: heart rate, respiratory effort, muscle tone, reflex irritability, and color. An Apgar score represents the general condition of the infant at 1 and 5 minutes after birth. Scores of 7–10 indicate absence of difficulty in adjusting to extrauterine life (Wong & Perry, 1998). Laura's baby is adjusting to extrauterine life.

2. Given all the above assessment data, what would you consider normal and/or abnormal?

   Pulse and respirations, milia, acrocyanosis, erythema toxicum, and Mongolian spots are all normal findings. Temperature is low and should be at least 97.8°F (36.5°C). Cephalohematoma is abnormal and should be monitored. Apgar score was normal, a few points were taken off, at least one for color or acrocyanosis.

3. If you find something abnormal, what are your nursing interventions?

   For decreased temperature, place infant under warmer or in an incubator and delay the bath time. For cephalohematoma, watch level of consciousness for any changes, observe for signs of increased intracranial pressure, monitor bilirubin because as the hematoma resolves, the bilirubin will increase. Look for any other signs of injury due to rapid delivery.

4. What interventions must be taken to ensure the safety of the infant?

   Use a warmer for controlling temperature, an ID bracelet and crib card for security, properly identify mother with ID bracelets each time they are separated, use a security bracelet, keep baby in crib and roll rather than carry them, and don't leave the baby unattended.

5. Why are Erythromycin and Aquamephyton given?

   Erythromycin ointment is placed in the eyes to prevent gonnorhea and chlamydia. Aquamephyton is used to promote clotting as the intestine is sterile and not yet producing vitamin K.

1315 Laura is in the recovery room. Nursing assessment reveals fundus at +3 above the umbilicus and deviated to the right. Lochia is large rubra with small clots. BP 90/50, P.120, R.24. She complains of being cold and is shivering and shaking. Her perineum is swollen, especially on the right side. An IV of 1,000 cc. LR with 10u. Pitocin is infusing into the right arm.

Focus Questions

1. What could be happening to Laura? Explain with pertinent data.

   The pulse is too rapid and fundus much too high and deviated, which could mean a full bladder and the inability of the uterus to contract well. Lochia is large and perineum is

swollen, especially on the right. Data could mean there is the development of a hematoma or possibly, with fundus high, pulse high, and low BP, the development of a hemorrhage from uterine atony. Shivering is a normal finding immediately after delivery.

2. What interventions should be done immediately and why?

   Have the patient void or catheterize the patient. Assess firmness of fundus and massage if flaccid and reassess for further signs of hemorrhage—check the perineum for further changes.

3. What are the practice standards of vital signs and checking the fundus in this stage? Why is this important?

   For the first hour check VS and fundus every 15 minutes; then check hourly for the next 4 hours. Check more often if there are any abnormal findings. Hemorrhage is a common complication immediately after delivery due to uterine atony, hematoma, vaginal lacerations, or retained placenta.

4. What is the Pitocin used for in this stage?

   It is used for smooth muscle contraction to keep fundus firm and contracted to prevent hemorrhage.

Reflective Writing

As you are leaving choir practice at church, an obviously pregnant woman is leaning over the hood of her car and yelling, "The baby's coming, please help me! I feel the baby's head coming out." No one is available except you! How will you help her?

- **remain with the patient. Ask help from someone to call 911.**
- **provide a clean environment for possible delivery; newspaper would work**
- **instruct mother to pant when head crowns; this prevents rapid expulsion of head**
- **rupture the amniotic fluid sac if it is still intact when head crowns**
- **apply gentle pressure to fetal head to prevent damage to the head and maternal perineum**
- **assist the head to deliver between contractions**
- **check for the cord and slip it over the infant's head if it is wrapped around the neck**
- **clear the airway by wiping mucous from mouth and nose and place infant on mother's abdomen prone and head in a slightly trendelenburg position**
- **cover and dry infant to prevent heat loss**
- **place infant skin to skin on mother**
- **double clamp cord and cut with sterile scissors or leave intact and keep placenta at same level as baby**
- **wait for placental delivery**
- **place infant to breast to promote uterine contractions**
- **massage the fundus if boggy**
- **transport to a medical facility**

Reference

Wong, D. & Perry, S. (1998). *Maternal child nursing care.* St.Louis: Mosby.

CASE #5 LISA LAWRENCE

Learning Objectives

1. Explain the diagnosis and treatment of the gestational diabetic.
2. Identify signs and symptoms of hypoglycemia and hyperglycemia.
3. Differentiate between NPH and regular insulin.
4. Explain blood sugar changes and insulin needs throughout pregnancy and postpartum.
5. Identify common complications of the gestational diabetic and her baby, as well as appropriate assessments and interventions.

Lisa Lawrence is a 32-year-old primipara. According to her EDC she is 24 weeks gestation. During this pregnancy she has experienced no complications except that her pre-pregnant weight was above normal. Her family history indicates that her maternal aunt and maternal grandmother have Type II or non-insulin dependant diabetes mellitus (NIDDM). There is no known history of birth defects or other chronic illness in the family. During her examination today she is told that her routine glucose challenge test was positive and that she will need to return for a 3-hour glucose tolerance test to rule out gestational diabetes. Lisa asks, "Does this mean I have to take those pills my aunt and grandma do?"

Focus Questions

1. How would the nurse respond to Lisa?

   The nurse could say something like, "The test may indicate that you need to be on a special diabetic diet and you may need to check your blood sugars. Sometimes insulin is required. You will not need to take pills, as they are harmful to the baby. By controlling your blood sugar through diet, insulin, if required, and exercise, babies do well. High blood sugars can harm the baby, and that is why we are doing the test to determine whether you have gestational diabetes." The nurse should know that stillbirth and congenital anomalies are possible problems associated with uncontrolled glucose levels (Wong & Perry, 1998), but it is too soon to discuss these complications as the diagnosis is not complete. These sequellae are important to discuss after diagnosis is confirmed.

2. How would the nurse prepare Lisa for the 3-hour GTT?

   The test will be administered after at least 3 days of unrestricted diet and physical exercise. Explain that she will need to have nothing by mouth after midnight. Blood will be drawn in the morning at the clinic. She will be asked to drink a sugary drink, and then blood will be drawn at hourly intervals for the next 3 hours. She should avoid caffeine and smoking. If two or more of the results are elevated, the test is positive.

Lisa's test shows that she has gestational diabetes. Since her blood sugars are high and uncontrolled, the physician has started her on 15 u. Humulin NPH insulin and 5 u. Humulin regular insulin this morning and a 2,000 calorie diabetic diet. Evening blood sugars (5 P.M.) are to be reported to the physician for an evening insulin order. The physician explains that she may be on insulin for the rest of her pregnancy. Later, Lisa asks the nurse, "How long do I have to follow these rules?"

Focus Questions

1. How should the nurse explain Lisa's insulin needs throughout her pregnancy and postpartum?

In early pregnancy the blood sugars are low or normal as the baby is growing and the mother is not eating as much due to morning sickness. As the pregnancy continues into the second and third trimesters, the hormones of pregnancy block the effectiveness of insulin. The effect is that the blood sugar rises during the second and third trimester. Extra insulin is needed to manage the rise in blood sugar. After birth, insulin is usually no longer needed as blood sugars return to normal values. She might expect to have multiple doses of insulin throughout the day especially in the second and third trimester to manage her blood sugars. Most gestational diabetics typically can manage their blood sugars with diet only and no added insulin. In Lisa's case her blood sugars are too high and that necessitates taking insulin throughout her pregnancy. Ten to 25% of gestational diabetics require insulin.

2. Explain how the nurse will teach Lisa to administer two types of insulin (NPH 15 u. and regular 5u.) together.

Steps of administering insulin are found in any textbook (Wong & Perry, 1998), but follow a procedure of wiping each bottle off, identifying the NPH, and gently rolling it to mix the cloudy mixture. With an insulin syringe, put air in the NPH bottle and then in the regular insulin bottle equal to the dose that is to be withdrawn. First draw up the 5 u. of regular insulin into an insulin syringe, then draw into the same syringe 15 u. of the NPH insulin (up to the 20 u. line). Lisa will need to practice getting air bubbles out when the regular insulin is first added as they notoriously collect in the syringe. Faculty will want to discuss insulin syringes and different types of insulin in more detail. Discuss the sites for injection, also. The leg is a good site to start with because of client dexterity and ease of injecting. Wipe off the skin with alcohol, pinch the skin up and, holding the syringe like a pencil, puncture the skin at a 45- to 90-degree angle and slowly inject the insulin. Cover the site and apply pressure with sterile gauze. Record the time and the site. Faculty could discuss possible experiences and variations in this method with clients having thin versus thick subcutaneous tissue.

3. What kinds of insulin have been ordered? How are they different and why are they both ordered?

The type of insulin ordered is usually biosynthetic human insulin. It has less antigenetic properties and therefore is more compatible. NPH is an intermediate-acting insulin and regular insulin is a fast-acting insulin. These two are usually combined and given prior to the breakfast and the evening meals to cover the client's food intake throughout the day. Insulin doses are adjusted to meet the blood glucose needs. Typically clients will need to test their blood glucose before meals and at bedtime, and sometimes physicians order blood glucose measurements 1 or 2 hours postprandial (Wong & Perry, 1998). Faculty should discuss onset, peak, and duration times of insulin as regular insulin works on the blood sugar rapidly and NPH, an intermediate-acting insulin, tends to regulate blood sugars for longer periods. Students should learn the peak times in order to anticipate when a low blood sugar is most likely to occur, although knowing the signs of hypoglycemia is essential in intervening in such cases.

4. When during her pregnancy will Lisa be most prone to hypoglycemia and hyperglycemia?

Early in pregnancy is the time when hypoglycemia is most common because of the developing fetus needs of and the poor intake of the mother related to morning sickness. Hypoglycemia can also occur in the postpartum period when the client is returning to the pre-pregnancy state. Hyperglycemia occurs in the second and third trimesters when insulin is blocked by the hormones of pregnancy (Wong & Perry, 1998).

5. Explain the signs of hypoglycemia and hyperglycemia and how each are treated.

Hypoglycemia	Hyperglycemia
shaky & anxious	**dry skin**
headache	**fruity breath**
clammy skin	**flushed skin**
tx. with juice/glucagon	**tx. with insulin, fluids, and electrolytes**

6. What other complications are possible for Lisa to encounter because of her diabetes?

   Babies tend to get larger in the gestational client; this causes a problem at delivery with malpresentation or cephalopelvic disproportion. Injury to the baby during delivery can potentially cause the mother to experience anxiety and fear. Failure to progress and thus a longer birth causes the mother to be prone to infection and hemorrhage. Trauma to maternal tissues can be caused from the size of large babies or the procedures necessary to help deliver them such as episiotomy, vacuum extraction, forceps, or cesarean section. Large babies put the mother at risk for uterine atony and subsequent postpartum hemorrhage as the tissues have difficulty contracting back down to size. Additional complications related to the mother's diabetes include pregnancy induced hypertension, premature delivery, and urinary tract infections.

Lisa's blood sugars have been elevated to 130–140 during her pregnancy. She complains that she always feels hungry. Lisa goes into labor at 37 weeks and experiences a difficult labor lasting 16 hours. She has a forceps delivery resulting in a fourth degree laceration, and she delivers a 12-lb. baby boy with evidence of paralysis of the left side of his face and left arm. Lisa is tired and upset and states, "My baby is fat and looks like he has been beaten up. I'm embarrassed to let my family and friends visit." She points to the baby in the crib next to her bed, "Look, his arms and legs shake funny, too."

Focus Questions

1. How would the nurse explain to Lisa why her baby weighed 12 lbs.?

   The fetal pancreas secretes insulin in response to maternal high blood sugars. The insulin acts as a growth hormone causing the fetus to become very large (Wong & Perry, 1998).

2. If Lisa had been a diabetic for 10 years, what could the baby be expected to be like in contrast to the gestational diabetic's baby?

   Diabetics of long standing who become pregnant have different problems related to their vasculature. Vascular problems can result in poorer oxygen and nutritional transfer to the baby as a result of compromised uteroplacental circulation. A small for gestational age baby or baby with intrauterine growth retardation (IUGR) could result (Wong & Perry, 1998).

3. What assessments of Lisa should the nurse make to monitor for potential complications after delivery and why?

   - **Hemorrhage: assess fundus, BP, P, lochia—possibly from uterine atony from an overdistended uterus**
   - **Infection: check temperature and episiotomy and watch for monilial vaginal infection r/t high sugar counts and increased growth of microorganism**

- **Hypoglycemia: monitor blood sugar and watch for postpartum due to changing hormones and drop in blood sugars**
- **Pregnancy induced hypertension: monitor BP and watch for seizures—frequently seizures associated with PIH and diabetes could occur in the postpartum period for up to 6 weeks.**

4. What complications does Lisa's baby have and what additional complications might the nurse anticipate? How might the nurse intervene?

   Lisa's baby has:

   - **Erbs palsy will usually resolve on its own—baby's arm must be supported. Follow-up with pediatrician is indicated.**
   - **Hypoglycemia, especially in first 2 hours of life—baby has signs of shaky arms or irritability, jitteriness, tachypnea, cyanosis; baby should be fed glucose water and formula and monitored for decreased blood sugar.**
   - **Macrosomia—watch for any further signs of injury r/t birth—monitor for fractured clavicle.**

   Other complications to anticipate include:

   - **Respiratory distress syndrome—watch for in babies who were premature or in mother's whose L/S ratios were less than 3:1.**
   - **Hypocalcemia and hypomagnesiumemia—detected through blood drawing; signs of hypocalcemia are similar to hypoglycemia.**
   - **Hyperbilirubinemia and polycythemia—watch the bilirubin level, especially if injury or bruising occurs.**
   - **Cardiomyopathy also occurs more frequently in IDMs and they need to be monitored for congestive heart failure or respiratory problems.**
   - **Other congenital anomalies (Wong & Perry, 1998).**

5. How will the nurse encourage maternal infant bonding?

   The nurse should point out positive aspects of baby, point out how baby responds to mother, role model appropriate behavior, point out temporary nature of his appearance, and encourage rooming in.

Reflective Writing

Lisa says to the nurse, "I'm sure glad this is all over and I won't have to deal with having diabetes anymore." How would you respond?

Educate her on her future health needs:

- **If blood sugar stays in control, you won't need to deal with this, but you are at risk for developing diabetes later in life due to gestational diabetes and your family history; obesity also plays a role in the development of diabetes**
- **If you get pregnant again, gestational diabetes may occur again**
- **Promote the health of you and your future babies by keeping your blood sugar in control especially prior to pregnancy; watch diet and intake of refined sugars; keep weight within normal limits; exercise often**
- **The infant of a diabetic mother is also at risk for obesity and diabetes later in life**

Reference

Wong, D. & Perry, S. (1998). *Maternal child nursing care.* St. Louis: Mosby.

CASE #6 TAMMY PETIT

Learning Objectives

1. Discuss physical and psychosocial nursing interventions appropriate for a mother experiencing a spontaneous abortion
2. Identify potential nursing diagnoses and interventions for clients experiencing spontaneous abortion.
3. List teaching priorities for a woman being discharged post-spontaneous abortion.
4. Describe and give the rationale and indication for McDonald's procedure.

Tammy Petit is a 34-year-old woman admitted to the hospital with complaints of cramping and bleeding. She has changed her pad 3 times in the last 2 hours. She has a history of 3 previous spontaneous abortions. She presents today crying, "I'm going to lose this one, too!" Chart data indicates she is married and has Aetna Insurance. Current pregnancy history: 12 weeks gestation, blood type 0 negative, Rubella susceptible. She and her husband have tried unsuccessfully to have children for the past 7 years. VS: 80/40, P. 120, R 32. , T.99°F.

Focus Questions

1. How can the nurse respond to help Tammy cope with this emergency?

   Use reflective therapeutic communication techniques and caring approaches, such as, "You must be feeling very sad." Let Tammy express her emotional distress. Use touch to convey caring. Get her support person there to help her. Give her information about what you will be doing to help her. According to Swanson (1999), enable Tammy to get through the event by informing, explaining, supporting, and validating her feelings. Stay with her, "being with" during this life transition can let her know the nurse cares. Faculty will recognize that using the caring framework in our approaches can help clients cope.

2. Analyze the data and determine the most immediate priority concerns for Tammy and why.

   - **Excessive bleeding with 3 pads in 2 hours, BP decreased and pulse increased could indicate that hemorrhage is imminent.**
   - **Anxiety r/t potential loss**

3. What additional signs would the nurse anticipate to indicate a worsening in client condition?

   Signs to observe would be:

   A change in level of consciousness, cool and clammy skin, decreased urine output, continued decreasing BP and pulse, and increasing bleeding.

4. List nursing diagnoses and appropriate interventions at this time for Tammy.

Nursing Diagnoses	Interventions
Fluid volume deficit	**Type and cross match for blood** **Start an IV with an 18-gauge needle** **CBC to evaluate hematocrit and hemoglobin** **Monitor the characteristics of the vaginal discharge; assess amount, color, odor, consistency** **Monitor VS for continued changes** **NPO**
Pain r/t contractions	**Position of comfort** **Analgesic medications as prescribed** **Comfort measures** **Breathing and focal point with contractions**
Anticipatory grieving r/t unexpected pregnancy loss	**Therapeutic communication** **Contact family, significant other to support** **Contact clergy of choice**

Tammy's doctor performs a D & C for an incomplete abortion. The nurse anticipates her recovery time will be complete by this afternoon, and that she will be discharged.

Focus Questions

1. How does her plan of care change now that she has aborted and is ready for discharge? Give specifics.

   Discharge teaching would include (Wong & Perry, 1998):

   - **Report any excessive bright red vaginal bleeding**
   - **Scant discharge will persist for one to two weeks**
   - **Antibiotics as prescribed to reduce risk of infection**
   - **Acknowledge that since she has experienced a loss she may have mood swings and depression; refer to support groups**
   - **Avoid pregnancy for 2–3 months**
   - **Intercourse, tub baths, tampons, douching should be avoided until bleeding stops**
   - **Iron supplements may be indicated**

2. What is the significance of her admission lab data and what is indicated on discharge?

   Rhogam and rubella vaccine are indicated. Rhogam is needed because of her Rh negative blood type, and a Rubella vaccine due to her non-immunity. With rubella vaccine, pregnancy should be avoided for 3 months.

Tammy returns to the hospital 8 months later. She is now 14 weeks pregnant and has been admitted for the McDonald's procedure.

Focus Questions

1. What is this procedure? Draw a visual explanation that could be used to educate Tammy prior to the procedure.

This procedure is performed to constrict the internal os and prevent premature delivery. McDonald's procedure (cerclage)—the student should draw a picture of the uterus with the cervix with a ribbonlike band placed around the cervix to constrict the internal os. The suture is left in place until close to term.

2. What are the discharge instructions that the nurse will provide for Tammy after the procedure?
   - **Monitor for contractions, signs of leakage of fluid, increased temperature, or foul odor**
   - **Bedrest may be recommended**
   - **Uterine monitoring may be implemented—she needs to know how to apply and transmit tracing to the monitoring center**
   - **Oral tocolytic drugs—if experiencing contractions and ordered by physician—importance of taking them on time and monitoring side effects (Wong & Perry, 1998)**

Reflective Writing

Is it professional and therapeutic for nurses to display their personal emotions regarding fetal loss when caring for this mother? Why or why not?

It's important to be caring and demonstrate empathy; however, it must be controlled. Do not share your personal birth losses with clients. Some tears are appropriate and can cause the patient to see that you care, but excessive crying would be inappropriate and may cause the client to feel she needs to comfort you. The role should be that you are supporting her. Take your emotions out of the room and release them with other staff members when they are excessive.

References

Swanson, K. (1999). Research-based practice with women who have had miscarriages. *Image, Journal of Nursing Scholarship,* 31(4), 339–345.

Wong, D. & Perry, S. (1998). *Maternal child nursing care.* St.Louis: Mosby.

CASE #7 MARILYN BARBIE

Learning Objectives

1. Differentiate between mild and severe symptoms of pregnancy induced hypertension (PIH).
2. List risk factors for PIH.
3. Discuss nursing interventions appropriate in caring for a client with severe PIH.
4. Explain the rationale for using $MgSO_4$ for clients with PIH.

Marilyn Barbie is a 16-year-old African American G1P0 diagnosed as a gestational diabetic at 24 weeks. Now at 35 weeks gestation, she presents to labor and delivery with blinding headache, abdominal pain, and complaints of seeing spots before her eyes.

Focus Questions

1. What could be happening to Marilyn?

   Marilyn most likely has pregnancy induced hypertension (PIH).

2. What places Marilyn at risk for PIH?

   Being an adolescent, primipara, and a diabetic makes her at more risk for pregnancy induced hypertension (PIH). Sources vary as to whether race is a risk factor (Oliveto, 1997; Patrick & Roberts, 1999; Wong & Perry, 1998).

3. Are these mild symptoms or severe symptoms?

   severe

4. What other data would confirm your suspicions? List the critical assessment data:

   - **BP increase to 160/110 or MAP of 127**
   - **Protein in urine more than 2+ on dipstick or 2g/liter in 24 hours**
   - **Excessive weight gain—more than a pound per week in second and third trimester or sudden weight gain of 4–4½ pounds per week at any time**
   - **Hyperactive reflexes 3+ and ankle clonus (Wong & Perry, 1998)**

Marilyn's vital signs are BP 160/110, P.120, R.32. She has facial edema and weight gain of 4 pounds since her visit last week to see the physician. Urine dip reveals a protein of 3+. The physician orders include a 6 gm. bolus of magnesium sulfate in 150 cc solution of LR over 30 minutes followed by 40 mg. $MgSO_4$ in 1,000cc LR at 2 gm./hr.

Focus Questions

1. Considering her symptoms and prescribed treatments, what specific interventions are necessary to promote safety?

   - **Seizure precautions**
   - **BP, P, R, reflexes every 15 minutes for an hour, every 30 minutes for 2 hours, and then every hour depending on institution protocol**
   - **Urine output of 30 cc is necessary every hour**
   - **Monitor for $MgSO_4$ levels for toxicity (especially with decreased urine output)**
   - **Calcium gluconate at the bedside**
   - **Darken room with decreased environmental stimuli**
   - **Monitor FHT**
   - **Monitor for abruptio placenta—vaginal bleeding, rigid boardlike abdomen**
   - **Bedrest**
   - **Daily weights**

Marilyn has a seizure prior to administration of the $MgSO_4$ drip. The nurse was only able to start an IV of LR maintenance line and had gone to prepare the drug solution. The nurse returns to find Sally, the patient care assistant (PCA), holding a tongue blade in the patient's mouth.

Focus Questions

1. What specific drug is most likely to be given to stop the seizure? What is the effect of this drug?

   Valium—anticonvulsant

2. What nursing interventions need to be instituted immediately?

   The nurse should remove tongue blade, place client on side to open airway, protect her from injury, monitor FHT; observe and chart duration of seizure, movements, responses of patient; administer prescribed Valium.

3. What should the nurse's initial response to Sally's actions be? How should the nurse address this issue with Sally later after the patient is out of danger?

   Take over and say nothing to Sally, but direct her actions, "Take out the tongue blade, help me keep her on her side." Meet with her privately regarding her actions and tell her that her actions were inappropriate and potentially dangerous in that she could have gagged the patient and caused her to aspirate. Tell her she needed to call for help as a first priority.

4. Considering the client's condition, what are potential sequella for the fetus?

   Fetal distress/demise. Marilyn may need an emergency C/S.

Reflective Writing

Managing client care in a crisis is particularly difficult. How do you plan to prepare yourself for these inevitable episodes?

- **Keep priorities straight**
- **Remain calm**
- **Keep abreast of crises that might occur in your area of expertise**
- **Talk about what you should do in crises situations with other experienced nurses and get their ideas**
- **Read and attend conferences r/t different kinds of crises**
- **Encourage mock crises situations to play out with other staff members**

References

Oliveto, T. (1997). Severe preeclampsia. *AJN* 97(7),47.

Patrick, T. & Roberts, J. (1999). Current concepts in preeclampsia. *MCN* 24(4), 193–200.

Wong, D. & Perry, S. (1998). *Maternal child nursing care*. St. Louis: Mosby.

CASE #8 BETH ANN CARSON

Learning Objectives

1. Discuss how nursing interventions might be altered if the client in labor were an adolescent.
2. Identify stages and phases of labor by looking at client assessment data.

3. Discuss comfort measures the nurse might initiate to help clients cope with labor.
4. Identify priority nursing assessments and interventions when spontaneous rupture of the membranes occurs prior to engagement of the fetal head.
5. Identify signs of cord prolapse and compression, as well as priority nursing interventions.

0800 Beth Ann Carson is a 16-year-old primipara at 40 weeks gestation who was admitted through the ER complaining of contractions every 5 minutes. She has had no childbirth classes. Nurse Judy's initial vaginal check shows that Beth Ann is 50% effaced, 3 cm. dilated, and at –2 station. FHT are 130 strong and regular. Contractions are every 5 minutes, lasting 30 seconds. Her mother has accompanied her to the hospital and is demanding that Nurse Judy give her daughter pain medication. The risk assessment and health history indicate no current problems. Her pregnancy has been normal to date. As Judy leaves Beth Ann's room, she comments to Sally, another nurse, "This one back in room six is a real whiner. These young girls need to realize this is not all fun and games!"

Focus Questions

1. Is this data congruent with normal findings for this stage of labor? List criteria to justify your answer.

   Yes it is congruent with Stage 1, latent phase—criteria are cervical dilation of 0–3 cm., contractions are 5 minutes apart lasting up to 45 seconds consistent with latent phase; intensity of contractions are probably strong as her mother is requesting medication, but the nurse needs to assess this further—it could relate to her age and lack of prenatal preparation for labor. The –2 station is not consistent for primiparas—most are engaged or at 0 station in latent phase.

2. What frequency and kind of monitoring is indicated for this stage of labor?

   Monitor VS, uterine activity, FHT, vaginal show, behavior, and energy level every 30 to 60 minutes or per unit protocol. Temperature is taken every 4 hours unless her membranes rupture. Vaginal checks are done only as necessary to identify progress of labor (Wong & Perry, 1998).

3. What nursing interventions should Sally suggest to Nurse Judy to help Beth Ann to cope with labor? Be specific.

   - **The adolescent will need additional support, especially since she has had no prenatal classes**
   - **Talk to the client not just her mother**
   - **Assign consistent caregiver to promote trust**
   - **Be honest with the adolescent, try to prepare her for each change**
   - **If possible allow her to participate in decisions**
   - **Don't treat her as being irresponsible just because she is young**
   - **Teach breathing techniques such as slow chest breathing**
   - **Use focusing techniques**
   - **Initiate relaxation coaching with mother supporting**
   - **Inform of progress**
   - **Praise efforts**
   - **Use comfort measures**

- **Offer fluids and ice chips**
- **Talk about when analgesics and epidural anesthesia could be started**

1700 Beth Ann is now 5 cm. dilated, having contractions every 3–4 minutes and is at a −1 station. FHT remain strong and regular at 130. While ambulating to the bathroom, Beth Ann's water breaks and she screams for help. Nurse Judy gets her back to bed.

Focus Question

1. Which of the following should Nurse Judy do *first* and why? What next?
   a. Call the physician/midwife
   b. Check FHT
   c. Turn her on her left side
   d. Check the color of the amniotic fluid
   e. Give her Demerol for pain

   First priority is to check FHT with ROM—the cord could prolapse especially since the fetal head is not engaged. If FHT has dropped significantly, call the physician or midwife next. If FHT are normal, next check color of fluid to determine if clear, which is normal, or meconium stained, green, indicating possible fetal distress. Faculty need to discuss various possibilities related to this situation and how nursing priorities will change.

The gush of fluid is clear. FHT shows a variable deceleration pattern, dropping abruptly to 50 beats per minute.

Focus Questions

1. What does the FHR pattern of variable deceleration mean, and what is most likely happening?

   Cord compression because of prolapsed cord into the vagina causes an abrupt drop in FHR or variable deceleration as a result of being compressed by the presenting part.

2. What are the nursing interventions that need to be instituted and why?
   - **Place her in Trendelenburg position, or knee chest, to relieve pressure off cord**
   - **Assess through a vaginal exam and feel for the loop of cord around the presenting part**
   - **Call for assistance; have someone call physician stat due to imminent cesarean section if FHR continues to decline**
   - **Place two fingers into the vagina to cervix and exert upward pressure against the presenting part to relieve compression of the cord**
   - **O_2 face mask 10–12 L./min. to support oxygenation of the fetus**
   - **Start an IV or increase the drip rate to support BP and blood flow to fetus**
   - **Continue to monitor FHT to evaluate changes r/t position change**
   - **Transport to operating room—if cord compression confirmed and fetus is in distress**

Reflective Writing

1. Considering Nurse Judy's comment on Beth Ann's admission, how could you best deal with a colleague like Judy?

   - **Relate your most recent positive experience with an adolescent**
   - **Help her to look at the situation from the adolescent's point of view (no childbirth classes, young age, lack of experiences, requiring coping skills)**
   - **Model caring interventions to the adolescent in Judy's presence, such as therapeutic communication techniques, "You must be very scared," or educational interventions "Watch me and breathe with me."**
   - **Don't agree with Judy or let her think her behavior is appropriate**

References

Copeland, D. & Douglas, D. (1999). Communication strategies for the intrapartum nurse. *JOGNN*, 28(6), 579–585.
Wong, D. & Perry, S. (1998). *Maternal-child nursing care*, St. Louis: Mosby.

CASE #9 MOTHER-BABY COUPLETS A, B, AND C

Learning Objectives

1. Analyze assessment data for 3 different infants and their mothers.
2. Discuss routine mother-baby nursing interventions (circumcision care, breast-feeding, and normal assessments).
3. Identify interventions for mother-baby couplets with common complications, such as diabetes, substance abuse, infection.
4. Describe delegation principles in mother-baby care assignments.

Today you are the nurse in charge of 3 mother-baby couplets.

Baby A is a male infant born at 37 weeks gestation to a diabetic mother. He weighed 10 lbs. 2 oz. and was a spontaneous vaginal birth. He is now 1 hour old. Baby A has a large caput, facial bruising, positive moro reflex, and Apgars of 6 and 8. Mom plans to bottle-feed. Baby A's vitals are T. 98°, P.130, R. 48.

Baby B is 3 hours old. Your assessment shows an SGA female infant of 42 weeks who weighs 5 lbs. and has small eye openings and a thin upper lip. Mom has a known history of alcohol and cocaine addiction. She also has a history of having hepatitis B. She is a chronic carrier. You note there are only two vessels on the umbilical cord. T. 96.8°, P.120, R. 62. The baby is jittery and has a positive clonus and a poor suck reflex. Apgars were 5 and 7.

Baby C is a 7 lb. 8 oz. male of 40 weeks gestation from a spontaneous vaginal delivery. He is scheduled for circumcision tomorrow morning. T is 98.2°, P.130, R.40. Mother plans to breast-feed. Apgars were 8 and 10.

Focus Questions

1. There are several routine procedures, lab tests, and treatments necessary for all newborns from birth to discharge. Discuss this plan of care, giving the rationale for all procedures and the treatments.

Eye prophylaxis is given at delivery with Erythromycin ointment to prevent gonnorhea and chlamydia. Aquamephyton IM is given to prevent hemorrhagic disease of the newborn from lack of vitamin K, which cannot be synthesized because of a sterile bowel. Identification is verified prior to mother or baby leaving delivery area. Apgar scoring at birth is to assess baby's adaptation to extrauterine life. Physical assessment of infant is to determine if there is any injury, abnormalities, or congenital anomaly. Gestational age assessment is to assess for risks of early or late gestation. State mandated newborn screenings are required such as PKU, etc. Ability of the baby to feed, eliminate from bowel and bladder, and attachment behaviors are also assessed. All newborns receive hygienic care such as bathing and cord care. Recent research shows natural drying is preferred over use of alcohol on cord (Dore et al., 1998). Varda and Behnke (2000) found that healthy newborns with axillary temperatures greater than or equal to 36.8°C (98.2°F) can be bathed after one hour of age when appropriate care is taken to support thermal stability. Old practices of bathing at four hours of age were believed to increase health-care workers' exposure to bloodborne pathogens and latex allergies.

2. What additional things would be indicated considering the histories for Babies A, B, and C?

   - **Baby A—blood sugars because of risk for hypoglycemia, bilirubin to assess for risk for hyperbilirubinemia if jaundice occurs, check for injury due to large size, blood work for calcium and magnesium may be done since infant is at risk for low levels. Watch for signs indicative of these abnormalities.**

   - **Baby B—watch temperature because it is low and monitor for hypothermia and cold stress; blood sugars for hypoglycemia associated with asphyxia r/t SGA and cold stress, because 2 vessels cord, check closely for congenital anomalies. Respiratory rate is increased, watch for hypoxia r/t meconium aspiration risk, check for meconium staining of cord or fingernails since she is postterm; jittery—watch for signs and symptoms of withdrawal from drugs/alcohol and report to physician. Check for signs of fetal alcohol syndrome as baby already has small eye openings and thin upper lip. Check mother and infant bonding r/t drug abuse. Infant will require HBIG and HBV within 12 hours of life due to mom's hepatitis B. Infant may need to be followed for infection due to hepatitis B and other possible maternal infections not identified, such as gonorrhea, chlamydia, and HIV (maternal lab work may be done).**

   - **Baby C—normal infant—nothing is needed except to monitor circumcision site for bleeding and infection.**

Baby A is doing well. His blood sugar is 80 and he fed well at his first feeding, taking 1 oz. of formula. The mother states, "I hope he does not have diabetes like me." Baby B's mother refuses to feed or look at her daughter. "I will have plenty of time to take care of her at home, let me rest." Baby C is returned to his mother after the circumcision and has Vaseline gauze wrapped around his penis and a small spot of bright red blood in the diaper.

Focus Questions

1. How should the nurse respond to Baby A's mother?

   He may not have diabetes at all, but he is at increased risk for it later in life.

2. How should the nurse document the interaction with Baby B's mother? List interventions the nurse might try to enhance bonding.

   - **Document the mother's statements in the chart. Use quotes and avoid judgmental remarks. Document mother's behavior towards infant (does she look at baby, feed and diaper, name infant, cuddle or talk to infant?)**

- **Nurse should: model appropriate behaviors, point out how the baby is responding to mother's voice, mother needs to understand the cues the baby gives her (French, Pituch, Brandt, Pohorechi, 1998), give her time to rest, tell her you will return—upon return hand her the baby and stay with her. Praise her efforts. Point out positive features of the baby.**

3. What teaching instructions are needed for Baby C's mother?

   Circumcision care: vaseline gauze was applied at time of circumcision; let it fall off naturally; if it doesn't, remove it for mother prior to discharge by getting it wet. Clean by showering penis with soap and water and avoiding touching or rubbing area, or follow standard procedures of hospital. Check for bleeding—a small spot is normal, but it needs to be monitored. Check for signs of infection such as pus or foul smell.

Mother A, a gestational diabetic, delivered a 37 week, 10 lb. 2 oz. baby boy vaginally one hour ago. You note the following data: mother's blood type 0+, rubella immune, fourth degree laceration, swollen perineum, fundus 2 cm. above the umbilicus deviated to the right and boggy, voided 50 cc, lochia large rubra with small clots, breasts soft and nontender (SNT), T 98.6, P.110, R. 20, BP 80/50, blood sugar 90. 1,000cc LR @ 125/hr. with 10 units of Pitocin infuses into R arm. Mother A complains of painful perineum, an 8 on a scale of 1–10.

Focus Questions

1. What nursing intervention is a priority considering the data given, and why?

   Need to assess for site of potential bleeding and stop it. Her pulse is slightly elevated and BP on low side, which could indicate bleeding. Fundus is elevated above normal and is deviated, which indicated a full bladder. Her output may mean she is not emptying sufficiently. With a full bladder, the fundus does not contract well. She also has a large rubra lochia. First massage the fundus to help it contract. This alone could correct the problem. Assess the bladder also as she may need to void or to be catheterized. Inspect other areas for signs of bleeding, such as perineum for a hematoma, bleeding at the episiotomy site, or for continued vaginal bleeding with clots bigger than an egg. This bleeding could suggest vaginal lacerations or retained placenta. Early postpartum hemorrhage is usually the result of uterine atony. The Pitocin in the IV bag will help the uterus to contract. If bleeding continues, call the physician for assistance.

2. What is the meaning of a blood sugar of 90 (use pathophysiology of gestational diabetes to describe your answer)?

   Her blood sugar is normal and reflects the return to her more normal blood sugars from the pre-pregnancy period.

3. Give three nursing interventions that might help to relieve the client's pain.

   Ice packs to perineum, tucks and dermoplast spray to perineum, and analgesics prescribed by physician.

Mother B delivered a 5-pound baby girl at 42 weeks gestation yesterday morning by a spontaneous vaginal delivery. Apgar scores were 5 and 7. Mother B has a history of alcohol and cocaine use as well as a history of hepatitis B. During report today you learned that she refused to feed her baby and asked for the baby to be returned to the nursery. Mother B's temperature at noon is 100.8°, P. 110, R. 32. She complains of chills and severe after-pains and has a foul smelling, rubra lochia. The next morning her temperature is 101°F, and she is asking for more pain medication.

Focus Questions

1. What postpartum care is standard for all mothers who have delivered, and what is the rationale for this routine?

   Immediately following delivery in fourth stage, vital signs, fundus, lochia, voiding, activity level, level of consciousness, and color are assessed every 15 minutes for 1 hour, then every 30 minutes during the second hour or as institution protocol demands. Temperature is checked every 4 hours unless elevated. The assessments continue every shift unless a change has been detected or a cesarean section was performed, in which case the frequency of assessments would increase. These routine assessments usually include vital signs and functional health pattern assessment with an additional focus on the obstetric concerns, for example breasts, uterus, bowel, bladder, lochia, episiotomy, homan's, coping. Protocols regarding assessments may vary according to institution but are generally done frequently in the early postpartum period to prevent hemorrhage, a hazard of the fourth stage of labor.

2. What additional interventions will Mother B need?

   Her temperature elevation after 24 hours was greater than 100.4° and has persisted and increased, which could indicate an infection. The nurse should assess potential sites for infection. Data shows that she also has chills, uterine cramping, and foul smelling lochia, classic signs of endometritis. The physician should be called and informed of her symptoms. It is likely antibiotics will be ordered. The woman may need pain medication, increased fluid intake, and to be positioned in a Fowler's position to help the infection drain from the uterus. It is also a concern that this mother is refusing to feed or care for the baby. The nurse should observe and document bonding behaviors. Possibly the mother is not responding well because she herself does not feel well. Once the infection is under control, a more careful assessment of her interaction with the baby should take place. Social service consult is indicated and a follow-up by public health nursing would be warranted because of her drug history. Referral to substance abuse treatment programs may be necessary.

Mother C, a G1P1, calls the nurse into the room and says, "I'm about ready to give up on breast-feeding. He does not seem to be very interested and does not latch on. What am I to do?"

Focus Question

1. How would you respond to this mother initially and what help could you give her?

   - **Initially the mother needs to be given encouragement to breast-feed. Fear can cause problems with the letdown reflex, so she needs to be calm and relaxed. Examine her nipples to determine if flat or inverted nipples are the problem. If they are or if latching has been a problem, she may need to pump her breasts. Failure to latch and nurse causes milk production problems because of a lack of stimulation. She may need to pump her breast every 2–3 hours and offer pumped breast milk. With support and perseverance, the newborn can begin to suckle appropriately at the breast. Pumping can bring out flat or inverted nipples, thus helping the newborn with the latching problem. Sometimes mothers just need help in waking a sleepy baby. Parents should be instructed to look for subtle cues that a newborn exhibits before achieving a fully awakened state, such as rapid eye movements under the eyelids, sucking movements of the mouth, stretching, small sounds, and restlessness. The newborn with these cues often latches well to the breast. Make sure the baby is also positioned well and maintains a consistent suckling pattern. The parents should understand the length of breast-feeding is about 10–20 minutes per breast, feeding**

every 2–3 hours around the clock for 8–12 feedings a day. To keep the infant interested, the mother switches breasts two or three times during the feeding. To assess if infants are getting an adequate amount, counting wet diaper and stools are helpful tools.

- **Home visits on breast-feeding mothers can also help for problems. Nurses making home visits can assess newborns weight (they may have as much as a 10% loss of weight from the birth weight), amount of output (6 wet diapers are good), presence of jaundice or hyperbilirubinemia, or signs of dehydration (fever, no wet diapers) (Locklin & Jansson, 1999).**
- **Some institutions use breast-feeding tools. Riordan (1998) has found that breast-feeding tools are not currently reliable but assessing breast-feeding problems is essential to identify and intervene with early feeding problems. LATCH is a tool used in some institutions and is in need of further research to establish valid and reliable breast-feeding assessment. The L stands for how well the infant latches onto the breast. Mothers may need a lot of help with directing the nipple into the mouth so that baby's mouth and mom's nipple are in direct alignment; A is for the amount of audible swallowing noted. Getting the baby awake enough to feed is a frequent problem in the early phases. The nurse may need to unwrap the baby to stimulate and awaken him/her. Getting the nipple with the whole areola well into the baby's mouth is really important. Tongue tie can be a source of this problem. T is for the mother's nipple type. Look for inverted nipples or problems of the nipple not protruding well. The mother may need to roll or stimulate the nipple first, or use shields or a breast pump; C is for the mother's level of comfort. Does feeding cause her pain? It should not. If it does, inspect the nipples well for cracks or engorgement. H is for the amount of help the mother needs to hold her infant to breast. Does the mother pull the baby to the nipple rather than the reverse, which is hard on the nipples? Does she need help in maintaining her position? Get pillows and help her support the baby. Other risks to assess r/t mom are support from family or friends, confidence level, ambivalence in breast-feeding, history of breast surgery, or education level. Risk factors in baby could be preterm birth or absence of suckling behaviors such as grasps breast eagerly, tongue down, vigorous and rhythmic sucking (Riordan, 1998).**

Reflective Writing

You are assigned the three mother-baby couplets described in the case today. Megan, a patient care technician (PCT), is paired with you. What tasks would you delegate to Megan and what tasks would you complete yourself? Why?

The answer will depend on the skills and competency of the patient care technician (PCT) as determined by the nurse and the institution. The PCT must be provided orientation and training by the institution and perform the tasks delegated according to the established standards, policies, and procedures of the institution. Examples of the tasks to be delegated to the PCT are hygiene, simple treatments, and simple diagnostic testing (VanCura & Gunchick,1997). On babies, Megan could do baths, vital signs, and PKUs, while the nurse assesses using functional patterns, teaches mom care of the baby at discharge, gives medications and IV therapy. On mothers, Megan could assist with baths, vital signs, bed making, obtaining supplies, and transporting the mother on discharge. The nurse would be responsible for teaching, assessments, monitoring of bonding, and feeding evaluation, as well as IV therapy or medications. The PCA has been trained to do lab work and routine tasks and report any elevations of vital signs to the nurse. The nurse is responsible for any type of assessment, teaching, judgment, or evaluation of the client care. Supervising, monitoring, and evaluating are the role of the nurse. When delegating, the nurse must be aware of what can be delegated to the

PCA in a particular situation, determine if the PCT is competent to perform the task, assure accountability and acceptance of the task by the PCT, supervise the performance of the task, intervene if necessary, and evaluate the entire delegation process (VanCura & Gunchick, 1997).

References

Dore, S., Buchan, D., Coulas, S., Hamber, L., Stewart, M., Cowan, D., and Jamieson, L. (1998). Alcohol versus natural drying for newborn cord care. *JOGNN*, 27(6), 621–627.

French, E., Pituch, M., Brandt, J., Pohorechi, S. (1998). Improving interactions between substance abusing mothers and their substance exposed newborns. *JOGNN*, 27(3), 262–269.

Locklin, M. & Jansson, M. (1999). Home visits: Strategies to protect the breastfeeding newborn at risk. *JOGNN*, 28(1), 33–39.

Riordan, J. (1998). Predicting breastfeeding problems. *AWHONN Lifelines*, 2(6), 31–33.

Stevenson, A. (1999). Immunizations for women and infants. *JOGNN*, 28(5), 534–544.

Van Cura, B. & Gunchick, D. (1997). Five key components for effectively working with unlicensed assistive personnel. *Medsurg Nursing*, 6(5), 270–274.

Varda, K. & Behnke, R. (2000). The effect of timing of initial bath on newborn's temperature. *JOGNN*, 29(1), 27–32.

CASE #10 ANNA RHODES

Learning Objectives

1. Collect and analyze appropriate assessments on pregnant client admitted with vaginal bleeding.
2. Differentiate between abruptio placenta and placenta previa.
3. Identify signs and symptoms of fetal distress and pathophysiology related to these responses.
4. Identify nursing interventions appropriate prior to and after an emergency C-S.
5. Explain problems of prematurity, their underlying causes, and nursing interventions.

Anna Rhodes is a 23-week-gestation white female, age 33, G4P3, presents in the labor and delivery suite. Her current pregnancy has been uneventful until this morning when she noticed two spots of bright red blood about the size of a nickel in her panties. She has no pain, FHT 140, strong and regular. BP 130/80, P.88, R. 20. No other vaginal leakage has been observed. Anna is concerned about being dilated and asks the nurse to check her.

Focus Questions

1. How would the nurse respond to Anna's request?

   The nurse should explain that a vaginal exam is contraindicated until an ultrasound can determine the source of the bleeding. An exam could cause more bleeding.

2. What data will the nurse need when reporting to the physician?

   The nurse will need: VS, FH pattern and rate, estimation of blood loss, history and current data on pregnancy, such as duration of pregnancy, gravida and para, contractions or leakage of fluid, any abnormalities during this or previous pregnancy.

3. Draw a complete placenta previa and a complete abuptio placenta showing uterus, fetus, placenta. Label the signs and symptoms showing the differences in the two conditions.

Complete Previa	Complete Abruptio
Painless vaginal bleeding	Painful vaginal bleeding
Bright red bleeding	Rigid boardlike abdomen
Changes in BP and P reflect the degree of bleeding	Massive shock

In a previa, the student should draw the placenta covering the opening to the cervix or completely covering the internal os. In abruptio, the student should draw the placenta in the fundus area but completely pulling away from the uterine wall. The faculty should discuss the variations in these two conditions.

4. Compare assessment data typically observed with placenta previa and abruptio placenta. What might the nurse anticipate knowing the differences in these two bleeding disorders of pregnancy and the data in this case?

   The data suggest, so far, that a placenta previa might be the cause of the bleeding. Currently the bleeding is only a few spots, and previa bleeding tends to begin this way. The client could stop bleeding only to be admitted again during pregnancy with another episode of bleeding that is a little heavier. If it were determined that the client had an abruptio placenta, bleeding would continue. In both cases the nurse should anticipate that a cesarean section may need to be performed depending on how much blood is actually lost and fetal responses. Assessments will be essentially the same, however, because bleeding is the primary problem. The nurse will observe characteristics, amount and color of the vaginal discharge, and assess the vital signs, paying particular attention to pulse and BP. Observe for any signs of labor contractions, pain, or tender uterus and the tenseness of the abdomen. Assessments for signs and symptoms of shock are required as well. The nurse might anticipate getting lab work to evaluate hemoglobin and hematocrit, type and cross match.

Tests confirm a complete placenta previa. Anna is sent home and returns the following month. The frequency of Anna's episodes of bleeding increased during the past month as well as the amount. She states she has saturated two pads within the last hour. The FHT are 180 and have a decreased variability. Scalp pH results are declining.

Focus Questions

1. Interpret the fetal data in the above paragraph and anticipate what could occur if these signs progress. What other clinical signs might the nurse anticipate?

   Fetus is showing signs of distress with the increased heart rate and decreased variability. The fetal heart rate could decrease, show decelerations, and decreased variability, and, if bleeding is continuous, acidotic scalp pH readings. Signs of meconium staining and fetal demise could ensue. The physician should be informed at the first sign of fetal distress and, in this case, should be fully aware of the amount of bleeding that has been occurring.

2. What interventions does the nurse need to implement, considering the data? Be specific and show priority of actions.

   The nurse could anticipate an emergency C-S because of signs of fetal distress. The client should have a type and cross match that is done with the H&H, an IV started with a #18 gauge needle, permit signed, NPO, insert a foley catheter, and prep the abdomen. Preparing the client is important throughout the process. Some of these things may have already been implemented.

An emergency C-S is performed resulting in a baby girl with a weight of 2 pounds and with meconium staining of the amniotic fluid. Apgar scores are 2 and 3. The baby is sent to the neonatal intensive care unit (NICU) in critical condition.

Focus Questions

1. What does meconium staining indicate? Describe the pathophysiology.

   It is usually an indication of fetal distress. The infant relaxes the bowel when stressed, which releases the meconium stool into the amniotic fluid. A green color appears. As the fetus is more stressed, meconium in amniotic fluid may look thicker.

2. What problems and interventions with this baby should the NICU nurses be anticipating and why?

Ineffective breathing patterns	**Immature respiratory center and lack of surfactant**	**Support respiratory efforts with ventilator Keep warm to avoid cold stress Conserve energy through TPN and Lipids feeding Decreased stimulation**
Thermoregulation ineffective	**Large surface area Decreased brown fat**	**Incubator Dry thoroughly at birth Continuously monitor temperature**
Altered nutrition less than body requirements	**Weak, absent sucking reflex prior to 32 weeks gestation**	**TPN & Lipids Gavage feeds**
Impaired skin integrity	**Lack of subcutaneous fat; the need for multiple monitor lines secured to the skin results in tissue damage**	**Frequent position changes, Reshape ears Soft bedding Monitor skin redness and breakdown**
Risk for infection	**Immature immune system Invasive procedures**	**Sterile procedures Wash hands Keep out visitors with colds**

3. What postpartum interventions will Anna require in addition to routine postpartum needs? Why?

   - **All the interventions necessary for client's recovery from a surgical procedure:**

     —coughing and deep breathing

     —turning in bed, progressing to dangling, and then ambulation

     —incentive spirometer

     —foley catheter

     —wound care

     —pain management, e.g., PCA

     —NPO until BS, then clear liquids and advance as tolerated

- **Emotional care and support r/t critically ill infant—often an up and down course**
  - **—take to see infant**
  - **—explain all tubes**
  - **—explain infant behavior, inability to respond**
  - **—encourage to touch if infant stable enough**
  - **—help to begin care taking**
  - **—support group**
  - **—facilitate interactions between parent and physician—need support in asking questions**

Reflective Writing

Discuss the pros and cons on withholding or withdrawing treatment to babies in the NICU, such as the one in this case, who seem to have little chance of quality of life.

- Pros

  Baby may become a financial burden to parents; baby may be disabled or mentally retarded and become a burden for family with constant care required; child may not experience bonding necessary for development of trust and could be abandoned by parents unable to cope or accept child's condition

- Cons

  Outcomes of the infant cannot be accurately predicted. It may be good; only God determines who dies. Nurses duty is beneficience, not doing harm.

Reference

Kavanaugh, K. (1997). Parents' experience surrounding the death of a newborn whose birth is at the margin of viability. *JOGNN*, 26(1), 43–51.

CASE #11 PEGGY PRICE

Learning Objectives

1. Identify risk factors in pregnancy from a nursing history and assessment.
2. List signs and symptoms differentiating true and false labor.
3. Discuss the rationale for and nursing interventions involved in administering tocolytic drugs to a client in premature labor.
4. Discuss the rationale for and nursing interventions related to the use of glucocorticoid drugs to a client in premature labor.
5. Identify signs and symptoms of aburptio placenta.
6. Discuss nursing interventions appropriate for clients experiencing abruptio placenta.
7. Explore nursing interventions appropriate for the client experiencing fetal loss.

8. Explore personal feelings or biases related to the care of the pregnant client who is a substance abuser.

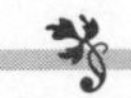

1200 Monday. Thirty-seven-year-old Peggy Price is a G3P2 woman who has a history of recurrent urinary tract infections during this pregnancy. She is a known cocaine addict and has been treated for gonorrhea in her second pregnancy. She currently has poor weight gain and anemia. Today, now 28 weeks gestation, she presents to the labor and delivery unit with abdominal cramping.

Focus Questions

1. Identify the risk factors in this case.

   Cocaine history, history of STD, poor weight gain, anemia, recurrent UTI during pregnancy, age over 35, current abdominal cramping at 28 weeks

2. What assessments should be collected? Which ones will confirm her labor?

   The nurse should assess dilation, effacement, station, status of membranes, VS, FHT, and duration, frequency, and intensity of uterine contractions. Dilation and effacement of the cervix will confirm labor.

3. What will determine whether the physician will try to stop the labor or let her deliver spontaneously?

   If there is over 4 cm. dilatation or fetus is dead, physician will not stop labor.

4. If the physician tries to stop the labor, what medication(s) would typically be ordered, and what are the actions and side effects of these drugs?

   Tocolytic drugs (Wong & Perry, 1998) will first be started intravenously, then by mouth or by subcutaneous route. Some typical drugs are the beta adrenergic drugs such as Terbutaline and Ritodrine, which inhibit uterine muscle activity. Side effects (SE) of Terbutaline or Ritodrine are: tachycardia, hypokalemia, hyperglycemia, and pulmonary edema, especially when used with Celestone. Magnesium sulfate decreases uterine activity. SE of magnesium sulfate are depressed or absent deep tendon reflexes, decreased respiratory rate, decreased level of consciousness; toxicity is enhanced with decreased urine output. Calcium gluconate should be placed at the bedside as an antidote for magnesium sulfate toxicity. Procardia, a calcium channel blocker, is also being used. SE of Procardia are tachycardia and bradycardia; it lowers BP, causes headache, fatigue, and possible pulmonary edema.

5. If delivery is planned, what medication would be given to Peggy to help the fetus? How does this medicine help the fetus?

   Celestone or Betamethasone is a glucocorticoid that enhances fetal lung maturity. It is usually given within 24–48 hours of delivery. When taking Celestone, the client should be observed for pulmonary edema (Wong & Perry, 1998).

1230 Monday. Peggy's contractions are of strong intensity, occurring every 3 minutes and lasting 45 seconds. Peggy's abdomen is as hard as a board. As the nurse prepares to do a vaginal check, dark red blood gushes out. The nurse stops and checks for a fetal heart rate with a doppler and finds none. Peggy's blood pressure is 90/60; P.120, her skin is pale, cool, and moist.

Focus Questions

1. What do these signs mean and what should the nurse do?

   Signs could mean she is experiencing an abruptio placenta; this is an emergency situation in which both mother and baby could die. The nurse should recognize that decreased BP, increased pulse, boardlike abdomen, and dark red bleeding are classic signs. Additional signs of profound shock could occur, such as cool and clammy skin and decreased level of consciousness. Notify the physician stat, plan for an emergency C-S.

2. Should a vaginal check have been done to measure labor progress? Justify your answer.

   No. It is unclear where the bleeding is coming from until an ultrasound can be done. A vaginal check could augment bleeding.

1245 Monday. Peggy's emergency C-S results in delivery of a 2-lb. stillborn baby boy with microcephaly and a right arm shorter than his left.

Focus Questions

1. What interventions are necessary to assist Peggy with the grieving process?
   - **Offer support through caring techniques of being present and sharing the experience.**
   - **Use and therapeutic communication, listen, and touch.**
   - **Get her family to support her.**
   - **Call the clergy to visit.**
   - **Let her see the baby and take a picture, footprints, and a lock of hair for remembrance.**
   - **Counsel her about the grief process and what to expect regarding her own responses and others.**
2. What referrals should be in the discharge plan of care?
   - **Grieving support group**
   - **Social service consult**
   - **Encourage treatment in a drug abuse program**
   - **Individual counseling or family counseling services**

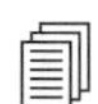

Reflective Writing

What are your feelings or biases about women who are substance abusers during pregnancy? How might this affect the care of this client?

Students may respond with a variety of feelings, beliefs, and biases, which may include:

- **The woman shouldn't do this; it is child abuse to knowingly take drugs that are harmful.**
- **She knew what she was doing and will have to carry the burden of the loss.**

- **Cocaine is very addictive, and she could not stop what she was doing. She may have really cared for the baby but couldn't overcome the addiction.**
- **In examining their own feelings, students could determine that they could not give the client good care because of their anger toward her, or students may feel they have a lot of empathy for the client and could be very caring.**
- **The faculty should ask them what is the nursing role in this case and reflect on the nurses' code of ethics.**
- **Faculty should help students see the role of addiction (Jessup, 1997) and the nurse's role of advocating for harm-reduction programs, such as enforcement of drunk driving laws, provision of Methadone as a legal substitute for heroine users, provision of clean needles and safe sex instruction to injection drug users, amnesty from loss of child custody in exchange for full participation in prenatal care. By welcoming all women into care settings and avoiding lecturing and threats, pregnancy complications can be identified and treated promptly (Kearney, 1997).**
- **Legal definitions of child abuse and neglect and agency protocol defines what nurses will do in their respective settings. Information gained regarding drug and alcohol abuse must be collected for a therapeutic purpose, not with a punitive or prosecutorial intent (Jessup, 1997).**

References

Flagler, S., Hughes, T. , Kovalesky, A. (1997). Toward an understanding of addiction. *JOGNN*, 26(4), 441–448.

Ruiz, R. (1998). Mechanisms of full-term and preterm labor: Factors influencing uterine activity. *JOGNN*, 27(6), 652–658.

Jessup, M. (1997). Addiction in women: Prevalence, profiles, and meaning. *JOGNN*, 26(4), 449–457.

Kavanaugh, K. (1997). Parents' experience surrounding the death of a newborn whose birth is at the margin of viability. *JOGNN*, 26(1), 43–51.

Kearney, M. (1997). Drug treatment for women: Traditional models and new directions. *JOGNN*, 26(4), 459–467.

Wong, D. & Perry, S. (1998). *Maternal child nursing care.* St. Louis: Mosby.

CASE #12 JUANITA GUITTEREZ

Learning Objectives

1. Discuss PIH and the usual medications administered for PIH.
2. Describe an incident report.
3. Relate to cross-cultural issues in the care of the obstetric client.
4. Discuss discharge plans and referrals.

Twenty-year-old Juanita Guitterez is a gravida 1, para 1, Mexican migrant worker. She had a spontaneous vaginal delivery (SVD) 12 hours ago following a labor of 18 hours. Pregnancy was complicated by pregnancy induced hypertension (PIH), which was diagnosed 2 weeks ago at her first prenatal visit to the clinic. Labor was induced at 38 weeks because of increased symptoms of PIH. She still has 3+ pitting ankle edema, her face and hands appear puffy, and she has deep tendon reflexes (DTRs) 2+. She is receiving IV Lasix. Her second dose of Lasix was given by the last shift. Nurse Kellie is coming on duty and making rounds. Kellie notes that her output has not significantly increased (100 ml total postpartum).

Focus Questions

1. What are the critical nursing interventions Kellie needs to do to care for Ms. Guitterez?

   Kellie needs to consider key assessment findings in order to give safe care to her client. Her assessment will be multifactorial:

   - **routine postpartum assessment**
   - **assessment of her client's PIH**
   - **assessment of the impact that language and/or culture will have on her client's care**

   Kellie will do a complete postpartum assessment that includes vital signs, fundal tone and location, perineal and breast check, amount and character of lochia, pain level, infant bonding behaviors, and infant care activities. Kellie will also monitor her client's PIH: she will check urine for quantity, protein, and specific gravity q1h and monitor DTRs and blood pressure. Kellie will be aware of previous vital signs and medication administration (drug, dose, and time). In addition, Kellie will assess her client's understanding of her condition, especially in regard to a possible language barrier. She will also assess the family's support and understanding of her client's condition.

2. Why is Ms. Guitterez still experiencing edema and having decreased urine output?

   Possible reasons for the persistent edema and decreased urine output may be postpartal eclampsia with worsening of her condition. Other reasons may include delayed postpartal diuresis or the possibility that the previous nurse did not administer the Lasix.

3. Develop a nursing care plan incorporating pertinent nursing diagnoses and interventions.

   - **Nursing Diagnosis: Fluid volume excess is related to retention and impaired sodium excretion secondary to impaired renal function.**
   - **Expected Outcome: The client will experience diuresis and decreased edema.**
   - **Nursing Interventions: Be strict regarding intake and output, encourage oral fluids and high protein diet, monitor blood pressure, administer prescribed medications (Lasix has been ordered for Ms. Guitterez), provide seizure precautions, monitor DTRs, monitor for pulmonary edema, maintain IV fluids as ordered.**
   - **Nursing Diagnosis: Altered social interaction.**
   - **Expected Outcome: Client will receive support from family and/staff.**
   - **Nursing Interventions: Assess understanding of English, utilize resources: common Spanish phrases listed in nursing resource books, hospital staff person who speaks Spanish, or family member, obtain Spanish language teaching guides, ensure discharge medication instructions are written in Spanish, obtain chaplain support if client wishes.**
   - **Nursing Diagnosis: Fear/anxiety related to condition and distance from home and extended family.**
   - **Expected Outcome: Client will experience decreased anxiety.**
   - **Nursing Interventions: Provide calm environment, educate client about procedures and nursing interventions, encourage verbalization of fears, keep client and family informed of condition.**
   - **Other nursing diagnoses may be listed: Altered urinary elimination, impaired verbal communication altered family processes, fatigue, sleep pattern disturbance, knowledge deficit.**

4. What are the maternal and fetal risks of PIH?

   - **Maternal risks of PIH: PIH can affect most of the mother's organ systems with resultant serious complications. Approximately 1% of women will develop seizures that result from cerebral edema. Cerebral hemorrhage or heart failure can lead to death in women with PIH. Retinal detachments can occur due to increased intraocular pressure. Vasoconstriction of the renal vessels can lead to acute tubular necrosis, and increased capillary permeability can lead to pulmonary edema. Thrombocytopenia is thought to be the result from platelet consumption. Hemolysis of red blood cells is manifested by a low hemoglobin and hyperbilirubinemia. In severe PIH the mother may experience the HELLP syndrome: hemolysis—H, elevated liver enzymes—EL, low platelet count—LP.**
   - **Fetal risks of PIH: Perinatal mortality is high and may approach 10–20%. Maternal vasospasm can cause some degree of an abruptio placenta and/or fetal hypoxia. As a result the infant may experience intrauterine growth retardation (IUGR). Development of dire maternal complications may necessitate early infant delivery with the concomitant risks associated with a premature infant. Infants may also experience untoward effects from maternal medication, namely sedatives and magnesium sulfate.**

Kellie discovered that the last dose of Lasix was not given. She administers the Lasix before she leaves. Jaunita's edema is decreasing and her urine output is 800 ml.

Focus Questions

1. Should Kellie complete an incident report (IR)? Why or why not? What data needs to be included in Kellie's documentation? What is not documented? Write an IR for the missed Lasix.

   - **Kellie should complete an incident report because the missed Lasix dose is an error of omission. An incident report should be completed for any event that is uncommon, abnormal, or inconsistent with the routine process.**
   - **Incident report data: patient's name, date of incident, date of report, location of incident, factual details of incident, name and signature of person completing report, and followup information as per agency policy (physician notification, client/family notification, Risk Management Department protocol).**
   - **No documentation of the initiation and completion of the incident report is included in the patient's chart. The incident report does not contain any subjective assessments of the incident, it is only a statement of facts and not conjecture.**
   - **Sample statement for incident report:**
     Patient identification and other information on form as per agency policy; then the factual statement:

     Missed medication, Lasix 40 mg IV, at 0900, date. Attending physician ____________

     notified at______________.

     Signed________________________________ Date and time__________________

2. Ms. Guitterez has received Pitocin for labor induction, Magnesium Sulfate, and Lasix. What is the action, usual dose, and side effects of these medications? What are the signs of Magnesium Sulfate toxicity and its antidote?

Medication	Action	Usual Dose	Side Effects
Pitocin (Oxytocin)	Stimulates smooth muscle of uterus and blood vessels. Increases strength of muscle contraction. Initially oxytocin lowers blood pressure but increases blood pressure with prolonged administration. Doses of 20 mU/minute or greater can cause decrease in urine output	Labor induction: 10 units/1,000 ml of IV solution = 10 mU/1ml IV fluid. Start at 1–2 mU/minute and increase by 1 mU/minute q 15 minutes until good contraction pattern reached.	Uterine hypercontractility: Abruptio placentae, fetal hypoxia, rapid labor, uterine rupture, tachycardia, fetal trauma d/t rapid birth, maternal hypotension, fetal arrythmias, maternal water intoxication, hyponatremia
Magnesium Sulfate ($MgSO_4$)	CNS depressant thus reduces possibility of seizures. Relaxes smooth muscle thus may decrease blood pressure. Decreases frequency and intensity of contractions.	For PIH: loading dose: 4–6 g IV as 20% solution in 15–20 minutes; maintenance: 1–2 g/hr IV	Sweating, flushing, nasal congestion, n&v, blurred vision, headache, slurred speech
Lasix (Furosemide)	Diuresis and mobilization of excess fluid, lowers blood pressure	20–40 mg q8h	Dizziness, headache, nervousness, tinnitus, hypotension, dry mouth, blood dyscrasias, metabolic alkalosis, hypokalemia, hypomagnesemia

- Signs of Magnesium Sulfate toxicity: decreased respirations less than 12/min, hyporeflexia or absence of reflexes, decreased urine output less than 30 mL/hour, toxic serum levels more than 30 mL/hour, fetal distress, significant drop in maternal pulse or blood pressure. Calcium Gluconate is the antidote for Magnesium Sulfate toxicity.

3. Review the pathophysiology of PIH and describe the signs and symptoms.

- Pathophysiology: Decreased placental perfusion, vasospasm, and endothelial cell damage due to decrease in circulating plasma volume and increase in maternal hematocrit. This pathophysiology is related to the physiologic changes of pregnancy.

Signs and symptoms:

- Hypertension due to generalized vasoconstriction
- Proteinuria, increase plasma uric acid and creatinine, oliguria, and sodium retention due to glomerular damage
- Facial, hand, abdominal edema, pitting edema after bed rest
- Headache, hyperreflexia, seizures due to cerebral edema and cerebral vascular spasms
- Dyspnea due to pulmonary edema
- Blurred vision and retinal pathology due to retinal vasospasm
- Decreased hemoglobin and hyperbilirubinemia due to hemolysis of red blood cells

- **Elevated liver enzymes, nausea, vomiting, epigastric pain, hypoglycemia, due to liver pathology (emboli)**
- **Thrombocytopenia (DIC) due to platelet aggregation and deposition of fibrin**

4. Describe some ways Kellie might foster inclusion of the family in Ms. Guitterez' care.

   Sit down and talk with family members about her condition, what is being done at present, and what the plans are for her recovery. Obtain a Spanish language translator if necessary. Provide Spanish language information guides. Encourage family members to care for the infant while in the hospital. Provide appropriate videos on infant care.

   Listen to family's concern, especially regarding the geographic mobility and living arrangements for migrant farmworkers. Obtain social service consult for hospitalization costs and continuity of care for both mother and infant after discharge. Ask family what they would like to do to care for Ms. Guitterez and the infant.

Ms. Guitterez is ready for discharge. She will be returning to her migrant farmworkers' community, which is now 200 miles north of here.

Focus Question

1. Write a bulleted list of all essential elements needed for Ms. Guitterez's discharge summary. How might Kellie ensure that Ms. Guitterez and her infant receive the necessary follow-up care after discharge?

   - **Routine postpartum discharge: report any warning signs to hospital or health care provider accessible to migrant farmworker community. Stress importance of seeking attention for warning signs. Provide written material that is understood by Ms. Guitterez and evaluate understanding. Warning signs: fever, foul smelling or irritating vaginal discharge; excessive lochia, return of bright red lochia after lochia has changed to serosa or alba; painful, red, or hot area on leg; painful, hot, or swollen area on breast; painful urination or inability to urinate; pelvic or perineal pain.**
   - **Stress importance of rest, diet high in protein, gradual return to activities, no strenuous activity for next 6 weeks.**
   - **Obtain social service consult for continuity of care for mother and infant in probable community.**
   - **Care of infant: ensure approved infant seat is available (family's own or hospital/service agency provided). Make arrangements for PKU testing. Provide thermometer and ensure mother knows correct use procedure and how to read the thermometer. Review normal physiologic adaptation: respirations, heart rate, skin, fontanels, color, activity, umbilical cord care, circumcision care, voiding and stooling, sleep patterns, feeding. Provide verbal, demonstration, video, and written material about breast-feeding, bottle-feeding.**
   - **Provide information about Women, Infants, and Children (WIC) and how to obtain this service.**

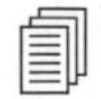

Reflective Writing

If you were in a foreign country with the same diagnosis as Juanita, what would your expectations of the medical system and the nurses be? What steps by the nurse would help you handle the communication obstacle?

- **Expectations: Medical and nursing staff should demonstrate respect of the client. This can be accomplished by listening to the client's questions, fears, and verbalizations about the situation and the care provided. There would be concern for the quality of the care received. Equipment, medications, even the physical environment may create a sense of competence or unease.**
- **Communication: Talking to a staff person fluent in my own language would do a great deal to lessen anxiety. If this is not possible, I would like to be able to point to common phrases in my language. Hopefully the hospital unit would have such a phrase book. I would also want understandable written instructions, especially for medication administration.**

References

Callister, L. V. (1995). Cultural meaning of childbirth. *JOGNN,* 24 (4), 327–331.

Gwyther, M. & Jenkins, M. (1998). Migrant farmworker children: Health status, barriers to care, and nursing innovations in health care delivery. *Journal of Pediatric Health Care,* 12 (2), 60–66.

Lambert, M. I. (1995). Migrant and seasonal farm worker women. *JOGNN,* 24 (3), 265–268.

Lester, M. A. (1998). Cultural competence: A nursing dialogue. *American Journal of Nursing,* 98 (8), 26–33.

Weber, S. E. (1996). Cultural aspects of pain in childbearing women. *JOGNN,* 25 (1), 67–72.

Wong, L. & Perry, S. (1998). *Maternal child nursing care.* St. Louis: Mosby.

chapter **2**

Annotated Pediatric Cases

 CASE #1 CARA MILLER

Learning Objectives

1. Discuss symptoms and diagnostic tests related to cystic fibrosis (CF).
2. List appropriate nursing assessments and interventions for a child with CF.
3. Discuss issues related to having a child with a chronic illness and its genetic impact.
4. Describe appropriate teaching strategies for instructing parents in the care of a nasogastric tube and medport.
5. Discuss the application of developmental approaches with the toddler and the adolescent.

Two-year-old Cara Miller is admitted to the pediatric unit with pneumonia. This is Cara's second admission with pneumonia in the past six months. Her history revealed a meconium ileus at birth. Clinical assessment reveals decreased breath sounds on the right side at the bases, rhonchi scattered in the upper lobes, respirations 32 and shallow, temperature 101°F. Thick secretions are suctioned after a nebulizer treatment and chest physiotherapy (CPT) per respiratory therapist. Cara's weight is 20 lbs. She has decreased subcutaneous tissue in her extremities. Her sweat chloride is 65 mEq/L. The mother states Cara tastes salty when she kisses her skin. Cara is started on IV Piperacillin.

Focus Questions

1. Describe the significance of the sweat chloride test in relation to the above assessment data.

   The test detects abnormally high sodium and chloride concentration in the sweat; greater than 60 mEq/l is diagnostic of cystic fibrosis. The physical assessment data that correlates with a diagnosis of cystic fibrosis (CF) is meconium ileus at birth, low weight and thin extremities, recurrent pneumonia with thick secretions, fever, and respiratory distress. A salty taste is a common sign that parents report.

2. Using a functional pattern framework, list the nursing assessments with rationale and interventions indicated for this child. Include priority.

   Activity exercise pattern is important to assess due to the thick mucous that obstructs the respiratory tract and becomes a medium for infection to develop.

   Assess respiratory rate and rhythm, use of accessory muscles, color, adventitious sounds, retractions, cough, alertness, activity tolerance (instructor could describe progression as the child ages, i.e., barrel chest, clubbing, emphysema);

	administer chest physiotherapy (CPT), postural drainage, aerosols with bronchodilators, DNase to decrease mucous viscosity, breathing exercises, administer antibiotics. Special devices to open airways. Cluster nursing activities to promote rest and schedule regular rest periods. Do CPT prior to meals.
Nutrition-Metabolic is important to assess because of obstructed pancreatic ducts, which leads to malabsorption syndrome of fats, proteins, and to a lesser degree carbohydrates	**Administer pancreatic enzymes with meals such as Pancrease and Cotazym-S, vitamin supplements especially water soluble forms of the fat soluble vitamins A, D, E, K, iron, diet high in calories and protein with fats as tolerated. Increase salt during hot weather or febrile periods. Often parents will need to be taught how to insert an NG tube and manage an infusion pump for nutritional supplements.**
Elimination is important to assess because malabsorption syndrome is common and marked by diarrhea, large frothy foul smelling stools, abdominal cramping and distention, weight loss. As nondigested food is excreted it causes increased bulk of stools and subsequent prolapsed rectum. Intestinal obstruction due to thickened mucous also causes abdominal distention and constipation.	**Teach parents to assess for intestinal obstruction and rectal prolapse. Interventions to prevent these problems are lower fat diet and enzymes. For treating intestinal obstruction: Go-LYTELY, laxatives and stool softeners. For prolapse, teach reduction with gloved finger.**
Role relationship is important to assess because of the family adjustment to the child with a chronic, life threatening illness that was genetically transmitted.	**Offer support and educate about the disease, encourage ventilation of feelings such as guilt, give anticipatory guidance, refer to counseling and CF Foundation.**

Cystic fibrosis (CF) is confirmed by the sweat chloride test. The physician has ordered Pancrease to be given with Cara's high-protein and high-carbohydrate diet with liberal use of salt. She was placed on water miscible vitamins A, D, E, K, and supplemental iron. Chest physiotherapy (CPT) after aerosol treatments with DNase is to be implemented. Cara's mother and father are overwhelmed with the diagnosis and the fact that the doctor has recommended genetic testing. They ask if there is anything they can do to prevent this from happening again. Both parents are working full time, and Cara is currently in day care.

Focus Questions

1. How should the nurse respond to Cara's parents question?

   Explain that CF is inherited in families. The risk of having another child with CF is 1 in 4. Encourage them to go for genetic counseling.

2. What are the issues related to having a child with a chronic illness?

   Several treatments daily will place a strain on the family and affect their employment and current day care arrangement. Parents will feel guilty and grieve over the loss of a perfect child. Both parents and child will go through a process of adjusting to having a chronic

illness. They will have day-to-day stresses related to constant care giving, the effect of the illness on their marriage and social lives, the effect of the illness on their other children, and the reactions of others. They will have stresses, such as finances, housing, and transportation. They will have worries about the future, especially any future children, and schooling for Cara. All family members will experience stress throughout the life of the affected child, such as entering school, adolescence, career issues, and death of the child.

Cara recovers from this episode of pneumonia. For long-term care of this child's chronic illness, the doctor orders nasogastric (NG) feedings nightly with the supplement Vital and plans to insert a central line for long-term antibiotic care. Cara remains on her current oral medications and CPT qid. Cara is to be discharged tomorrow.

Focus Questions

1. How might the nurse instruct the mother to insert the NG tube and administer the feeding?

   The nurse should assess if the parent can adequately perform the procedure. The nurse could use demonstration and return demonstration to teach the procedure and give the mother written guidelines with pictures and step-by-step instruction. The mother should be given a number to call if she has any problems. (The faculty may want students to role-play appropriate teaching using a doll.)

2. How would the nurse deal with teaching the mother about the future central line?

   Assess if the parent is capable and confident in performing this procedure, and plan an appropriate time in which to conduct the teaching sessions once the central line is inserted. The nurse will need to decide if home care nurses are needed to supervise initially or if discharge may have to be delayed for the parents to become confident in caring for Cara. Describe what the central line is and show visual diagrams of its insertion. Plan teaching of the care of the central line, such as changing the dressing, administering antibiotics, troubleshooting problems, and knowing the warning signs of infiltration, air embolus, clotting, etc. (Faculty will want to review these skills with students using models and role-play.)

3. Cara is resistant to taking her medications. What strategies could the parents use?

   The parents could use play and rewards. They could allow Cara to help if she is developmentally able or hide medication in food. Other strategies include keeping security items with child and informing parents that children frequently regress. Parents could hold Cara on their lap in a comfort hold, touch and talk when giving meds, prepare Cara immediately before any painful procedure, and make med time a consistent time.

Reflective Writing

Children with CF may live to adolescence and early adulthood. They have lived their lives dealing with frequent hospitalization, medications, treatments, and invasive procedures. How can the nurse best approach an adolescent CF client in the hospital for an acute illness episode?

The nurse must realize the adolescent is dealing with the life transition of adolescence as well as dealing with the chronic illness. The adolescent needs independence, privacy, and positive peer relationships. Concerns are related to body image and a sense of control over their lives. Like other adolescents, they are prone to risk-taking behaviors such as alcohol, drugs, and sexual activity. The chronic illness and acute visit to the hospital can trigger fear related to imminent death and anxiety related to loss of control. Every hospitalization can evoke these feelings. Nurses need to promote self care, allow privacy, promote peer involvement with liberal visiting hours, encourage leaving their clothes on even at bedtime, and allow them to control the situation when possible. Encouraging

goal setting and future planning is especially important since new treatment modalities may extend their lives (i.e., lung transplantation). Nurses should create normalcy in the child/adolescent's daily routine while hospitalized, such as school and peer activities. Some adolescent units have a pool room or other areas in which teens can interact.

References

Wong, D. (1999). *Whaley & Wong's nursing care of infants and children.* 6th edition. St. Louis: Mosby.

Christian, B., D'Auria, J., & Moore, C. (1999). Playing for time: Adolescent perspectives of lung transplantation for cystic fibrosis. *Journal of Pediatric Health Care,* 13(3)Part 1,120–125.

CASE #2 JESSE JAMES

Learning Objectives

1. List the immediate nursing interventions for a child who has experienced a fall from a significant height.
2. Describe the routine assessments and nursing interventions related to care of a child in 90–90 traction after surgical pinning of a compound fractured femur.
3. Discuss the impact of hospitalization on the development of a preschool child.
4. Describe action and side effects of common drugs used for children in traction.
5. Discuss specific discharge teaching for a preschooler going home in a spica cast.
6. Discuss the nurse's legal responsibility in suspected child neglect.

Four-year-old Jesse James fell out of a second-story window onto a concrete landing. A nurse is walking by and sees him fall. Jesse is unconscious. There is a bone protruding from his left thigh, which is oozing a small amount of blood.

Focus Question

1. What should the nurse's immediate interventions include (state priority)?

   First, the nurse should look to see if Jesse has an open airway and is breathing. The nurse should take care in assessing this to make sure the head and spinal column is not moved because of possible spinal injury. Stabilize the neck and the spine. Call for help. Stay with the patient. It is important to check circulation to make sure blood loss is not excessive. The nurse should assess for head injury by assessing level of conscious, pupil size and equality, and bleeding from nose or ears. Be sure to stabilize the leg where the bone is protruding. Do not attempt to reduce fracture; use the other leg as a splint if no splint is available. Check the 5 P's (pain, pulselessness, pallor, paresthesia, and paralysis). If available, cover open wound with a sterile or clean dressing.

Jesse is taken by ambulance to the hospital emergency room and admitted to the orthopedic unit. Jesse arouses easily to stimulation and responds to verbal commands. The CAT scan of his head is negative. He sustained a compound fracture to his left femur. It was surgically pinned, and he is placed in 90–90 traction. The physician orders: Tylenol with Codeine 1 tsp. q 4 hours po prn, Pericolase 1 qd. po, pin care every 8 hours.

Focus Questions

1. What routine assessments and interventions would be important in Jesse's case and why?
   - **continue to assess for signs of head injury: LOC, PERRLA;**
   - **maintain the traction: check amount of weight, hanging freely, bed position, ropes in center of tract;**
   - **assess pain and medicate as needed. Muscle spasms might require an order for Valium;**
   - **maintain alignment: shoulder, hip, and leg in proper position;**
   - **check pin sites for bleeding and infection, cleanse and dress pin sites, antibiotic ointment to pin sites;**
   - **prevent skin breakdown: use special mattress, check skin for redness, especially bony prominences, wash and dry skin, stimulate with massage, and change position every two hours;**
   - **prevent complications: check 5 P's, assess pedal pulses for circulation (foot color, nail bed color) with boot application, check skin around boot, encourage lung expansion with deep breathing, passive and active ROM with uninvolved joints, check for objects in the bed or in the boot, prevent constipation with fluids, fiber, and stool softener.**
2. What are developmental issues that Jesse's nurse will need to manage?

   Jesse is a preschooler. Children of this age are physically active and immobilization will be difficult for him. Provide physical activities that he could do in bed, such as coloring, playing with clay, video games, Nerf basketball, punching bag, etc. Pain will be an issue related to the traction, the fracture, and muscle spasms. Pain assessment, management, and documentation are important. A common fear of preschoolers is body mutilation and pain. Preschoolers experience more fears and may need a parent to be present, a nightlight, a sitter or volunteer to read to him, and play to help him play out his fears and give him a sense of control.
3. Explain the rationale for and potential side effects of Jesse's medications.

   Tylenol with Codeine combines an opiate and a nonopiate analgesic. It is used to manage his pain. Medicate him prior to pin care and well before he becomes uncomfortable. Nurses should use pain assessment tools, such as the FACE'S scale, and document findings so that evaluation of pain relief and effectiveness of pain management strategies can be assessed (Jacob & Puntillo, 1999). One of the side effects of Codeine is constipation. Pericolace is used in this case to prevent the problem of constipation caused by immobility and the use of Codeine for pain control.

Jesse is placed in a spica cast and is due to be discharged tomorrow. Jesse is alert and has resumed his normal behaviors indicating no residual concerns regarding a head injury. His mother is here to learn home care instructions related to his cast.

Focus Questions

1. What information about Jesse's mother and home situation will need to be assessed prior to teaching?

   Assess her educational level, her ability and confidence in managing the care of Jesse, as well as her prior knowledge of cast care. In addition, the nurse needs to assess the home environment. Is there a constant caregiver available for Jesse? Is there access to the home? Are there plans for dealing with Jesse's daily needs, eating, toileting, sleeping,

and clothing? Are there adequate resources available, or will they need community assistance?

2. Describe specific strategies the nurse could use in teaching (1) cast care, (2) medication administration, (3) strategies for meeting activities of daily living, such as toileting, eating, sleeping, bathing, and diversional activities, (4) follow-up medical care.

   The instructor should detail each of these areas, such as cast care—checking for circulation, relieving itching with ice packs, keeping small items out of cast, and preventing skin breakdown by changing position. (The instructor could divide students into groups for this question, letting each group deal with one aspect and then reporting to the entire class.) Pros and cons of different teaching strategies (demonstration, use of written instructions, etc.) could be discussed prior to a decision being made regarding teaching Jesse's mother.

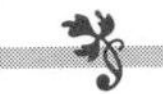

The public health nurse is scheduled to make a follow-up visit to Jesse's home. As the nurse enters the home, she notes trash and clothing strewn over the floors and dirty dishes piled everywhere. Jesse is lying on a couch in front of the television. Pop cans and candy wrappers are lying around him. The windows are wide open with no screens and flies are everywhere.

Focus Questions

1. What might the nurse conclude after visiting Jesse in his home?

   The nurse could conclude there is neglect present in the home. The condition of the home with poor housekeeping, absent screens on the windows, and presence of junk food all lead the nurse to think of neglect. The nurse should be concerned about Jesse's nutrition, safety, and hygiene.

2. What other data does the nurse need to collect?

   The nurse should do a physical assessment of Jesse to determine if the mother is taking proper care of the cast, assessing circulation, managing pain, and providing adequate nutrition. Check to see if medical appointments have been kept. Look around to see if food is available. Ask Jesse where he sleeps and what he does during the day. Find out if he uses other positions besides just lying on the couch. Examine the perineum for excoriation and cleanliness. Are there any family support systems for Jesse and his mother? Is there evidence of drug or alcohol abuse with the mother?

3. What is the nurse's legal responsibility?

   The nurse should report and document findings to the public health agency and report the incident to Child Protective Services. Schedule follow-up visits. Educate Jesse's mother where deficits are identified. Offer parenting resources. Encourage her to seek family support.

Reflective Writing

The neighbors next door to you have been your friends for years. You observe the mother using discipline techniques that you feel border on child abuse. For example, she jerks her children, aged 10 months and 2, by the arms roughly and shakes them, uses a fly swatter to smack them on the legs and arms when they are misbehaving, and screams and yells at them frequently. Should you intervene? If yes, how would you intervene. If no, give your rationale.

Legally the nurse is responsible for reporting child abuse to the Child Protective Services (CPS). CPS will make the determination whether the child should be removed from the situation or remain with the family. The students will want to discuss the dif-

ferences between abuse, discipline, and the issue of knowing the people in the case. If the nurse is unsure, as the students might be in the case above, they can look for more definitive signs of abuse in the child, such as bruises, welts, burns, lacerations, poor hygiene, inappropriate dress, or risk factors in the parent, such as job stress, psychiatric problems, drug/alcohol abuse, poor impulse control, and a low tolerance for frustration. In addition, the nurse must educate the mother immediately about shaking her child as this could cause shaken baby syndrome. She needs to be educated on normal child behavior for various age levels. A 10-month-old and a two-year-old should not be hit with fly swatters or jerked and shaken roughly. A common finding in abuse is that the parents lack knowledge of normal child behavior. Also, the nurse could model appropriate nonviolent discipline methods such as time out and distraction. Not intervening could result in the children's injury or even death.

References

Carlson, K. (1998). Selected resources on pediatric pain. *Journal of Pediatric Nursing*, 13(1), 64–66.

Chiocca, E. (1998). Child abuse and neglect: (Part 1) A status report. *Journal of Pediatric Nursing* 13(2), 128–130.

Chiocca, E. (1998). The nurse's role in the prevention of child abuse and neglect: Part II. *Journal of Pediatric Nursing*, 13(3), 194–195.

Cowan, P. (1999). Child neglect: Injuries of omission. *Pediatric Nursing*, 25(4), 401–418.

Jacob, E. & Puntillo, K. (1999). Pain in hospitalized children: Pediatric nurses beliefs and practices. *Journal of Pediatric Nursing*, 14(6), 379–388.

Wong, D. (1999). *Whaley and Wong's nursing care of infants and children.* 6th edition. St. Louis: Mosby.

CASE #3 ANGEL CHRISTMAN

Learning Objectives

1. Discuss assessment data and nursing interventions appropriate for ketoacidosis.
2. Explain the underlying pathophysiology of ketoacidosis.
3. Analyze the impact normal development has on self-care behaviors of adolescent diabetics.
4. Discuss assessment data and nursing interventions appropriate for hypoglycemia.
5. Compare insulin needs of the diabetic experiencing illness to the well diabetic.
6. Devise a career plan outlining goals for attainment of a clinical nurse specialist.

Angel Christman is a 17-year-old known diabetic since age 5. She is admitted to the emergency room with a blood sugar of 450 and with flushed dry skin. Her mother found her on the bathroom floor nonresponsive and has brought her to the hospital.

Focus Questions

1. What do you think the problem is, and what other assessment data would help confirm your suspicion?

   It could be diabetic ketoacidosis (DKA). DKA is identified by high blood sugar, flushed skin, loss of consciousness, acetone breath, dry skin, acidosis, and glucosuria.

2. Explain the underlying pathophysiology of this problem.

   It is an autoimmune, metabolic disorder, characterized by hyperglycemia from absent or deficient insulin secretion. Fats are used as a source of energy when glucose cannot

be utilized. Fat breakdown leads to ketones in the urine, elimination of ketones through the lungs resulting in acetone breath, and ketones in the blood or ketonemia, which lowers the pH. Hyperglycemia causes shifting of fluids (osmotic diuresis) into the blood and elimination through the kidneys with resultant dehydration.

3. What classic treatment is indicated? (include meds and IV solutions)

   Regular insulin is used intravenously through a pump to reduce the hyperglycemia and fluids of normal saline and electrolytes of potassium, magnesium, and phosphate are replaced. Insulin, fluids, and electrolyte replacement is the standard therapeutic management. The blood sugar is monitored hourly in the acute phase. Potassium should be given as long as renal function is adequate (urine output at least 30 cc/hr.) and cardiac monitoring is employed to assess alterations in potassium concentration. (The instructor might want to emphasize to never give potassium as an IV bolus as cardiac arrest will result.)

Angel was diagnosed with diabetic ketoacidosis (DKA). She has stabilized with IV fluids, electrolytes, and insulin. She has resumed her 2,100-calorie diabetic diet and insulin doses and is preparing to be discharged tomorrow. She reveals to the nurse that this whole thing happened because she did not feel well yesterday and did not take her insulin. Her mother tells the nurse that Angel has not been in good control for some time now since she has been dating and hanging out with friends. Her mother suspects that Angel has also been experimenting with alcohol.

Focus Questions

1. What specific information do diabetics such as Angel need to know about in caring for themselves during illness and infection?

   Angel needs to monitor her blood glucose and urinary ketones every 3 hours; use of a sliding scale of regular insulin during sick days in place of regular doses is recommended. Angel should stay in contact with her health care provider during illness. She should never omit insulin during an illness. Infections tend to raise the glucose level. If she vomits more than once or if blood sugars exceed 240 and urine ketones are high, notify the physician. Fluids are important to encourage hydration and flush out the ketones. Simple carbohydrates can be used as tolerated. It is possible that in Angel's case, it is an issue of adolescent rebellion, not lack of knowledge.

2. How should the nurse address Angel's suspected behavior? How does the period of adolescence influence Angel?

   The nurse needs to have a discussion with Angel regarding her mother's suspicion, and she should seek to develop a trusting relationship with Angel rather than lecture to her. Nurses must convey caring and be honest and nonjudgmental. Ask Angel how she would help if her best friend had diabetes. Think about how to make the treatment regimen fit her daily routine. The nurse must be knowledgeable about the development of the adolescent and consider how development affects her disease. The teenager does not consider the consequences, conforms to peer pressure and rejects authority, lives in the present, does not have mature thinking, and focuses on self-concept and body image. Encourage Angel to discuss the consequences and alternatives. Make her a partner in the decision making. Establish a contract with her and set goals together. She needs to feel a sense of control. Encourage her to share with her friends. Having a safety net of friends can help Angel feel supported. Adolescents also frequently experiment with alcohol, and adolescents with diabetes are often unaware that alcohol ingestion leads to episodes of hypoglycemia. While abstaining is best, taking a snack prior to drinking alcohol can reduce these episodes. The nurse should discuss dieting behaviors common to adolescent girls because they can also trigger hypoglycemia or

hyperglycemia. Insulin manipulation or omission has been identified as a weight loss method. Menstruation can lead to hyperglycemia a few days before the onset due to hormonal fluctuations (Wong, 1999; Muscari, 1998; Christian, D'Auria, & Fox, 1999).

Angel is referred to the diabetic clinical specialist. Two months later the nurse is working in the diabetic clinic and Angel arrives for her scheduled appointment. During her interview Angel reports she has been having frequent episodes of low blood sugar. Currently she just takes orange juice and has not required emergency medical intervention.

Focus Questions

1. What are the classic signs of hypoglycemia?

   Classic signs are nervousness, headache, shakiness, anxiety, and clammy skin. Seizures, and even death could occur.

2. What questions should the nurse ask or what other data is needed to find out why the episodes are occurring?

   Both open- and closed-ended questions can reveal data. Is there documentation of her blood sugars, and if yes, what does it reveal? What have you eaten for the past 3 days? Tell me about your eating patterns before or after exercise. Do you drink alcohol? Tell me about the amount of insulin you have been taking. (The faculty might want to discuss the true dawn phenonmenon or the Somogyi effect when discussing the evaluation of blood sugar documentation. Also, discuss the value of the HgbA1C result.)

3. What basic information does Angel need to know to treat hypoglycemia?

   She should know the signs and always keep hard candy on her person. Four ounces of orange juice or glucagon can be used as treatment. She should wear a medic alert bracelet.

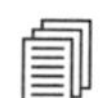

Reflective Writing

After completing your basic nursing degree, you decide you want to become a clinical specialist dealing with adolescents who have diabeties. What do you need to plan to realize your goal?

In developing a career plan you need to:

- **assess the trends—is there a need for a diabetic clinical specialist in your area, and if not, are you willing to relocate?**
- **evaluate your priorities and skills—do you have requirements for being a clinical specialist—if no, what additional education and experience will you need?**
- **develop a career plan and time line to meet your goal—plan to get your B.S.N., if not your basic degree, and then your M.S.N. Where can you get these degrees? How long will it take? Will you go full-time or part-time? Meanwhile how will you get experience in that area? Where will it be best to work? Realize this is a long-term goal that will take several years. Focus on your goal, keep a positive attitude, build your knowledge, join professional organizations, talk with other clinical specialists, and utilize continuing education (Hobbs, 1998).**

References

Christian, B., D'Auria, J., & Fox, L. (1999). Gaining freedom: Self responsibility in adolescents with diabetes, *Pediatric Nursing*, 25(3), 255–260.

Freeland, B. (1998). Diabetic ketoacidosis, *American Journal of Nursing*, 98(8), 52.

Hobbs, B. (1998). Taking charge of your career. *American Journal of Nursing*, 98(1), 36–40.

Muscari, M. (1998). Rebels with a cause, when adolescents won't follow medical advice. *American Journal of Nursing*, 98(12), 26–30.

Wong, D. (1999). *Whaley & Wong's nursing care of infants and children*. 6th ed. St.Louis: Mosby.

CASE #4 TRACEY JONES

Learning Objectives

1. Describe the causative factors implicated in cleft lip and palate and the expected treatment employed.
2. Describe how the nurse promotes maternal infant bonding when the child has a cleft lip and palate.
3. Write expected outcomes and nursing interventions related to nutrition preoperatively in a child with a cleft lip and palate.
4. Determine nursing diagnoses and interventions for the infant with cleft lip postoperatively.
5. Document attainment of goals of priority nursing diagnoses in a narrative note.
6. Communicate effectively with an adolescent mother having a child with a birth defect.
7. Analyze interventions required immediately postoperatively for cleft palate repair.
8. List postoperative instructions the parents will need to know to care for the child with cleft palate.
9. Describe the long-term needs of the child with cleft lip and palate.
10. Discuss the educational needs of nurses caring for mothers of children with cleft lip and palate who are breast-feeding.

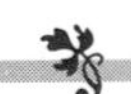

Tracey Jones was born today at 12:30 P.M. Immediately upon her birth, it was noted that she has a cleft lip and palate. Her mother is extremely upset and is convinced she is to blame because she did not drink milk during pregnancy. Tracey's mother appears very young and the nurse learns that she is only 17 years old. When the nurse brings Tracey to her mother, her mother states, "I can hardly stand to look at her. When can this be fixed?" Tracey's cleft lip and palate are unilateral right side.

Focus Questions

1. From your knowledge of cleft lip and palate, what is the expected therapeutic management?

   Surgical correction of the lip is completed as long as the child is free of infection, weighs over 10 lbs., has a hemoglobin more than 10, is over 10 weeks old, and is stable. The palate is repaired between 6–18 months. Several operations may be required. Prior to palate repair some physicians use a special dental device to pull the palate together (Mitchell & Wood, 2000).

2. How should the nurse respond to the mother's feelings of guilt? How should the nurse respond to the mother's comments related to having difficulty looking at Tracey's defects?

First, the nurse might convey that there is no evidence to support her fear of having caused the cleft lip and palate because of inadequate intake of milk. The causes include genetics or heredity, environment, or teratogenisity. Increased parental age, infections during pregnancy, use of anticonvulsants or steroids, and smoking is implicated in some cases. The child may also have other syndromes that include the defects of cleft lip and palate. Second, the mother's reaction is to be expected and accepted. Parents may have strong feelings and express negative reactions when they first see the defect. Be aware that the defect itself may place Tracey's mother at risk for failure of maternal attachment. Her verbal remarks support this risk. Nurses must seek to encourage bonding and help the mother cope.

3. What strategies should the nurse use to promote maternal infant bonding?
   - **Model caring behaviors toward the infant; talk to infant, cuddle and demonstrate acceptance in the presence of the mother.**
   - **Encourage the mother to express her loss of the perfect child.**
   - **Offer her hope by showing her pictures of children with good repairs, and connect her with parents who have coped well with this same experience (if mother is receptive to this idea).**
4. Identify nursing outcomes related to nutrition and possible nursing interventions the nurse could employ preoperatively in this newborn during the first week of life.
   - ***Outcome:* The newborn will consume 2–3 oz. of formula every 3–4 hours. *Interventions:* offer formula at specified intervals; feed in upright position, demonstrate feeding techniques; stay with the mother during first few feedings; use flanged nipple and soft pliable bottle (special feeding devices); place nipple between tongue and palate; burp frequently.**
   - ***Outcome:* The newborn will gain weight (specify amount and remember to expect up to 10% loss of birth weight in the first days). *Interventions:* Assess weight daily; analyze if birth weight and current weight are within expected parameters and infant is steadily gaining.**

Tracey has returned today at 10 weeks of age from surgery for a unilateral cleft lip repair (cheiloplasty). She has been wearing a dental appliance to facilitate closure of the palate, and the suture line has steri strips applied on the lip. Her physician has ordered half-strength hydrogen peroxide and water to cleanse the suture line, application of elbow restraints, feeding using the cleft palate nipple/bottle, and giving Tylenol 15mg/kg of weight per dose q 4 hours p.r.n. pain (no more than 5 doses in 24 hours). The mother comes to the nurse's station and says, "Tracey just won't stop crying, and I have to go now. I can't stand this."

Focus Questions

1. What top three nursing diagnoses, in order of priority, and interventions are applicable to Tracey at this time?

Risk for injury trauma to suture line	**Position supine or side; use elbow restraints; keep objects out of bed; do not use pacifiers; prevent crying episodes with medications and anticipate infant needs; cleanse suture line per physician's order after feedings**
Pain r/t surgery	**Comfort, cuddle, employ analgesics, remove restraints and assess skin and massage arms**

Risk for altered nutrition less than body r/t difficulty eating postoperatively	**Feed upright; use special devices for palate and feeding; burp frequently; medicate.**

2. Write a narrative note describing how the goals of the nursing diagnosis of first priority in focus question number 1 have been met?

   1000 2/2/2000 Nursing Note. Suture line is clean, dry, and approximated with steri strips. Infant positioned supine, elbow restraints intact, restraints removed every two hours, arms exercised and massaged. Cried at intervals. Medicated with Tylenol for crying unresolved by diaper change or feeding. Suture line cleansed with 1/2 strength hydrogen peroxide and water after feeding. K.Bennett, S.N.

3. How might the nurse respond to Tracey's mother? Give rationale.

   The first priority would be to help Tracey's mother learn how to stop the crying so as to prevent injury to suture line. Tracey's mother may be feeling very overwhelmed because she is an adolescent with a child who is crying and has a major surgical incision. The nurse might respond, "Let's go see why Tracey is crying," and then proceed to help the mother problem solve what could be done in this situation. The nurse needs to determine when the last pain medication was given. The nurse could help the mother change the diaper, feed, or encourage her to pick up the infant. It could be that the mother is afraid of picking Tracey up and needs assistance in picking up the infant in such a way as not to hit the suture line (not over the shoulder). It could be that Tracey needs a stronger pain med and the nurse may need to call for a different analgesic order. Perhaps, due to mother's age and lack of life experience, she may need the nurse to role model proper problem-solving skills and resultant interventions appropriate to Tracey's care.

At 13 months old, Tracey has a cleft palate repair. As the nurse enters the room, she observes the transporter from surgery placing Tracey in her bed, flat on her back. The mother is at the bedside and strokes Tracey's head as Tracey is crying.

Focus Questions

1. What immediate actions should the nurse take and why? Show priority of interventions.

   The nurse should assess Tracey's airway and breathing as she will now breathe differently through her nose. Assess the level of consciousness and the vital signs for stability. Assess the suture line for intactness and bleeding. Place Tracey on her side or abdomen postoperatively to encourage drainage of secretions.

2. List the most important instructions the nurse should give the mother regarding protection of the suture line postoperatively.

   Tracey needs soft foods, no hard items such as toast and chips, no forks or spoons (only wide bowl type to dump food into mouth), or cup only. (Tracey should have been weaned prior to surgery.)

3. What long-term care will Tracey need?

   The risk for middle ear infection could lead to hearing impairment, so hearing evaluations will need to be planned; there is a risk for speech impairments, so follow-up with a speech therapist will be needed. Dental follow-up for long-term impact on dentition.

Reflective Writing

You are caring for a mother on the postpartum unit who wants to breast-feed her baby who has a cleft lip and palate. Another nurse tells you she thinks the mother will be unable to nurse because of the decreased ability of the infant to suck. How would you respond to this nurse and educate her to the benefits of breast-feeding an infant with cleft lip and palate?

This line of thinking by the other nurse is totally false. The mother could use special feeding devices to cover the palate area and aid in suction, use a breast pump or manually express some milk prior to feeding to encourage let down and free flow of milk, or pump milk and bottle feed using special bottles and nipples. Breast-feeding (BF) has many benefits to the infant with cleft lip and palate. BF enhances the facial muscles and benefits speech. Also, the immunity gained from breast milk helps with the problems of otitis media and respiratory infections. Breast-fed infants are able to regulate the flow of milk and are less prone to choking, and BF infants gain weight and are discharged earlier than bottle-fed infants (Wong, 1999).

References

Mitchell, J. & Wood, R. (2000). Management of cleft lip and palate in primary care. *Journal of Pediatric Health Care,* 14(1), 13–19.

Wong, D. (1999). *Whaley and Wong's nursing care of infants and children.* 6th edition. St. Louis: Mosby.

CASE #5 SHAUNA BRYANT

Learning Objectives

1. Describe clinical findings associated with pneumonia.
2. Determine nursing diagnoses and interventions of priority in a child with pneumonia and sickle-cell anemia.
3. Analyze play activities or toys appropriate for the school-age child with sickle-cell anemia.
4. List interventions appropriate to giving Penicillin intravenously.
5. Analyze the implications of an increase in pain for the child with sickle-cell anemia.
6. Describe collaborative problems associated with sickle-cell anemia.
7. Determine supplies and protocol to use when giving a blood transfusion.
8. Discuss educational discharge needs of the client with sickle-cell anemia.
9. Analyze the pros and cons of having children when one or both parents carry the sickle-cell trait.

Shauna Bryant, a 10-year-old African American client, was admitted today coughing productively thick, white, mucous, and having a temperature of 101.6° F, rapid and shallow breathing, and chills. Shauna begins to cry and says, "I don't want another IV, they hurt too much." Her mother reports that she has a history of sickle-cell anemia, and she is upset that Shauna must be hospitalized. She states, "It is Shauna's fourth admission. I'm afraid I'm going to lose my job if I miss anymore work. Can't you do something to prevent her from hurting?" Her physical exam reveals diminished breath sounds on the right side in the lower quadrant of her posterior lung fields and rhonchi scattered throughout the remaining lung fields. A chest x-ray confirms the diagnosis of pneumonia. When assisting Shauna to the bathroom, the nurse notes weakness with ambulation.

Focus Questions

1. In addition to the above clinical findings, what other signs could the nurse expect to see in a child with pneumonia?

   Fine crackles, dullness to percussion, chest pain, retracting, nasal flaring, rapid respiratory rate, cyanosis, headache, vomiting, diarrhea, abdominal pain, irritable behavior, and anorexia could be expected.

2. What are nursing diagnoses and interventions that would be most expected with her symptoms?

Ineffective airway clearance	**Assess VS, lung fields, elevate head of bed, change position, humidify environment (aerosols or nebulizers), encourage deep breathing and coughing, use incentive spirometer, suction, give expectorants, employ chest physiotherapy, force fluids, monitor I & O, administer pain medications and antibiotics, observe for deterioration in condition (bloody sputum, pallor, cyanosis, dyspnea)**
Activity intolerance	**Promote bedrest, organize activities for uninterrupted sleep, assist in activities of daily living, assess tolerance to activity as child improves and ambulates, create diversional activity**
Body temperature, altered	**Monitor trends in temperature, assess every hour and, if elevated, administer antipyretics; evaluate effectiveness of antipyretics. Force fluids. Change linens if diaphoretic.**
Fear	**Explain procedures, be calm, stay with patient in respiratory distress, use toys or attachment items, create diversional activities, use interventions to improve breathing**
Altered family process	**Explain therapy, procedures, orient to environment, encourage family involvement, provide information**

3. What kinds of play activities would the nurse provide while Shauna is on bedrest?

   The nurse could use board games, reading, art projects, and organizing collections in a scrapbook as long as child's tolerance to activity permits.

Shauna is given Penicillin intravenously as per physician's orders. She is continued on her usual home dose of 30 mg of MS Contin bid p.o. At 1500 today the nurse finds no change in respiratory assessment, and Shauna rates her pain as an 8 on a scale of 1–10. Her pain is located in the chest and joints of the arms and legs. Shauna is getting a blood transfusion this afternoon.

Focus Questions

1. What nursing interventions are indicated when giving Penicillin intravenously?

   The nurse should check allergies prior to initiating; check the medication five rights; obtain any specimens for C & S prior to initiating drug; monitor for signs of anaphylaxis (rash, itching, respiratory distress); discontinue and manage emergency of ana-

phylaxis (epinephrine); watch for signs of superinfection (black, furry tongue, vaginal itching). See pharmacology text for additional signs.

2. Shauna's pain level is increasing. What could be precipitating this pain? Describe the pathophysiology of pain in the client with sickle-cell. What top two nursing interventions are needed? Be specific.

   Shauna is susceptible to developing a sickle-cell crisis when her body is stressed with an infection. Her RBC's are sickled, occlude her blood vessels and cause ischemia. Pain develops in the area in which ischemia exists. Perhaps she is experiencing a crisis. Opiods, such as MS Contin are used to manage the pain in clients with a sickle-cell crisis. However, Morphine Sulfate IV could be used instead because of its rapid effect. Other drugs could be used as well, such as Toradol. Fluids and electrolytes are important to cause hemodilution and prevent sickling.

3. If she develops a sickle-cell crisis, what are possible complications for Shauna?

   Sickle-cell crisis can lead to ischemia. It has diverse effects on the body, such as leg ulcers, hematuria, cerebral vascular accident, chest pain syndrome, retinopathy and blindness, abdominal pain, enlarged spleen with hemorrhage, or enlarged liver.

4. What supplies will the nurse need to administer the blood transfusion, and what protocol should the nurse follow?

   The nurse will need a Y-type inline filter tubing, an IV access with a 22 to 24 gauge needle, depending on size of child, normal saline solution, and labels per institution policy. Some institutions may require an infusion device. The nurse must check Shauna's blood type to assure the right type blood is being administered. The nurse must check the patient's requisition form that includes the blood type and Rh factor, chart number, the number on the blood bag, and Shauna's ID band with another R.N. to verify correctness. If any information does not match, notify the blood bank and do not administer. Both nurses must sign the form prior to initiating appropriate therapy. Protocols vary but usually involve beginning the infusion slowly and taking the vital signs frequently, such as every 5 minutes for the first 15 minutes, every 15 minutes 4 times, every half hour until 1 hour after infusion is complete. The nurse must assess for transfusion reactions (dyspnea, rash, fever, chills, back pain, nausea, vomiting, tachycardia) and stop the infusion if reaction occurs. Sometimes Tylenol and Benadryl are given prior to giving the blood to minimize minor reaction.

Shauna is recovering from her pneumonia and her pain has subsided. Today she will be going home. She is to be discharged on oral Penicillin and her usual dose of MS Contin.

Focus Question

1. In planning for her discharge, what educational needs could the nurse address concerning Shauna's medications, her dietary needs, and how she can promote her own health?

   - ***methods to avoid infection*—practice good nutrition, wash hands, stay away from others who have infections, implement prophylactic PCN and know dosage and side effects, seek medical care at first sign of infection, encourage sound nutrition with folic acid supplements**

   - ***methods to minimize tissue deoxygenation*—avoid high altitudes or nonpressurized airplanes, avoid infection, avoid strenuous activity, avoid cold environmental temperatures, force fluids to 1600 ml/m^2/day**

- *educate on sickle cell anemia/crisis*—**teach how to manage pain and importance of fluids; teach signs of complications such as blood in urine, vomiting, diarrhea, fever, joint pain, abdominal or chest pain, swelling and redness, cough, retractions, jerking or twitching of face, legs, or arms, seizures, weakness or inability to move arms or legs, severe headache; carry medic alert; avoid use of cold remedies and decongestants with Ephedrine (promotes vasoconstriction) and avoid Demerol (promotes seizures); refer to National Association for Sickle Cell Anemia (Simon, Lobo, & Jackson, 1999; Wong, 1999).**

Reflective Writing

As a nurse you will care for clients who carry the sickle-cell trait and are trying to decide whether to have children or not. It is your role to support and educate clients, not make judgments on their choices. To prepare yourself for these situations and help you gain perspective on their decisions, what would be good arguments in support of and against having children, knowing that the risk is 1 in 4 of having a child with the sickle-cell disease.

- **An argument in support of having children is that the chance of having a child with the disease is 25%. As screening and diagnoses are made earlier, the disease can be managed, and as technology increases, new treatments such as bone marrow transplantation or even a cure can be anticipated.**
- **An argument against having children is pain and suffering an afflicted child will have and the guilt and burden that the parents may suffer as a result of having an afflicted child. In addition, the parents may decide against having children because their children may in turn produce children with the disease.**

References

Mitchell, R. (1999). Sickle cell anemia. *American Journal of Nursing*, 99(5), 36.

Simon, K., Lobo, M., & Jackson, S. (1999). Current knowledge in the management of children and adolescents with sickle cell disease: Part 1, physiological issues. *Journal of Pediatric Nursing*, 14(5), 281–295.

Wong, D. (1999). *Whaley & Wong's nursing care of infants and children.* 6th Edition. St. Louis: Mosby.

CASE #6 TOMMY HILL

Learning Objectives

1. Describe the pathophysiology of asthma.
2. Identify asthma triggers.
3. Discuss the benefits and effects of anti-inflammatory and bronchodilator medications for asthma clients.
4. Discuss treatment of status asthmaticus.
5. Identify teaching strategies useful for cognitively impaired clients.
6. Explain the correct use of inhalers.

Eight-year-old Tommy Hill was admitted last night with wheezing, difficulty in breathing, and coughing. He was anxious and restless. He was accompanied by his mother who stated, "This always happens when he gets a cold." Tommy has had numerous lung related illnesses requiring hospitalization during the last two years. This is his third visit this month to the emergency room with an asthma attack. His mother has remained with him all night, but as the nurse enters the room today, she says, "I'll be back in a second, I have to have a cigarette."

Focus Questions

1. What data does the nurse need today during the interview and the initial morning assessment?

   - **Physical Assessment: (a) VS including O_2 saturation, temperature, respiratory rate, pulse, blood pressure; (b) peak flow meter measurements; (c) activity tolerance; (d) lung sounds—wheezing, rales, rhonchi, tight feeling; (e) use of accessory muscles for breathing-intercostal retractions; (f) check for shortness of breath and coughing; (g) check skin color for circumoral cyanosis.**
   - **Interview: History of breathing problems: How often? What are the triggers? How long do they last? What are the symptoms? What helps?** ***Medications used routinely.***
   - **Knowledge base of child and mother: What do Tommy and his mother know about the disease? Pathophysiology? Treatments? Does he do the peak expirations flow rates? Triggers? Does his mother understand her smoking is a trigger?** *Past testing:* **Has Tommy had allergy testing? What other tests/results?**

2. What are possible asthma triggers Tommy and his mother need to be aware of?

   Asthma triggers include: smoking, allergies (pollen or food), household products (solvents, paint vapors, dust), weather (cold or humidity), air pollution, exercise, infection, and emotions

Aerosol Ventolin treatments have been decreased from every hour to every four hours. Oral Prelone: 1 tsp. t.i.d. p.o. is started this morning. O_2 saturation is 94% on room air. Rhonchi are scattered throughout the lung field.

Focus Questions

1. What effect do Ventolin and Prelone have on Tommy's lungs, and what side effects should the nurse be watching for?

   - ***Ventolin aerosol*****—bronchodilator—to relieve symptoms by relaxing the airway and opening it so breathing is easier. Side effects: tachycardia, jitteriness, tremors, headache, and nausea.**
   - ***Prelone*****—oral corticosteroid and anti-inflammatory—this drug prevents and reverses airway inflammation to decrease symptoms. Side effects: nausea, mood changes, increased appetite, flushed cheeks, and headache. There are more serious effects with long-term use.**

2. What evaluation criteria would indicate improvement in his condition?

   Some criteria could be disappearance of rhonchi in lung field; decreased coughing, wheezing, and chest tightness; easier breathing (decreased rate) without use of accessory muscles; increased O_2 saturation.

3. If improvement does not occur and he progresses to status asthmaticus, what should the nurse anticipate would be done?

Status asthmaticus is a condition in which the asthma symptoms do not subside and is an emergency situation. The child may go to ICU. There should be emergency equipment at bedside; endotracheal intubation and assisted ventilation may be necessary; administer oxygen, elevate head of bed to ease breathing, check respiratory status and level of consciousness frequently, administer Epinephrine, nothing by mouth.

Tommy improves and is ready for discharge tomorrow. The nurse has scheduled a time with the mother to discuss how she can help Tommy prevent future attacks and better care for him as he learns to cope with this disease. In working with Tommy's mother during hospitalization, the nurse learns that his mother is a visual learner and appears to be somewhat slow in grasping material. Tommy will be on Ventolin and Intal inhalers, and daily monitoring of his peak expiratory flow rates (PEFR).

Focus Questions

1. Create a visual diagram that explains the pathophysiology of asthma that could be used with Tommy's mother, since she is a visual learner.

   Student needs to draw an outline of a person showing the trachea, bronchial tubes, and lungs. They should show a normal person, and then show that the airways narrow and that muscle walls tighten, and then the walls of the airway swell. The swelling produces mucus, which further clogs the narrowed airways.

2. How could the nurse best teach Tommy's mother about his medications, asthma triggers, and care during his attacks?

   Since she is a visual learner and appears to be slow grasping material, the nurse should use diagrams and pictures to illustrate how meds work and what triggers symptoms. Care should be taken that care instructions are simple, to the point, and bulleted in the written material she takes home. Repetition is important. Also, giving her the pictures, etc., to use will help remind her of how to take care of Tommy. Tommy and his mother should do a return demonstration after teaching.

3. How much responsibility can Tommy assume for his own disease management?

   At eight, Tommy can begin to assume responsibility for his own care, especially in view of his mother's limited abilities. Tommy can remind his mother to give him his meds, probably be taught about triggers to avoid, do his own inhalers and daily measurements of his peak expiratory flow rate (PEFR). Tommy could be in on teaching sessions with his mother, so he can help her remember what was taught. It would be important to find a family member other than his mother to periodically monitor his treatment regime. The school nurse could also be involved in monitoring his asthma at school.

4. How might the nurse teach Tommy to use an inhaler correctly?

   Use demonstration and return demonstration. Have pictures that show steps and send it home with him. Tell him to tape it to the inside of his closet or on the refrigerator, etc., so he can refer to it as he uses his inhaler. (Faculty might have inhalers available for practice in correctly teaching clients.)

Reflective Writing

Often in your career as a nurse, you will be faced with children experiencing emergency situations, such as an asthma attack. If you call the physician to report respiratory distress in the child and he or she responds, "Handle it, I'm busy." What would you do?

- **Before hanging up with the physician on phone, verify with the physician measures that could be implemented. Take verbal orders.**
- **Take measures to ensure safety of the child, such as raise HOB, start O_2, call respiratory therapy for prescribed treatments, or call a Code Blue if necessary.**
- **Call your supervisor and ask him or her to come to the unit (follow chain of command).**
- **Call another physician or telephone again the same physician.**
- **Document responses of child.**
- **Document interactions with physician and supervisor.**

References

Middleton, A. (1997). Managing asthma: It takes teamwork. *American Journal of Nursing, 97*(1)39–42.
Wong, D. (1999). *Whaley & Wong's nursing care of infants and children.* 6th edition. St.Louis: Mosby.

CASE #7 DYLAN BANKS

Learning Objectives

1. Discuss pathophysiology of a ventricular septal defect.
2. Give the rationale for critical nursing interventions postcardiac catheterization.
3. Discuss route, dosage, effect and side effects of two cardiac medications (Lasix and Lanoxin) including drug calculations.
4. Reflect on the impact of the child with Down syndrome on the family.

Three-week-old male infant, Dylan Banks, diagnosed with Down syndrome and ventricular septal defect (VSD), is admitted for cardiac catheterization. Dylan is in mild congestive heart failure. His birth weight was 7 lb. 9 oz. He has a history of tachypnea (50–70/minute), poor feedings, a recent onset of diaphoresis, and decreased urine output (3–4 wet diapers/day). Dylan has just returned to the unit, status postcardiac catheterization. Today's weight is 7 lb. 10 oz.

Postcatheterization orders:

- Admit to cardiac unit
- Diagnosis: Down syndrome, VSD
- Status postcatheterization
- Condition: stable
- Diet: as tolerated, breast-feeding
- Daily weights
- I&O
- O_2 @ 2–4 L/min per NC

- Furosemide 1 mg/kg p.o. stat and q 12 h (stock: 10 mg/mL)
- Digoxin 8 mcg/kg p.o. stat and qd (elixir stock: 50 mcg/mL)
- Routine nursing postcardiac catheterization

Dylan is placed in a crib by the OR transporter. He is accompanied by his parents. Nasal flaring and mild substernal retractions are apparent.

Focus Questions

1. What assessment data needs to be obtained? Explain the rationale for the assessment data.
   - **Check catheter site: assess for bleeding, swelling, and hematoma formation.**
   - **Maintain affected limb in straight position to prevent movement and subsequent trauma to the site possibly causing dislodging of clot at site.**
   - **Check vital signs: heart rate is taken for full minute to assess for dysrhythmias or bradycardia; peripheral pulses, especially below catheter site, for equality and intensity as compared to opposite leg; color and temperature of affected extremity for signs of arterial occlusion; blood pressure for signs of hypotension that may indicate cardiac hemorrhage or hemorrhage at site.**
   - **Compare data to precatheterization baseline data: to assess changes in condition.**
   - **Assess IV/po intake: hydration and status of blood glucose after period of time NPO.**
2. Identify pertinent findings in Dylan's history that are indicative of a VSD. How might the pathophysiology of a VSD be explained to his parents?
   - **Pertinent findings: Symptoms exhibited by Dylan include failure to thrive, excessive sweating, and fatigue.**
   - **Parental explanation: The heart has four areas or chambers. Dylan has an opening between the two lower chambers of the heart where there is not an opening expected. Dylan's heart condition is one of the most common cardiac conditions seen. (Use of a picture or model should be used as a teaching aid.)**
3. What equipment will Dylan need? Why? What position should Dylan be in? Why? After the nurse's initial assessment postcatheterization, what will he/she tell the parents?

   The nurse needs to obtain the following equipment: Nasal cannula for oxygen administration, pulse oximeter to assess blood oxygenation, sterile dressings available if necessary for catherization site reinforcement, medications from unit stock or pharmacy. Dylan should be maintained in a position with his leg straight to avoid clot dislodgment from the catheterization site by using sandbags. The nurse will inform and reassure the parents of Dylan's condition. The nurse will instruct the parents to keep Dylan's leg straight and explain the reason for this. The nurse will explain the equipment used for Dylan.
4. Calculate the medication dosage. Discuss furosemide and digoxin: action, side effects, parent teaching.

   Furosemide:

   Infant weight: 7 lb. 10 oz. = 3.4 kg

   mg : kg = mg : kg

   1 : 1 × x : 3.4

   x = 3.4 mg

mg : mL = mg : mL

10 : 1 = 3.4 : x

10 x = 3.4

x = 0.34 mL

Digoxin:

Infant weight: 7 lb. 10 oz. = 3.4 kg

mcg : kg = mcg : kg

8 : 1 = x : 3.4

x = 27.2 mcg

mcg : mL = mcg : mL

50 : 1 = 27.2 : x

50 x = 27.2

x = 0.54 mL

Medication	Action	Side Effects	Parent Teaching
Furosemide (Lasix)	Rapid acting diuretic, inhibits reabsorption of sodium, increases potassium excretion	Headache, tinnitus, deafness (can be permanent), vertigo, orthostatic hypotension, irregular or weak pulse, hepatic dysfunction, profound diuresis, hypokalemia, hyponatremia, thrombocytopenia, neutropenia, anemia	Give at same time every day with food. Do not discontinue unless instructed by physician. Report signs of electrolyte imbalance (weakness, thirst, anorexia, fatigue, muscle cramps). Serve potassium-rich foods. Discard oral solution bottles 60 days after opening.
Digoxin (Lanoxin)	Acts on heart to increase myocardial contractility. Inhibits activity of enzyme that transports sodium across cell membranes (sodium may be retained and potassium lost)	Weakness, headache, confusion, facial neuralgia, parasthesias, bradycardia or tachycardia (especially in children), arrhythmias, hypotension, blurred vision	Teach parent to take pulse for full minute and record. Report abnormalities to physician. Give at same time every day. If nausea and vomiting occur, withhold dose and notify physician. Teach correct measurement and administration. Teach signs of congestive failure. Keep med locked up and keep syrup of ipecac and poison control number on hand. Medic alert identification should be worn.

0900—Assessment data for Dylan is as follows: Equal bilateral pedal pulses, good capillary refill, toes warm, no edema, dressing D&I, infant awake, rooting. Apical pulse: 140, respirations 40, T 96.8. 0930: Infant is crying weakly and refusing to nurse. Serosanguinous oozing noted at site, legs cool to touch, affected leg color is slightly mottled. Infant has not had a wet diaper for 3 hours. Pulse in affected limb is 120, unaffected 132, apical pulse is 132.

Focus Questions

1. How will the nurse handle Dylan's feeding? (position for breast-feeding)

   Instruct mother to keep affected leg straight while in crib and while feeding. A rolled towel may help positioning. Assist mother with positioning.

2. Analyze vital signs and physical findings and their progressions. What is their significance and what should the nurse do?

   Apical pulse and respirations: WNL for age. T of 96.8°: cold stress. Double wrap infant; cover head with a hat. Reassess temperature after approximately 1 hour.

   Assessment thirty minutes later:

   Oozing at site: Control the bleeding, put pressure above the catheterization site. Assess color and amount of blood on dressing, outline and date. Notify physician if bleeding continues despite interventions.

   Leg color and pulse in affected leg: pulse may be weaker for a few hours after catheterization, but there should be a gradual increase in strength: continue to monitor pulses and if difference continues, notify physician. Coolness and mottling of affected extremity may indicate an arterial obstruction. In light of other factors, consult with physician. No voiding for three hours: infant has been NPO: continue to monitor output.

3. List and explain appropriate nursing interventions for Dylan at this time.

   - **Pulse oximetry: monitoring of oxygenation**
   - **Maintenance of IV fluids: prevent dehydration and hypoglycemia**
   - **Assessment data: vital signs, pulses especially below catheterization site for symmetry and equality, temperature and color of affected extremity, dressing site**
   - **Assess for any cardiac dysrhythmias due to catheter in heart during procedure**
   - **Keep accurate record of intake and output**
   - **Keep parent informed about nursing care and infant's response**
   - **Begin discharge teaching if appropriate at this time**

Dylan is to be discharged this evening if everything is stable (no further bleeding, vital signs WNL, good perfusion, and instructions given to parents).

Focus Question

1. Prepare a general Parent Education Sheet outlining pre and postcardiac catheterization care for the unit's Education Manual. Pay careful attention to important information that parents need.

   - **Be aware of the parents' educational/reading level as a pamphlet is selected or prepared. Pamphlets should be written two to four grade levels below the literacy level of the audience (Bernier, 1993).**

- **One example might be this: Your child has just had a test to find out more information about his heart. This test is a cardiac catheterization. A tube, called a catheter, was placed in a blood vessel in his groin. The doctor then guided this tube through the pathway of the blood vessel and eventually to the heart. Important information about your child's heart was gained and your doctor will be able to give you what this information means.**

When you take your child home, you should follow the instructions below:

- **Take off the bandage tomorrow and replace it with an adhesive bandage for about 3 days; keep the area in the groin clean and dry. Sponge bathe and do not give tub baths; look at the area every day for the next 4–5 days. Call your doctor if you see any redness, swelling, bleeding, or fluid (drainage) coming from the area; call your physician if your child has a fever; your child may attend school but may not do heavy exercises; your child may eat a regular diet; if your child has any pain, you can give Acetaminophen or Ibuprofen. Follow the label directions for the dose you will give; keep your follow-up appointment.**

- **Faculty may want to have students analyze their own education sheet or an already prepared sheet to check for reading levels using SMOG (Mc Laughlin, 1969) or other readability formulas.**

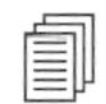

Reflective Writing

Dylan's mother is only three weeks postpartum, and, in addition to her physical and emotional needs, she has to cope with the extraordinary needs of a child with Down syndrome and congenital heart disease. She may experience postpartum "blues" or postpartum depression. Discuss and describe the blues and depression. How might the nurse identify these conditions? What (if any) referrals should be made? How can the nurse be of the most help to this mother?

- **Postpartum blues: Usually occur within 1 to 5 days after childbirth and last about 1 to 4 days. Common symptoms include mood swings, feeling low, anxiety, feeling overemotional, tearfulness, fatigue, confused thinking. Postpartum depression: Symptoms include severe anxiety, panic attacks, crying after the usual 1 to 4 days of postpartum blues, disinterest in the infant, insomnia, negative feeling toward the infant. These symptoms last longer than the blues and the mother may have either a weight gain or a weight loss and have difficulty in taking care of her own activities of daily living (ADLs).**

- **Postpartum depression is a serious condition and the nurse should institute prompt referral to appropriate practitioners. These practitioners can include the mother's own family practitioner, obstetrician, or psychiatrist. The mother may also benefit from community resources, such as support groups. The nurse can help Dylan's mother by sitting down and listening to her. The mother may not be aware of community resources, either for herself or her child with Down syndrome. The mother, at this time, is in the mode of gathering information. The nurse should provide the information that the mother needs now and sources of information particularly for use as Dylan grows.**

References

Beck, C. T. (1998). A checklist to identify women at risk for developing postpartum depression. *JOGNN*, 27(1), 39–46.

Beck, C. T (1995). Perceptions of nurses' caring by mothers experiencing postpartum depression. *JOGNN*, 24(9), 819–825.

Bernier, M. J. (1993). Developing and evaluating printed education materials: A prescriptive model for quality. *Orthopedic Nursing*, 12(6), 39–46.

McLaughlin, G. H. (1969). SMOG-grading: A new readability formula. *Journal of Reading*, 12, 639–646.
Wong, L. & Perry, S. (1998). *Maternal child nursing care.* St. Louis: Mosby.
Zickler, C. F., Morrow, J. D., & Bull, M. J. (1998). Infants with Down syndrome: A look at temperament. *Journal of Pediatric Health* Care, 12(3), 111–117.

CASE #8 JUSTIN BENNETT

Learning Objectives

1. Identify preoperative assessments for a two-year-old child going to surgery for inoption of a foreign body.
2. Analyze nursing priorities postoperatively for the recovery room nurse and later as the child is transferred to the Short Stay Unit (a unit where children are taken care of for a 24-hour period or less).
3. Develop a content outline to present to parents of toddlers regarding child safety issues.
4. Discuss the nurse's role in dealing with parents who do not observe child safety practices.

Joan Bennett brought her 2-year-old son Justin into the emergency room because he had swallowed a nickel. He appears to be in no respiratory distress and is playing with his truck. X-rays reveal a coin lodged in his lower esophagus. The physician determines that if Justin does not pass the coin by tomorrow, surgery to remove the coin will be indicated. Justin is transferred to the Short Stay Unit for overnight observation.

Focus Questions

1. In preparing for the surgery, identify essential assessment data the nurse needs to gather and document on the surgical checklist for a possible morning surgery. Include any developmental issues.

   Although institutions' surgical checklists vary, nurses will need to identify if the child has allergies, loose teeth, a labeled security item, parental consent; see that lab work if ordered is complete and on the chart, fingernails clear of nail polish; record current vital signs, if client voided, list of any medications, pertinent history and physical, NPO; check for gown and underpants on, documentation of preoperative teaching, ID band; remove jewelry, etc.

2. How should the nurse prepare Justin for this procedure?

   The nurse should address the things that Justin will see, hear, smell, and feel. Use a book designed for surgery that includes pictures of equipment, stretcher, mask and gowns, syringes, and anesthesia equipment. Take Justin on a tour, let him experience being on a stretcher, allow him to play with syringes without needles, masks and gowns. Be careful about the terminology used with Justin. Avoid words such as, "put to sleep"; use instead words like "special sleep."

3. How should the nurse prepare the mother for this surgical procedure?

   The parent in most cases is allowed to accompany the child to the surgical area where they can also wait for the child's return. Some institutions will allow the parent to stay for induction of anesthesia. After anesthesia the physician will remove the foreign body with a special instrument. After surgery, the child will be placed in a high-

humidity environment and antibiotics may be used to prevent a secondary infection. Inform the parent of the room to which the child will return. Include the parent in the discussion of surgery with Justin, showing the parent the pictures as well.

Justin did not pass the coin, and it was removed by a physician using a lighted scope through the mouth under general anesthesia. The procedure took only minutes and Justin recovered from the anesthesia. He is now in his room with his mother at his side.

Focus Questions

1. What were the nursing priorities during the recovery period in the postanesthesia care unit?

   Priorities are airway, breathing, and circulation. Priority of attention to airway and breathing is followed by monitoring for vital signs frequently, including temperature. As the child awakens, the parent is allowed to be with the child. The nurse collaborates with anesthesia physicians and the surgeon for any problems.

2. When Justin returns to the Short Stay Unit, what supplies will the nurse need to have ready, what physical signs, and what regarding the chart will the nurse check?

   The nurse needs: suction equipment, oxygen flow meters and cannula/mask, pulse oximeter and routine cardiac monitoring equipment, IV therapy pump, and a clean crib. Physical assessments to make are: airway, breathing, level of consciousness, level of pain, temperature and vital signs, mouth for bleeding, skin color, bowel sounds, and breath sounds. Review orders and check to be sure essential preoperative routine medications were also reordered.

The preschool teacher at the hospital's on-site child care facility has asked the nurse from the Short Stay Unit to develop and present to interested parents a program on safety for toddlers.

Focus Questions

1. Devise a topical outline for this program.

Prevention

a. **motor vehicle safety**

b. **drownings**

c. **burns**

d. **poisoning**

e. **falls**

f. **choking and suffocation**

g. **bodily injury**

2. Under each topic, list at least three specific suggestions to offer parents.

   - ***motor vehicle safety*—use car seat restraints that are federally approved; properly follow directions on how to secure the child; do not allow child to play at the curb or behind cars that are parked; supervise toddlers when riding toys (only on sidewalk, never in street).**

- ***drownings*—supervise around any water no matter how small; keep bathroom door closed and toilet shut as toddler is top heavy and can fall in; fence pools and keep gates locked.**
- ***burns*—store matches and lighters in locked area; keep electric cords out of reach or to back of counter; cover electrical outlets with protective devices.**
- ***poisoning*—keep all medications locked and out of reach; keep Syrup of Ipecac available; keep telephone number of poison control by telephone.**
- ***falls*—keep screens on windows secure; keep gates at the top of stairs; avoid use of walkers.**
- ***choking and suffocation*—avoid hot dogs, hard candy, nuts, grapes, and pop corn; discard old refrigerators or take off doors; keep blind cords out of reach, keep latex balloons out of reach.**
- ***bodily injury*—do not allow play with scissors or knives; teach personal safety such as name, address, phone number; teach not to go with strangers; if firearms in home, keep them locked and out of reach.**

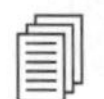

Reflective Writing

As professional nurses, we often encounter situations in which we observe parents failing to follow child safety practices. For example, you might see a child riding in a car without a seat belt or a toddler in a baby pool as the mother sunbathes. What is your reaction to this? Is your response effective and appropriate as a professional nurse? How could you make the most impact on parents?

Students may react in many different ways, but usually their response is one of anger toward the parent. Anger is not the best response to use when trying to reach a parent. Sometimes the parent underestimates the child's probability of being injured, underestimates the danger, or lacks knowledge related to the child's growth and development and prevention of injury. Toddlers are frequently prone to injury due to their curiosity, unawareness of the danger, and their increased mobility. Nurses can be most helpful to parents by providing anticipatory guidance regarding growth and development, as well as by educating parents on the hazards children of this age encounter.

Reference

Wong, D. (1999). *Whaley & Wong's nursing care of infants and children.* 6th ed. St. Louis: Mosby.

CASE #9 CAREY NESTOR

Learning Objectives

1. Discuss clinical signs of cerebral palsy (CP).
2. Describe feeding techniques used for children with CP who have feeding problems.
3. Discuss pain assessment and management in a child with CP.
4. Discuss teaching related to cast care post heel cord lengthening.

Carey Nestor is a 9-year-old male who has cerebral palsy and is accompanied to the hospital by his foster mother. He lives with a foster mother and father and seven brothers. He is currently scheduled for a heel cord lengthening. The nurse is assigned to this child and will do an initial assessment and admit the child.

Focus Questions

1. What is the most significant underlying cause of cerebral palsy?

   Anoxia

2. If Carey were only 9 *months* old and undiagnosed, what assessment data would the prompt the nurse to report his or her findings to a clinical nurse specialist for possible specialized treatment programs?

   Data would include persistence of reflexes, failure to achieve developmental milestones, spasticity or involuntary movements, abnormal postures, increased or decreased muscle tone, or varying degrees of paralysis.

3. From your knowledge of cerebral palsy, what key clinical signs would you expect Carey to exhibit?

   The nurse might see spasticity related to the leg muscles or orthopedic problems like hip dislocation, scoliosis, or joint contractures, which would cause mobility problems; possibly speech, swallowing, or eating problems, mental retardation, seizures, or attention deficit hyperactivity disorder.

4. When admitting Carey to the Short Stay Unit, what information will the nurse collect? Give some examples on how to word the questions using therapeutic communication.

   Questions should be worded positively and sensitively to obtain information regarding Carey's functional ability. The nurse could use therapeutic communication and ask about the child's functional abilities and daily routines. For example, "Tell me about Carey's eating, toileting, bedtime routines, special devices, and ways to interact with Carey."

The foster mother was a valuable resource for the nurse during the interview. The nurse found out that Carey was born prematurely and had a difficult delivery with meconium aspiration. Carey was not easily adopted because of his disabilities, and was placed in foster care. Assessment reveals a child with significant developmental delay: his motor abilities are hampered by leg spasticity and he is unable to be mobile without assistive devices, speech and hearing deficits are present, feeding deficits have been improved with the foster mother providing manual jaw control, there is mild mental retardation and associated seizures. Tomorrow Carey is scheduled for the heel cord lengthening. He takes Baclofen 5 mg. b.i.d. p.o. and Phenobarbital 25 mg. b.i.d. p.o. Carey weighs 55 lbs. The foster mother must leave at 3 P.M. today to care for her other children.

Focus Questions

1. What are the top three nursing problems that concern the nurse this evening when Carey's mom is absent?

   The top three problems are risk for injury r/t physical disability or seizures; risk for altered nutrition less than body requirements r/t lack of jaw control; and impaired verbal communication r/t cognitive impairments, speech and hearing deficits.

2. The nurse is preparing to send Carey to surgery. What things will the operating nurse want to know specifically about Carey in order to provide optimum care? Describe Carey's needs in terms of the functional patterns. (Your instructor may ask you to role-play this conversation between the transferring nurse and the OR nurse.)

   - **Activity and exercise—current vital signs and temperature, allergies, any loose teeth, activity abilities and needs**
   - **Cognitive perceptual—need to know how Carey can communicate verbally, his intellectual ability, how he responds to pain, when he was last medicated**
   - **Nutrition metabolic—NPO status, when last ate, current IV fluids**
   - **Elimination—when Carey last voided, any problems r/t to continence**
   - **Coping—how he responds to new situations, security items**

3. Describe how you will feed Carey today while the mother is at home caring for the other foster children.

   Since Carey is 9 years old and weighs 55 lbs., feed him in an upright sitting position with arms forward. The middle finger of the nonfeeding hand is placed posterior to the body portion of the chin, the thumb is placed below the bottom lip, and the index finger is placed parallel to the mandible. Feed slowly and observe swallowing movements while keeping the head from hyperextending (Wong, 1999).

Carey returns to your unit following surgery. Your unit is a 24-hour short stay area of the hospital. Carey has bilateral lower leg casts below knees to the toes. He is crying and has facial grimacing upon arrival to the unit. The foster mother is here assisting with his care, but she will need to leave soon to care for her other children at home. His medications are Morphine Sulfate 0.1 mg/kg. IV q 4 hours p.r.n., Tylenol with Codeine elixir 1 tsp. Q 4 hours p.o. p.r.n., Valium 1–2 mg. p.o. q6 hours p.r.n., and Phenobarbital b.i.d. p.o.

Focus Questions

1. What assessment data will you use to determine a need for pain medication?

   The nurse needs to check when the last dose was given, assess crying and facial grimacing, check vital sign changes such as increased heart rate, and heed mother's request as she is more sensitive to Carey's needs.

2. Give the rationale for each of the drugs in the case and the side effects you will monitor. Are there any problems in the orders as written?

   Both Morphine and Tylenol with Codeine are given for pain and the side effects are respiratory depression, hypotension, and constipation. The Codeine in Tylenol with Codeine also causes nausea and vomiting. Tylenol has side effects of liver toxicity with overdosage. Valium is a muscle relaxant given to decrease the incidence of muscle spasms and seizures. Side effects of Valium include lethargy and drowsiness, as well as respiratory depression. Phenobarbital is given to prevent seizures. Side effects of Phenobarbital are hangover and lethargy. The Phenobarbital order lacks a dosage. The Morphine dose is not worked out according to the weight.

3. List instructions that the nurse will provide the foster mother in managing the care of the casts.

   Teach the mother to turn Carey so casts dry evenly; check circulation in toes using 5 P's (pain, pallor, pulselessness, paresthesia—lack of sensation, paralysis—lack of move-

ment); check skin around cast for excoriation and pedal cast; and ice and elevate cast to decrease edema.

4. What are the responsibilities of the short stay (less than 24 hours) nurse when following the minimum standards of care?

   Protocols will vary. Generally the nurse will assess clients on admission and every 4 hours or more often if indicated; ensure client takes fluids and advances to a diet as tolerated; assess client voiding pattern and pain control; educate parents on discharge instructions regarding home care; assure that client demonstrates improvement in condition and if not, client is transferred.

5. What would be one major difference in the plan of care for the PACU (post-anesthesia care unit or recovery room) nurse versus the short stay nurse?

   Although both nurses would have similar concerns postoperatively, the PACU nurse would have the most immediate concern of oxygenation related to removal of the endotracheal tube. Monitoring for responsiveness and stability of respirations, O_2 saturation, and vital signs is critical as well as ruling out problems of shock related to surgery or anesthesia reactions. See focus question number 4 for short stay nurses's responsibilities.

Reflective Writing

What are your beliefs about sterilization of individuals who are mentally retarded?

Students could respond in a number of ways, such as:

- **Mentally retarded individuals should be sterilized as it is morally wrong to allow individuals to produce children who may be mentally deficient and a burden to society.**
- **Mentally retarded people should be allowed to procreate as it is their right to do so. They may need assistance from others to care for their children.**
- **Some mentally retarded individuals should be sterilized and others allowed to reproduce, based on the degree of their mental retardation. Some would be competent and others would not (Wong, 1999). (The instructor might want to discuss the etiologies of mental retardation as the cause may not be of genetic origin and children produced could be normal.)**

Reference

Wong, D. (1999). *Whaley & Wong's nursing care of infants and children.* 6th edition. St.Louis: Mosby.

CASE #10 MEG LONDON, PEDIATRIC NURSE PRACTITIONER

Learning Objective

1. Identify teaching appropriate for pediatric clients and their families regarding colic, asthma, adolescent birth control, obesity, home safety and febrile convulsions.

   Instructor may assign a small group of students to a single client, then bring students together for a total class discussion of all of Meg's clients.

Meg London is a pediatric nurse practitioner working in a clinic. This morning she has six clients to see in rooms 1–6 prior to the physician's examination. (This is a variation of unfolding cases, which highlights how a day might "unfold" for a pediatric clinic nurse.)

Room 1. Eight-week-old Ashley is here for a well baby check. Ashley is Ellen's first baby. Ellen has many questions as Ashley is a colicky baby and sleeps very little. Ellen states, "I'm so tired! I want to be a good mother, but I just cannot seem to satisfy her at all—no matter what I do!"

Room 2. Connie is a 17-year-old student who is getting ready for a new adventure, moving away (300 miles) for college. Connie has come today to get her "shots" up to date and get a physical for college. She confides to Meg "I'd like to also get some birth control pills. My mom cannot know this, but I want to be ready for the college party scene."

Room 3. Bobby is a 10 year old with newly diagnosed asthma. Bobby has been prescribed an Intal inhaler to be used 3 times daily and a Proventil inhaler to be used prn. He is very upset because he can no longer play soccer, as the night air causes him to wheeze. He says he'll have to be a "nerd" and not play sports now. Sandy, his mother, is very concerned about him and tells Meg he purposely "forgets" his inhaler and has refused to tell his friends he has asthma.

Room 4. Peggy is a 13 year old who weighs 180 pounds and is 5 feet tall. Her mother, Sue, has tried to get her to lose weight with no success. Peggy has "no friends" and says, "Everyone calls me Miss Piggy—I hate school—why do I have to be fat?" She is here to see if the physician will give her diet pills.

Room 5. Debbie is frantically chasing Andy, her 2 year old, around the exam room as he opens cupboards, climbs on the furniture, and is generally into everything. She tells Meg that last week he got into the medicine cabinet and had the bottle of Tylenol open when she found him. Andy is here for a postantibiotic ear re-check. Debbie confides to Meg that she is worn out chasing and worrying about Andy's safety.

Room 6. Scott is 18 months old. His mother, Kellie, brought him here for a normal well child checkup. Kellie tells Meg that she is afraid Scott is going to be epileptic because last month he had a high fever and had a convulsion after getting an ear infection. "I'm so scared!"

Focus Questions

Room 1—Ashley

1. What additional information does Meg need to get during her interview?

   Meg might ask some of the following questions: Is Ashley formula or breast-fed? How often and how much? Does she tolerate feedings? Any spitting up? When is she colicky or is there no pattern? How does Ellen respond to her crying and what helps? Is her weight increasing? Dehydration? Who are Ellen's supports—husband, parents, friends? Physical assessment findings on Ashley.

2. Providing Ashley is just colicky and is otherwise doing well, how can Meg teach Ellen?

   Reassure her that she isn't at fault. If Ashley is breast-feeding—eliminate cow's milk from Ellen's diet; Ashley could be allergic to her mother's diet (eliminate and then wait 5 days to see if it makes a difference). If on formula may want to switch formulas (physician will decide this), for example (no soy). Possible drugs for the infant: sedative (Phenobarbital or Atarax), antispasmodics, antihistamine, or antiflatulents. Overstimulation (too much bouncing or movement) may upset the infant. Don't smoke in house or around baby. To help colic, lay baby face-down across your forearm, with her abdomen on your palm. Have someone else watch the baby for a few hours, so Ellen can get away for the sake of her own sanity. Colic will go away in about three months. Eileen could place Ashley on her tummy on top of a hot-water bottle (not too hot). The heat and pressure provide relief. Try a swing or a rhythmic motion (car ride).

Room 2—Connie

1. What additional information does Meg need to get during her interview?

   Find out what Connie knows about sexually transmitted diseases (STDs) (birth control pills won't prevent them). Is she sexually active? How many partners? If she is a virgin, why has she decided to have sex? Has she ever had a gynecologic exam? Breast exam?—(will need to do them today). What is her knowledge of birth control pills?

2. What kind of teaching/counseling should Meg give to Connie today prior to her physical and gynecologic exam?

   Teach her about the pelvic and breast exams to allay her fears. Teach relaxation techniques during exam. Enumerate benefits of abstinence. Educate on prevention of STDs and use of condoms. Explain contraception—methods available and the pros and cons of each. Review hygiene—washing front to back, no douching. Stress importance of follow-up care and regular exams.

Room 3—Bobby

1. What additional information does Meg need to obtain during her interview?

   Find out Bobby's and his mother's knowledge of asthma including how it is best managed. Is he compliant with the use of his two inhalers, and do they help? Talk with Bobby as to why he feels he can't tell his friends—why is he ashamed?

2. How might Meg help Bobby and his mother, Sandy, cope with his asthma?

   First, Meg needs to convince Bobby to use both his Intal and Proventil inhalers to prevent attacks (Intal) and relieve symptoms if he has an attack (Proventil). He may well be able to play soccer if he is compliant. She also needs to explain why it is important he carry both inhalers—asthma can be dangerous and if he has an attack, he needs to use Proventil immediately. Perhaps she can make a contract with Bobby: he is compliant for two weeks and then she will reevaluate his condition. The Intal may prevent his attacks and allow him to participate in soccer. Sandy needs to know that Bobby is very concerned about peer acceptance (normal development) and needs to feel "normal." Perhaps his best friend could be educated on the symptoms and treatment of asthma and serve as a buddy to Bobby and an advocate to educate others. Many athletes have asthma and still participate and excel in sports. Meg needs to caution Sandy regarding the harm overprotecting can cause. Bobby needs to learn to accept responsibility for his own care by allowing him to take his own medications, measure and monitor his peak expiratory flow rates (PEFR), and ultimately become in control of his own care.

Room 4—Peggy

1. What additional information does Meg need to get during her interview?

   Meg needs a diet history on Peggy—what does she eat? A three-day recall will help assess her problem areas. Is there a family history of obesity? Is she active? What does she like to do? How has she tried to lose weight before? Why does she feel diet pills will help?

2. How might Meg help Peggy work on losing weight without medication?

   First, obesity cannot be cured, only controlled. Peggy needs to understand this. Meg could suggest: Drink 4–6 glass of water each day; eat some fresh fruits and vegetables each day; eliminate "empty calories" (pop, candy, chips, etc.); eat smaller portions (use small plates to give the illusion of more food); exercise: walk, bike, dance. What else does she like to do? Any activity is good. Set realistic goals to lose no more than 2 pounds per week; get family support, keep fat foods out of the house, walk every night as a family. Reward weight loss with nonfood items; limit TV and sedentary activities; Refer her to self-help groups such as Weight Watchers and teens for support.

Room 5—Andy

1. What additional information does Meg need to get during her interview?

   Let Debbie vent her feelings—describe her typical day. What safety issues she is concerned about? What hazards are in the home: stairs, stove, low knobs, what else? What has she done so far to safe-proof the home?

2. How can Meg help Debbie cope, and what does she need to do to help Debbie child-proof her home for the future?

   Assure Debbie that Andy is normal and that curiosity is a part of normal development. She can try to discipline with "no" and distraction. Soon she could use "time out." Find acceptable outlets for his energy—gym set, tricycle, slide, etc. Debbie needs to be taught how to childproof her home (Locked cabinets, childproof caps, covered outlets, stove knobs high, handles not out so he can grab them—use gates, locks.) Constant supervision of a 2 year old is a necessity for safety. Keep phone number for poison control beside phone and Syrup of Ipecac on hand.

Room 6—Scott

1. What additional information does Meg need to get during her interview?

   Additional information on Scott's seizures—length, type, number of episodes. How was it treated? Why does she feel he might have epilepsy? Who told her this? Does she feel it was caused by ear infection? A physical exam needs to be done on Scott.

2. How might Meg educate Kellie?

   Provide information on febrile seizures (common in children 3 mo to 5 years; risk of developing epilepsy is low—1% without other risk factors). Epilepsy is not caused by febrile seizures. Fever can trigger seizures in children who have high cortical excitability and low seizure threshold. Fever is commonly associated with upper respiratory or gastrointestinal infections, and has been associated with immunizations, such as MMR or DPT. Encourage Kellie to discuss her concerns with the physician, who can discuss risk factors and further put her worries to rest (Sagraves, 1999).

Reflective Writing

How would you feel about giving birth control information to Connie without consent from her parents? What is the nurse's role?

The instructor will hear a variety of "feelings" concerning this dilemma. However, the nurse's role is one where one's own values and beliefs cannot dictate his/her response to this adolescent seeking help. One thing the nurse could do is urge Connie to talk to her parents about her desire for birth control. Connie is not yet at an age of majority, which is 18. In some states she can, however, consent to her own treatment based on the Mature Minor's Doctrine or Emancipated Minor. State laws vary and nurses need to be aware of their state's laws.

References

Hennigen, L., Kollar, L., & Rosenthal, S. (2000). Methods for managing pelvic examination anxiety: Individual differences and relaxation techniques. *Journal of Pediatric Healthcare,* 14(1), 9–12.

Muscari, M. (1999). Adolescent health: First gynecologic exam. *American Journal of Nursing,* 99 (1), 66–67.

Picciano, M. F., McBean, L., & Stalling, V. (1999). Nutrition & the life cycle—How to grow a healthy child. *Nutrition Today,* 34(1), 6–13.

Sagraves, R. (1999). Febrile seizures—Treatment & prevention or not? *Journal of Pediatric Health Care,* 13(2), 79–83.

chapter **3**

Annotated Mental Health Cases

CASE #1 CALLIE COZY

Learning Objectives

1. Analyze assessment data characteristic of clinical depression.
2. Assess suicide potential.
3. Apply principles of safe care for the client who is depressed.
4. Implement the nursing process for the depressed client.
5. Plan individualized discharge teaching for the client/family.

Callie Cozy is a 47-year-old Italian-American, Caucasian woman admitted to River City Hospital's Psychiatric Unit after a week of outpatient tests for gastrointestinal disturbances. Callie, a public school teacher, is married to Jake. They have two grown children, a son 24 and a daughter 22, who reside out of state. Callie's father is dead and her mother lives with Callie and Jake. Over the past two months, Callie's weight has declined from 145 to 120 pounds, she has difficulty falling asleep and awakens by dawn, and has vague abdominal pain. The admitting diagnosis is Major Depression.

Focus Questions

1. How do Callie's symptoms compare to the usual expected symptoms of depression?

   Depression is frequently manifested in physical complaints such as gastrointestinal disturbances. Depression may occur after a perceived loss. Callie may perceive a role change from a mother of dependent children to mother of adult children as a loss. The loss of her father may still be difficult. Weight loss, which may indicate lack of appetite, and sleep disturbance are significant signs of depression.

2. What further assessment data should the nurse gather?

   The nurse should discuss recent changes in energy level; circumstances surrounding father's death; suicide potential; relationship with mother, husband, children

3. What specific questions will the nurse ask Callie?

   How has your life changed recently? Describe your typical day? How do you feel about yourself? When and under what circumstances did your father die? How do you feel about your significant relationships? Have you thought about suicide?

Upon assessment, Callie states she has little energy or interest in things she formerly enjoyed. It takes all her strength to do her work as a fourth grade teacher, and after work she "collapses in bed." She started having stomach pain after working very hard to implement a district improvement plan with her students and then only received a mediocre evaluation from her supervisor. Callie stated she previously received high evaluations. She has been told she is a "perfectionist." When Callie's father died of heart failure four years ago, Callie's mother came to live with Jake and her. Callie is grateful that her mother is there to help her because, while Jake is a good provider and a loving husband, he is not very helpful around the house. While her children are living in a neighboring state, they call frequently, visit on holidays and participate in family gatherings. The nurse asks Callie how she feels about herself and she says, "Worthless, empty." When asked if she feels suicidal, she replies, " I think every day about ending this pain."

Focus Questions

1. What is the significance of the data the nurse has added to her assessment?
   - **Callie has experienced an assault to her self-concept, which may have been a factor in the development of her depression. However, if Callie had unrecognized depression, she may not have performed well because of the depression, resulting in the poor evaluation and the further deepening of her already existing depression. Either way she has a self-esteem disturbance.**
   - **Family relationships seem to be adequate although Jake may not realize what added emotional and physical support Callie needs now. He might not be used to negotiating their roles as is suggested by his lack of helping with household chores even though his wife also works outside the home.**
   - **Callie is having suicidal thoughts, which require further evaluation.**
2. How will the nurse reply to Callie's last statement?
   - **Are you experiencing thoughts of suicide?**
   - **Assess suicide potential. "Do you have a plan?" If so, "When do you plan to act?" "Do you have the means?" "What do you hope will happen?" "Can you contract one of the nurses or promise to let one of the nurses know if you are feeling like you are going to hurt yourself?"**
   - **Empathize and offer hope by giving positive expectations. " I hear that you are in pain now. You will feel better."**

Callie's primary nurse will plan her care and prepare for her discharge. Her physician orders Nortriptyline 75 mg @ 8 PM qd po. Callie attends groups but spends all free time in bed. When her husband Jake visited, he told a nursing assistant, "Callie needs to snap out of this and start eating more. Everyone has aches and pains as they age."

Focus Questions

1. What nursing diagnoses might the nurse identify for Callie?
   - **Risk for self-directed violence related to depressed mood and feelings of hopelessness.**
   - **Altered nutrition, less than body requirements, related to depressed mood.**
   - **Sleep pattern disturbance related to depressed mood.**

- **Self-esteem disturbance related to impaired cognition fostering negative view of self.**
- **Hopelessness related to perception of worthlessness.**

2. What nursing interventions should the nurse implement for Callie?
   - **Establish a therapeutic relationship.**
   - **Communicate the potential for suicide to team members.**
   - **Secure a no suicide contract.**
   - **Convey a message of hope.**
   - **Explain that depression is an illness and her feelings are related to the depression.**
   - **Teach stress management techniques including progressive relaxation.**
   - **Teach assertiveness techniques.**
   - **Administer and monitor medication as ordered.**
3. What is the advantage of Nortriptyline compared to a selective serotonin reuptake inhibitor?

   Nortriptyline tends to cause less agitation, insomnia, gastrointestinal distress, and weight loss, which are important considering the symptoms Callie experienced.
4. What are the advantages of Nortriptyline over a monoamine oxidase inhibitor (MAOI)?

   Nortriptyline does not have the restriction requiring avoidance of foods containing tyramine.
5. What nursing interventions address the three common side effects (dry mouth, sedation, nausea) that may occur with any antidepressant?
   - **dry mouth—Offer sugarless gum or candy, ice chips, or sips of water.**
   - **sedation—Request order for drug to be given at bedtime. Instruct client not to drive or use dangerous equipment while sedated.**
   - **nausea—Give medication with food to minimize gastrointestinal distress.**
6. What nursing interventions address the common side effects of tricyclic antidepressants?
   - **blurred vision—Offer reassurance that symptom is time limited and should subside in several weeks. Teach to avoid driving until vision clears. Remove items from pathways to prevent falls.**
   - **constipation—Encourage client to eat foods high in fiber, increase fluids, and perform physical exercise if not contraindicated.**
   - **orthostatic hypotention—Instruct client to rise slowly. Monitor lying and sitting blood pressure. Avoid long hot baths or showers.**
   - **urinary retention—Monitor intake and output. Instruct client to report hesitancy or inability to urinate. Stimulate urination by running water or pouring water over the perineal area.**
   - **tachycardia and arrythmias—Monitor and report changes.**
   - **seizures—Observe clients with history of seizures and institute seizure precautions.**
   - **photosensitivity—Teach client to wear sunscreen, protective clothing, and sunglasses outdoors.**
   - **weight gain—Teach value of nutritious, low calorie foods and increased activity.**

7. What nursing interventions are important when a client is taking an MAOI?

   Teach about foods containing tyramine that need to be avoided. Monitor for symptoms of hypertensive crisis such as severe occipital headache, palpitations, marked increase in blood pressure, fever, nausea and vomiting, nuchal rigidity, chest pain, sweating, and coma. If symptoms of hypertensive crisis occur, discontinue medication and notify physician, administer short-acting antihypertensive medication as ordered, and use cooling measures to decrease fever.

8. What are appropriate outcomes for Callie?

   Callie:

   - **has not physically harmed herself.**
   - **interacts willingly and appropriately with peers, staff, and family.**
   - **eats a well-balanced diet to prevent weight loss and maintain nutritional status.**
   - **sleeps 6–8 hours per night and verbalizes feeling well rested.**

9. How would the nurse approach Callie about the issue of including the family in discharge planning?

   Ask her permission to talk with Jake and possibly her mother about her diagnosis of depression, the importance of treatment for depression, and the desire to share discharge teaching with them. Her response should be documented in her chart.

10. What discharge teaching and planning must be implemented?

    - **signs of depression**
    - **contract to call a suicide crisis line or preferably her physician or clinical nurse therapist if she sees depression or suicidal feelings returning**
    - **medication teaching including name, purpose, side effects and which ones to report to doctor, dosage, schedule, importance of taking medication regularly and length of time it may take to be effective**

11. How should the nurse respond to Jake?

    "Callie can't 'snap out of this' because she has an illness that causes the sufferer to have physical and psychological pain, lack of energy, lack of appetite, and difficulty sleeping. With treatment, including antidepressant medication, she should begin feeling better within a month. She needs your patience and support." It is important to let Jake vent his feelings regarding his wife's illness and give him some support.

Reflective Writing

How has your understanding of depression changed after studying and discussing this material?

This will vary depending on how much accurate information a student has acquired prior to this case study. The important points include the idea that depression is an illness that can be life threatening and is treatable with various antidepressants and behavioral approaches. Assessment data including low self-esteem found in depression will be recognized. Medication is selected according to which side effects are most compatible with the client's condition.

Reference

Townsend, M. (2000). *Psychiatric mental health nursing: Concepts of care.* 3rd ed. Philadelphia: F. A. Davis.

CASE #2 TAMARA CLARK

Learning Objectives

1. Differentiate between objective and subjective patient assessment data.
2. Define assessment criteria for anorexia nervosa and bulimia nervosa.
3. Identify priority and goals of care for anorexia nervosa.
4. Discuss health promotion activities for eating disorders.
5. Identify communication strategies to explore feelings about treatment issues and patient control issues.
6. Identify personal feelings related to anorexia nervosa and treatment.

Tamara is a 20-year-old university student who has been brought to the ER by her roommate, Carrie. The admission record indicates Carrie found Tamara unconscious in their university condo. Tamara is 5 ft. 5 in. and weighs 94 lbs. Carrie says there are four girls living in the condo. The roommates share the rent, but they individually take care of their own meals. Carrie says she rarely sees Tamara eat. Recently Tamara has been borrowing clothes from two of the roommates who are petite because Tamara's clothes are too big for her. The ER physician has ordered serum electrolytes, EKG, BUN, creatinine, urinalysis, CBC, and thyroid tests.

Focus Questions

1. Summarize the subjective and objective assessment data available on Tamara. What objective data would support a possible diagnosis of anorexia nervosa?

   - **Subjective Assessment Data: Eating patterns are unknown, she is responsible for her own food, her clothes are too big, and she is borrowing clothes from the roommates.**

   - **Objective Assessment Data: Excessive weight loss (15% below expected range for age and height). Normal range for 5 ft. 5in. should be 117–156 lbs. Assessment data that validates the medical diagnosis of anorexia nervosa: Fat phobia, self-starvation, extreme weight loss, denial of weight loss, cessation of menstruation, dry skin with lanugo, complaints of feeling cold, dysrythmias from electrolyte imbalance, osteoporosis, feeling a need to be in control, perfectionistic.**

2. What additional data would the nurse need to collect in order to have a comprehensive nursing assessment of Tamara? How would the assessment data change if Tamara had bulimia?

   Additional data needed to assess for anorexia: menstrual cycle and irregularities, nutritional diary, feelings about her weight, skin appearance (dry lanugo), anxieties and fears, frustrations, sense of self, eating and purging experiences, motivation for treatment or ambivalence about treatment, and weight history. Different assessment data needed for bulimia: Find out if Tamara ever feels her eating patterns are out of control. Does she use fasting, bingeing, and purging to control her weight. Inquire about laxative abuse and misuse of other drugs (tobacco, cocaine) and medications. Inquire about self-induced vomiting. Check tooth enamel for erosion, check for cardiac irregularities, and find out if patient ever eats in secret and is dissatisfied with established eating patterns.

3. What is the priority of care for Tamara? What nursing orders could the nurse initiate to establish a physiological baseline and monitor Tamara's physical status?

   Priority of care for a seriously emaciated anorexic is restoration of physiological stability and nutritional rehabilitation of 1,200 calories per day to stop starvation. In addition the nurse must gain the trust and confidence of the patient and establish a balance of exercise that is not excessive for the individual. Increase self-esteem and improve assertiveness, promote more normal sense of body image, help client maintain weight and take charge of eating patterns, and assist with health maintenance plan after discharge. Nursing orders: I&O, daily weight, vital signs, documentation of weight gain.

Carrie indicates Tamara is very concerned about being too fat and has been defensive about her appearance and secretive about her diet. Carrie is unable to provide information about Tamara's family, but she states Tamara is concerned about making good grades to please her parents. In the past few weeks, Tamara has been very upset with one of the roommates. Tamara overhead this roommate discussing Tamara's weight and eating patterns with some sorority sisters. Carrie thinks Tamara was crying last night because she feared her sorority sisters would think bad things about her. Tamara told Carrie she was frustrated, hurt, and angry that the roommate was indiscreet about the use of her name and the discussion in general.

Focus Questions

1. The nurse wants to help Tamara sort out her thoughts and feelings about her roommate's behavior. What ways could the nurse focus the conversation to help Tamara sort out her feelings?

   Ways to focus the conversation: Recognize Tamara's thoughts and feelings are real to her. (She does feel hurt. She does feel out of control. She thinks she is fat.) Give feedback on distorted thoughts. (Her weight is too low to support her body life processes and is below normal for her height and age.) Focus on the here and now. (Today she was able to increase her caloric intake. She has control over what she selects to eat to meet her caloric needs.)

2. What health promotion activities could the nurse suggest to educate parents and school-age children about anorexia and bulimia?

   Suggested health promotion activities could include: a school educational program for female athletes and their parents and inservice programs for athletic coaches about the signs and symptoms of eating disorders, self-esteem programs for 8–10 year olds and their parents, show a movie about Karen Carpenter, and then discuss the disease and how one can prevent and/or recognize the problem.

Tamara has begun to gain weight and is in the normal weight range for her height. The nurse is suspicious that Tamara feels her weight is getting out of control.

Focus Question

1. How could the nurse address the issues of control with Tamara?

   Discuss Tamara's feelings about her weight gain. Reassure her the goal is to regain health not to promote excessive weight gain. Identify the normal range of weight for height. Reassure her ability to work with the dietitian to balance her diet and maintain her weight. Make a list of ways she can control weight. Make a list of alternate behaviors she can use when she feels out of control. Contract with her for a specific limit to her exercise.

Reflective Writing

Complete the following letter. Your instructor may ask you to share this letter with another classmate or respond to another student's letter.

Dear________:
I think Tamara and her roommates should____
____because______________
____
____

I (have/have not) known someone with anorexia or bulimia and therefore I
____
____
____
____

Sincerely,
Your Name

PS: If I were anorexic I would want someone to ______________________________
____
____

References

Bonwell, C. C. & Eison, J. A. (1991). Additional strategies promoting active learning—Writing in Class in *Active learning: Creating excitement in the classroom.* ASHE-ERIC Higher Education Report No. 1, 35–38. Washington, D.C.: ERIC Clearinghouse on Higher Education.

Hill, K. & Maloney, M. J. (1997). Treating anorexia nervosa patients in the era of managed care. *Journal of the American Academy of Child & Adolescent Psychiatry,* 36(11), 1632–1633.

McGown, A. & Whitbread, J. (1996). Out of control! The most effective way to help the binge-eating patient. *Journal of Psychosocial Nursing,* 34(1), 30–35.

Tiggemann, M. & Raven, M. (1998). Dimensions of control in bulimia and anorexia nervosa: Internal control, desire for control, or fear of losing control? *Eating Disorders: The Journal of Treatment and Prevention,* 6 (1), 65–71.

CASE #3 JOE FREDERICK

Learning Outcomes

1. Identify assessment data characteristic of a client with schizophrenia.
2. Analyze assessment data characteristic of a client with schizophrenia.
3. Explain rationale for treatment with antipsychotic medication.
4. Identify nursing interventions and outcomes for the client with schizophrenia.
5. Plan individualized discharge teaching for the client/family.

Day 1. Joe Frederick, age 26, an African American electrical engineer is married to Sally, a computer programmer. They have no children. Joe's only close relatives are his grandmother, who raised him, and an older sister. According to Sally, Joe has been having difficulty sleeping for the past month and has complained about the stress at work and headaches. At times Joe "talks to himself." Yesterday Sally received a call from Joe's boss stating that Joe has been "behaving

strangely" during the past month. Joe has been warning others in his work group about the dangerous forces controlling them on the Internet and refusing to use his computer. Two days ago Joe left the office after lunch and did not return for three hours. Yesterday Joe was absent from work without notifying the office. When Sally returned home she found Joe still in bed. He stated he had to protect himself from the "dangerous forces." After consulting with their HMO, it was decided that Joe should be admitted to the psychiatric unit for one week of stabilization. Admitting diagnosis is "Possible Paranoid Schizophrenia." Joe is started on Olanzapine (Zyprexa) 10 mg qd po.

Focus Question

1. Relate Joe's current clinical data to the common signs of schizophrenia.

   Difficulty sleeping **that may have occurred when Joe started experiencing** ***auditory hallucinations. Functioning at a level below premorbid state*** **is present. It is difficult to concentrate on job related tasks when hallucinating and Joe's** ***complaints of stress at work and headaches*** **could be a sign of anxiety, which would increase when trying to work while having** ***disorganized thinking.*** **However, it is important for the physician to evaluate other possible organic causes for the headaches.** ***Talking to oneself*** **is often a manifestation of hallucinations. Believing that there are dangerous forces trying to control him are signs of Joe's** ***paranoid delusions,*** **and the** ***bizarre behavior*** **and** ***withdrawing*** **to bed are attempts to cope with the frightening delusions. Joe is receiving intervention and treatment early in the course of his illness and hopefully will respond to treatment and maintain his ability to work. If he had been allowed to withdraw for a longer period of time, he would probably have shown symptoms that included poor grooming, decreased food intake, and increasingly bizarre behavior.**

Day 2. Joe has remained in his room, refused to eat meals with other clients in the day room or go to the nurses' station for his medication. Joe showered and groomed himself. He had juice and cereal for breakfast and ate half the food on his lunch tray but refused his supper tray, stating he was worried it might have too much radiation. While he took his Olanzapine the day he was admitted, today he refused to take it until Sally came to visit and told him it was important for him to take it, so he could come home soon.

Focus Questions

1. As his primary nurse, what nursing diagnoses do you identify for Joe?
   - **Alteration in thought processes related to possible panic anxiety and biochemical factors are evidenced by delusional thinking.**
   - **Sensory-perceptual alterations related to biochemical factors and withdrawal into the self are evidenced by talking to self, difficulty sleeping and poor concentration, suggesting auditory hallucinations.**
   - **Risk for violence: self-directed and directed at other; risk factors: hallucinations and delusions of persecution.**
   - **Sleep pattern disturbance, less sleep than required, is related to hallucinations and fear as evidenced by wife's and client's statements.**
   - **Noncompliance related to distrust is evidenced by refusal to take meds and participate in treatment milieu.**
   - **Knowledge deficit related to difficulty in trusting and lack of information about management of newly diagnosed illness is evidenced by failure to participate in treatment milieu and medication regime.**

2. What nursing interventions do you plan to implement with Joe?

   Develop trust by establishing a one-to-one relationship. Make brief, frequent contacts. Be accepting. Be sensitive to Joe's need for personal space. Do not touch without explaining. Maintain a low stimulus environment to decrease anxiety and monitor Joe frequently for dangerous behavior that could lead to violence to self or others. Be aware of Joe's tendency to misinterpret whispering or laughing by others who he can see but cannot hear. (ideas of reference) Do not argue with Joe about delusions, but do not confirm them. Relate to underlying feeling if possible (example: "It must be frightening to believe that forces are controlling you over your computer."). Observe for behaviors that may indicate hallucinations (talking to self, laughing, assuming a listening pose). Try to distract Joe when he is hallucinating. Let him know you do not share his perception. "I realize the voices are real to you, but I do not hear any voices." Focus on reality and on concrete, real people and events in discussions. Provide structure to help Joe focus on reality and gain control in his environment. Administer and monitor medication. Monitor sleep pattern and discuss sleeping difficulties with physician. Offer measures, such as relaxation techniques and soft music, to assist Joe in getting to sleep and decrease anxiety.

3. What is the rationale for medication treatment in Joe's condition?

   Schizophrenia is a brain disorder believed to be partially caused by an excess of dopamine. Antipsychotic medication decreases the positive symptoms of schizophrenia, such as delusions and hallucinations, by decreasing dopamine.

4. What are the advantages of Olanzapine over conventional antipsychotics such as Haldol or Thorazine?

   Olanzapine is a newer antipsychotic that is more specific in the dopamine receptors that it affects, and, therefore, it is less likely to cause bothersome side effects that are more likely with medications that unselectively target dopamine receptors (Thorazine, Haldol, etc.). A big advantage of the newer antipsychotics is their likelihood of improving quality of life and affecting negative symptoms of schizophrenia, such as decreased motivation, lack of enthusiasm, and decreased sense of purpose, by increasing motivation, enthusiasm, sense of purpose, and curiosity. However, the newer meds are more expensive.

5. What nursing interventions are important when a client is taking an antipsychotic?

   Monitor vital signs. Take blood pressure of client sitting and standing at least once every day. Monitor for signs of movement disorders. Monitor for signs of blood dyscrasias. Teach about importance of medication and side effects.

6. How will you respond to Joe's reluctance to take his medication?

   Initially wait and offer later in the day. Enlist the help of someone with whom Joe has a trusting relationship.

7. What outcomes do you expect Joe to accomplish?

   - **Participate in treatment with less expression of delusions.**
   - **Demonstrate ability to relate appropriately/satisfactorily with others.**
   - **Demonstrate trust in significant personal and caregiver relationships (wife, physician, one nurse).**
   - **Has not harmed self or others.**
   - **Differentiate between what is real and what is not real.**
   - **Problem solve by asking reality-based questions, particularly in regards to medications, work, hospitalization.**
   - **Maintain anxiety at a manageable level.**

Day 3. The psychiatrist who is seeing Joe tells Sally that Joe probably has schizophrenia. After talking with the physician, Sally asks you, "What is going on with Joe? When do you think Joe can return to work?"

Focus Questions

1. How will you reply to Sally?

   Considering that Sally may be experiencing an initial response of shock or disbelief as a family member has been diagnosed with an illness that has a stigma or is understood as serious, the nurse should ask Sally what she heard the physician say, what she knows about schizophrenia, and how she is feeling. Then the nurse will be supportive and relate to her with empathy as Sally needs support to cope with her husband's illness. The nurse will give simple, accurate information about schizophrenia but leave the majority of the teaching for discharge meetings with Joe and family education groups. When Joe returns to work is up to Joe, his physician, and his employer.

2. What community resources are likely to be helpful for Sally?

   The National Alliance for the Mentally Ill (NAMI) and many local affiliates are helpful sources of information and support for families with members who have a brain disorder. Many local groups give a series of classes to educate families about schizophrenia. They include topics such as cause, medications, and symptom management, community resources for treatment, and how to best respond to problem behaviors.

3. How would you approach Joe about the issue of including the family in discharge planning?

   Once Joe's anxiety is decreased to a moderate to low level and he is generally in reality, the nurse should ask if he wants his wife and possibly his grandmother and sister to meet with him as he learns about what is needed to manage his recovery. If he responds affirmatively, the nurse will reinforce his decision as an important way for him to receive support. If Joe is leery of having his family involved, the nurse would encourage him to let those close to him be involved so they can give him caring support and get accurate information about the treatment and management of the illness he is experiencing.

4. What discharge teaching and planning must you implement?

   Teach about the medication and possible common side effects. Teach when to report side effects to physician or clinical nurse specialist. Do not discontinue the medication. Discuss importance of taking medications even when not experiencing symptoms of illness. If bothersome side effects are a concern, discuss with physician. Teach about the importance of avoiding extremes of heat or cold. Discuss symptoms associated with schizophrenia and chronic nature of the illness. Supply information on family support groups.

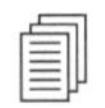

Reflective Writing

Imagine you are the parent or sibling of a person who has schizophrenia. How would you feel? What would be your greatest concerns? What would you want from nurses involved with caring for your family member?

Responses will vary. Grief reactions are likely. Once students learn about biological/genetic etiologies or predisposition they may be concerned about their own or their offspring's vulnerability. Hopefully students will empathize with family members' feelings and expect nurses to help family members vent and cope effectively with their feelings of fear and frustration. Nurses are in a key position to give accurate informa-

tion about the illness and available community resources to help family members learn how to help their loved one manage his or her illness.

References

Hartman, C. R., Knight, M., Glod, C. A. "Pharmacotherapy." 745–788. in Burgess, A. (1997) *Psychiatric nursing: Promoting mental health.* Stamford, Connecticut: Appleton and Lange.

Karch, A. M. (1998) *Lippincott's nursing drug guide.* Philadelphia: Lippincott. 834–835. (Olanzapine dosage)

McFarland, G. K., Wasli, E. L., & Gerety, E. K. (1997). *Nursing diagnoses and process in psychiatric mental health nursing.* 3rd edition. Philadelphia: Lippincott. 217–242.

Townsend, M.C. (2000). *Psychiatric mental health nursing: Concepts of care.* 3rd edition. Philadelphia: F. A. Davis.

Vallone, D. Schizophrenia. 503–517, in Burgess, A. (1997) *Psychiatric nursing: Promoting mental health.* Stamford, Connecticut: Appleton and Lange.

CASE #4 JOE GERMAINE

Learning Objectives

1. Describe physical signs and disease complications of alcoholism.
2. Explain the mental mechanisms of denial, manipulation, and rationalization in the disease of addiction.
3. Discuss appropriate responses to denial, manipulation, and rationalization.
4. Identify the signs and symptoms of delirium tremens.
5. Explain the role and approach of Alcoholics Anonymous (AA) in the treatment of addiction.

Joe Germaine, a 45-year-old thin, pale, worried-looking man, comes into the physician's office for complaints of stomach pains. In response to a question about his employment, he tells the nurse that he just lost his trucker's license because after a minor accident the police found a thermos of vodka in his truck. He states, "I don't think it's very fair. I didn't drink any of the vodka. They didn't even check my blood alcohol level." He also relates that he has a court date next week.

Focus Questions

1. What physical symptoms are often seen in an individual who has been drinking alcohol excessively for many years?

   Physical symptoms may include: wasting limbs, a fine tremor, nutritional deficits showing in skin, hair, and nails, ascites, liver enlargement, spider nevi over chest, face, and neck.

2. What disease processes are associated with excessive drinking?

   Disease processes may include: cirrhosis, esophageal varices, esophagitis, gastritis, duodenitis, gastric or duodenal ulcers, pancreatitis, and cardiomyopathy.

3. What are appropriate responses to Joe's statements about the unfairness of losing his license?

   Appropriate responses to Joe's statements about the unfairness of losing his license would be to make little comment pro or con about this event but rather to encourage him to talk about his story.

4. What is the rationale for the nurse's responses to his complaints of unfairness?

   The rationale for not commenting positively or negatively is that the nurse does not want to add to any rationalizations that Joe already uses, nor does the nurse want to confront or lecture at this point as little facts are known. The purpose is to get to know the patient and to increase trust so that he will want to stay for treatment.

5. What symptom of alcoholism is being demonstrated in the data?

   The symptom of denial is being demonstrated by the fact that Joe had a thermos bottle of vodka with him and he had the need to have it and to keep it hidden.

6. Typically the nurse makes notes on the patient's chart for the physician to see regarding the patient's presenting complaint. What information should the nurse record on the patient's chart? Why?

   The nurse should record, in the patient's words, what he has said about his pains, his losing his license and the reasons for it, and his court date. The reason for this is that he may indeed have gastrointestinal problems or illnesses, but recording the rest of the data will help the physician in the search for a diagnosis and its etiology.

7. What further information should the nurse gather from Joe regarding his drinking habits?

   Further information to gather would include questions from an alcohol screening test such as the DAST or the MAST: how much, when, how often, any DUI charges, do family or friends complain about his drinking?

8. How can the nurse ascertain if the answers being given are true?

   The nurse cannot know for certain if the answers given are accurate, but she or he can notice if the answers seem vague, or if Joe is trying to cover up by his manner of responding, which can help validate a problem with drinking.

Joe comes into the office the following week complaining again of stomach pain. His hands are shaky and he confides that he is to be admitted by court order to the community hospital for chemical dependency treatment tomorrow. He says, "I haven't had a drink for three days. Even though I know I don't need to go into the hospital, I'll do what I have to to get my job back."

Focus Questions

1. What could be happening to Joe's physiologic status in this situation?

   What may be happening is that Joe, because he stopped drinking three days ago, is experiencing alcohol withdrawal symptoms, which precedes delirium tremens.

2. What data are needed to support your conclusions?

   Data to support this would be fine tremors, hypertension, anxiety, restlessness, insomnia, tachycardia, possible nausea, and diaphoresis.

3. Are there any immediate concerns that need to be related to the physician?

   The nurse would need to relate to the physician Joe's symptoms and the fact that he has not had a drink for three days and is entering a treatment facility.

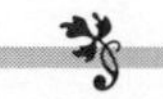

Three weeks later Joe returns to the physician's office. He reports he is out of the hospital and is now going to Aftercare groups once a week. He is also going to attend AA meetings. He says he wants to get some nerve pills like Xanax from the physician because he feels so nervous all the time. The physician hears this request from Joe and turns to the nurse and says, "Well, I don't suppose it could hurt anything, do you? As long as he goes to Aftercare and his AA meetings?"

Focus Questions

1. What is meant by the concept *manipulation?* How is Joe demonstrating this?

   Manipulation is defined as a long-standing pattern of behavior aimed at immediately satisfying one's own needs no matter what the cost to others. In chemical dependency treatment, Joe would have learned he is to abstain from alcohol and mood altering drugs, such as minor tranquilizers like Xanax. He is trying to manipulate the physician into prescribing the pills by pointing out how nervous he is, and explaining how he's doing all the things he's supposed to by going to AA and Aftercare. Then he can rationalize to himself that since the physician prescribed the medication, it's ok to take it, contrary to what the treatment facility said.

2. What would AA say about his using nerve pills?

   AA and most treatment facilities believe that total abstinence from any substances is necessary for a person to begin the recovery process from alcoholism and substance abuse.

3. How can the nurse respond in a manner that encourages problem solving among the three of them (Joe, the physician, and the nurse)?

   The nurse could respond by giving the facts about AA and the treatment approaches to alcoholism that abstinence from any mind-altering substances is essential. The nurse could also suggest that the treatment facility might have some input into Joe's concern about his nervousness.

Reflective Writing

When you first read Joe's statement that he didn't drink any of the vodka and the police didn't check his blood alcohol level, what did you think? What was your gut reaction to his statement of unfairness? Why did you feel that way?

Hopefully this exercise will help students identify the unconscious invitation from the client for the nurse to also deny the client has problems with alcohol. It may also help them identify any of their own experiences with alcoholics that have colored how they will work with clients with that disease.

References

Crigger, N. (1998) Defying denial: Clues to detecting alcohol abuse. *American Journal of Nursing*, 98, (8)20–21.
Kinney, J. (1996). *Clinical manual of substance abuse.* St. Louis: Mosby.
Sullivan, E. J. (1995). *Nursing care of clients with substance abuse.* St. Louis: Mosby.

CASE #5 JUNE JUNIPER

Learning Objectives

1. Explain why someone experienced a crisis, according to Aguilera's paradigm.
2. Differentiate between a crisis and someone exhibiting signs of anxiety and/or depression.
3. Apply the most important concepts in assessing someone who is experiencing a crisis.
4. Apply general principles of crisis intervention.

June Juniper is a 40-year-old woman who comes to the medical department of a large company. She appears anxious, is crying, and holds herself tightly as she sits in the chair of the waiting area, rocking slightly. She tells the nurse that she can't get her breath and she doesn't know what's wrong. "It just started this morning when I woke up. I've never felt like this. I feel like I might die. My heart is pounding out of my chest, and I'm so scared."

Focus Questions

1. What might be happening with June?

   June seems to be very anxious and perhaps is experiencing hyperventilation or an anxiety attack. She appears to fit the definition of someone in crisis, that is, a state of emotional dysequilibrium when the person's usual coping mechanisms have failed and that person feels as though they cannot cope.

2. What kinds of questions would the nurse want to ask June? According to crisis intervention theory, what questions *should* be asked?

   The nurse might ask: What has just happened to you in the last few days? What has changed in your life just recently? What is the meaning of what has just happened in the past few days? The nurse should assess if June is seeing the event realistically or in a distorted way. The nurse should determine who available support persons are to June, her usual coping skills, and if June is homicidal or suicidal.

3. What physical assessment data should be collected?

   Physical data to collect right now would be her vital signs (VS). Monitor VS for changes over time.

After a minute in the exam room with the nurse, June relaxes a bit, her vital signs are normal, and she says she can breathe better now. She continues to cry. She tells the nurse her 19-year-old daughter just moved out of the house this past weekend, and her teen-aged son who still lives at home is working a lot of hours and is busy with friends. When questioned about a husband, she says he died suddenly a year ago, last July. Now this year in July she finds that even with her job keeping her busy and having friends who care, nothing makes her happy. She says it was hard when her husband died, but "I coped. Now I feel like I'm falling apart. It doesn't make any sense. I feel empty and like there is nothing inside me."

Focus Questions

1. According to Aguilera's paradigm, what are the three balancing factors that determine whether someone experiences a crisis or not?

   The three balancing factors are perception of the event (daughter's moving out in June's case), coping skills available, and situational support.

2. What is the difference between a crisis and someone just being anxious or depressed?

   The difference between a crisis and someone who is just anxious or depressed is that someone in a crisis feels as though they are literally falling apart, they are panicked and cannot cope any longer, and they want to get relief *now*. Someone anxious or depressed does not feel the sense of urgency at this point and may continue to cope, even if it is marginally. The person in crisis feels a great emotional upset and that he/she is helpless to find a solution.

3. Why did June experience a crisis at this time? What was the precipitating event? What did this event mean to June?

   June experienced a crisis now because it is the anniversary of her husband's death, and she probably has not allowed herself to grieve over that loss. This made her vulnerable to her daughter's moving out, the precipitating event, which signified to her that her family had fallen apart. The son's being very busy with job and friends further reinforces this.

4. What coping mechanisms has June been using since her husband died? What were her situational supports? Was she using her supports at this time?

   The coping mechanism suggested by the data is that June has kept busy since her husband's death and has perhaps used some suppression. More data would need to be gathered to know more of her coping mechanisms. Her situational supports appear to be her friends, and perhaps her children. Her children are less available to her now, and because she is feeling the loss of her children as well as her husband, she is probably not using her friends well now as supports.

June and the nurse begin to discuss what steps June can take to make her feel better. She says she is tired of feeling depressed and sad and wants to do what she can to prevent any further attacks of anxiety like the one she just had.

Focus Questions

1. How could the nurse help June gain an intellectual understanding of her immediate problem?

   Help June look at how she has been coping since her husband died, and how her daughter's moving out has reawakened the grief of the loss of her husband, making her feel she could not cope and become very anxious. Help her verbalize what her daughter's moving out meant to her and look at how realistic or unrealistic her perception of that event was.

2. How would the nurse frame/state the cause of her anxiety, relating it to past and present events?

   "For the past year since your husband's death, you have coped fairly well by keeping busy with your job, family, and friends. When your daughter moved out recently close to the time of the anniversary of your husband's death, your feelings of loss were reawakened and it felt like your family had totally broken apart. Thus you became very anxious, couldn't stop crying, and felt like you were going to die with the anxiousness."

3. How would the nurse help her improve her coping mechanisms right now to help her get through her days?

   Encourage her to identify past coping behaviors that helped her when she was anxious and depressed so that she can reestablish some of those behaviors. Help her problem solve new coping behaviors that fit within her lifestyle and values.

4. What situational support can June use to help her deal with her depression and anxiety?

   In terms of situational support, she needs to identify at least one friend with whom she can talk freely about the changes in her life. She can establish times with her children when they will all get together for a meal or an activity so that she feels she is continuing to be in contact with them appropriately. The nurse may also serve as a situational support.

5. What feelings does June need to explore in more detail?

   June needs to discuss her grief in more detail, especially in regard to the loss of her husband, and also to discuss the changes in her family with her children beginning to move out of the home. To get June to talk about her husband, the nurse should ask about specifics of his death, the aftermath, the funeral, how she and the children handled it, etc.

This allows her to re-experience some of the grief while she has some support. She may also find it helpful to go to a widows support group or to join some other support group.

6. Outline a plan the nurse could use to specifically address June's present circumstances.

   Given the present circumstances of June presenting to the medical department, she can perhaps arrange to stop by to see the nurse a couple more times in the next few days to "see how she is doing" and to gain support. Interventions that should be done *today* include: helping June attain an intellectual understanding of the crisis, identify and agree to try one coping behavior in the next few days, and find one situational support to talk with. In the *next two to four weeks* she needs to work more on her grief regarding her husband and changes in the family. She needs to identify new coping behaviors to use and new ways to relate to her children who are becoming adults.

Reflective Writing

Everyone has had a time when they experienced a crisis, sometimes for a brief period, other times for longer periods. Write a paragraph about when you experienced a crisis. Why did it become a crisis?

The purpose of this assignment is to help students realize that experiencing a crisis is a normal part of life. It should help them to internalize the concepts by applying them to a personal situation.

References

Aguilera, D. C. (1997). *Crisis intervention: Theory and methodology.* St. Louis: Mosby.
Johnson, B. S. (1997). *Psychiatric-mental health nursing.* Philadelphia: Lippincott.

CASE #6 JULIE POLAR

Learning Objectives

1. Identify assessment questions specific for abused clients with post-traumatic stress disorder.
2. Identify content recommended for psychoeducation of abused clients.
3. List nursing diagnoses for abused clients with post-traumatic stress disorder.
4. Identify nonpharmacological interventions for abused clients with post-traumatic stress disorder.
5. Discuss actions, side effects, dosage of Prozac.
6. Identify client outcomes that indicate positive response to specific treatment plan.
7. Discuss the nurse's role in prevention of date rape and education of others about date rape drugs.

- **Instructor may want to use cases 6, 7, and 8 together, assigning a small group of students to each case. A general class discussion regarding similarities and differences of the clients could follow.**

At a local university, a busy walk-in mental health clinic employs nurses who see a variety of clients with mental health disorders. Today Mary Smith, R.N., is working the evening shift. Julie Polar, a 20-year-old freshman, comes to the clinic. Julie fills out the patient history and current health assessment form. Julie's patient information indicates she works in a local nightclub and lives with her mother. Her responses to the abuse assessment screening questions indicate she has a history of repeated sexual abuse by her uncle and she is afraid of her current boyfriend. Her major complaint is difficulty sleeping. After reading these data, Mary enters the examining room.

Focus Questions

1. What assessment questions should Mary ask?

   Tell me what happens that makes sleeping difficult. Have you ever had this problem before? Has something happened recently that has triggered a painful memory? Tell me about your relationships with other people in your life. Are you taking any medications?

2. What topics of information should be included in the psychoeducation of abused clients?

   Some topics are cycles of violence, access to shelters, legal services, government benefits, support networks, signs and symptoms of anxiety, dissociation, and post-traumatic stress disorder, escape plan, relaxation techniques, adequate nutrition and exercise, and sleep hygiene.

Julie states that she came to the clinic today because she is having vivid images of sexual assault that cause intense anxiety. The last few weeks she reports having nightmares of her uncle coming into her bedroom. She has difficulty sleeping, and even the slightest sounds make her jump. Her uncle sexually abused her as a child, and now she has difficulty in relationships with the opposite sex. Her boyfriend has been pressuring her to have a more intimate relationship. This week she found out her boyfriend was unfaithful, and she told him she doesn't want to see him anymore. Julie said, "Breaking up was all my fault. I shouldn't have resisted his affections, but I was not ready."

Focus Questions

1. Julie's emotional responses are characteristic of post-traumatic stress disorder. What are potential nursing diagnoses for Julie?

   - **Anxiety (severe to panic)/fear**
   - **Powerlessness**
   - **Sleep pattern disturbance**
   - **Coping, ineffective individual**

2. What nonpharmacological interventions might Mary use to help Julie?

   Encourage a consistent time to go to bed and to arise. Encourage not to nap during the day or use caffeine. Teach relaxation techniques and schedule a relaxation time before retiring. Explore the use of deep breathing and counting to ten to decrease stress. Identify past and present coping methods that are positive and reinforce them. Assist to identify when feelings of powerlessness and loss of control began. Identify personal strengths and the things in her life she can control. Encourage sharing of feelings and letting go of anger to enable rebuilding future relationships.

Julie has been taking an aerobics class but recently has not been motivated to attend. The physician prescribes Prozac (fluoxetine) for her symptoms of post-traumatic stress disorder.

Focus Questions

1. Describe the action, side effects, and dosage of Prozac.

   Prozac is a selective serotonin reuptake blocker. Usual dosage is 20–80 mg/qd. The most common side effects include headache, anxiety, insomnia, transient nausea, vomiting, and diarrhea.

2. Determine what outcomes would indicate a positive response to treatment?

   Julie sleeps through the night, and nightmares decrease. Julie returns to aerobics class. Julie states use of one stress reduction technique. She identifies a plan to resolve unexpressed feelings and emotions.

Reflective Writing

While you are finishing your charting, a group of male university students are seated in the waiting room prior to their physical exams. You hear their conversation about the big dance Friday night after the football game. One of the students says he has big-time plans for after the dance. He says he has some Rohypnol, the sedating drug used for date rape. Suddenly the student looks over at you and maintains eye contact with you. How will you respond to this situation. What is your responsibility as a nurse?

Rohypnol is illegal in the United States. It is on the list of scheduled drugs, which means there are requirements to document its distribution. It is a crime to give a controlled substance to anyone without their knowledge with the intent of committing a violent crime such as rape. Violation of this law is punishable by up to 20 years in prison and a fine of $250,000. Legally, no crime has been committed, except possession of an illegal substance. You may check with the policy and procedure for handling student misconduct on campus, before this student sees the physician. Proper authorities may need to be notified. You could begin an increased media blitz on campus regarding precautions to take to prevent date rape. You could post a description of the drug throughout the campus. You may wish to counsel the student. To ignore the incident would be inappropriate behavior.

References

Boyd, M. A. & Nihart, M. A. (1998). *Psychiatric nursing contemporary practice.* Chap. 33, Biopsychosocial aspects of caring for abused persons, (pp. 1062–1074) Lippincott: Philadelphia, PA.

Johnson, L. (September 25, 1998). Obliteration 'date rape' drug. Steps taken to end Rohypnol misuse. *Imprint Online: Human,* 21 (10). University of Waterloo Student Newspaper. Available online at: *http://imprint.uwaterloo.ca/issues/092598/4Human/features03.shtml.*

CASE #7 FRANNIE CATZ

Learning Objectives

1. Identify assessment questions specific to panic disorder.
2. Identify assessment data relevant to panic disorder.
3. Identify nursing interventions for clients with panic disorder.

4. Identify educational interventions for clients on Xanax.
5. Discuss how positive self-talk can help one manage thoughts and feelings of panic disorder.

- **Instructor may want to use cases 6, 7, and 8 together, assigning a small group of students to each case. A general class discussion regarding similarities and differences in the clients could follow.**

Shannon Cassidy, R.N., is sitting at the front desk of an urgent care center when a young woman and her husband appear. He says he thinks his wife, Frannie, is having a heart attack. He wants Shannon to help her. Frannie complains of being short of breath and dizzy. She states she has chest pain and she does not want to die. Her hands are trembling. Shannon alerts the physician and places Frannie on the cardiac monitor in holding room number 1. Frannie has no signs of cardiac symptoms as the cardiac monitor shows no irregularity.

Focus Questions

1. It is determined that Frannie is not experiencing a life-threatening event. Shannon suspects Frannie is having a panic attack. What questions would give Shannon more specific information to support her assumption?

   Shannon might ask: When did your symptoms begin? Did your symptoms appear during a period of activity or rest? (Students may not be aware that panic attacks tend to occur at rest, while heart disease related chest pain is likely to occur during activity.) What was happening in your life just prior to the onset of your symptoms? What were your most recent thoughts about what was happening in your life? What were you feeling about the time you had your attack? Have you ever had these types of thoughts, feelings, or symptoms before? Have you had situations when all of a sudden you felt frightened and others with you did not? How have these attacks interfered with your daily life? What changes have your family and loved ones had to make because of these attacks?

2. What additional assessment data should Shannon obtain?

   Inquire about the use of substances that are panicogenic, such as sources of caffeine, pseudoephedrine, amphetamines, cocaine, or stimulants. Consider smoking and withdrawal from alcohol or barbiturates. Binge drinking will exacerbate panic attacks. Assess sleep patterns for disturbances such as awakening during the night. Determine if poor eating patterns are creating low blood pressure and hypoglycemia. Inquire about degree of physical activity and physical fitness. Ask Frannie if the frequency of her symptoms increase in the days before her menstrual cycle. Assess her fears of losing control and feeling trapped. Assess how attacks impair mobility and identify what coping strategies Frannie has used to manage her symptoms.

Frannie is 30 years old and married to Dale. They have four children. She reports that she fears being unable to care for her children. She admits to being afraid to drive the car or ride on the train. Recently she has been having headaches. Dale canceled their vacation this morning because Frannie collapsed and said she felt like she was going to die. Dale insists that Frannie take one of her Xanax. Her husband frantically searches through Frannie's purse and finds a bottle of Xanax. Frannie tells Shannon, "I took the last Xanax I am going to take last night. I'm not taking anymore of it. There must be something else I can take." Dale reports that Frannie has been using Xanax for these panic attacks for some time now.

Focus Questions

1. Considering the data, what nursing diagnoses are appropriate for Frannie?
   - **Fear**
   - **Anxiety (severe to panic)**
   - **Knowledge deficit: Xanax withdrawal**
2. What action should Shannon take regarding Frannie's statement about her Xanax? What other medications are effective for panic disorders?

   Inquire about usage of Xanax, including dosage, frequency, and Frannie's compliance with Xanax treatment. Inquire about her knowledge of Xanax and the importance of not stopping the drug abruptly. The selective serotonin reuptake inhibitors, especially paroxetine (Paxil) and sertraline (Zoloft), are effective for panic disorder.
3. What nursing interventions could be used with Frannie?

   Encourage her to verbalize about phobias. Provide safety. Substitute positive thoughts for negative thoughts. Gradually teach to stop, wait, don't run away from fearful situations encountered. Teach to use relaxation exercises and visual imagery. Explore what may decrease fear and make it manageable, such as positive self-talk, singing, and counting. Educate patient on the dangers of withdrawing from Xanax abruptly. Stress importance of consulting with physician before discontinuing Xanax.
4. Frannie and Dale said the doctor indicated he will treat Frannie's panic attack with Paxil, anxiety management techniques, and cognitive restructuring. They want you to explain what he means by cognitive restructuring. Your response is:

   There are a variety of cognitive behavior techniques that help you monitor your body for signals of anxiety and stress. You will learn how your thoughts connect with your emotional responses and behaviors. You will learn new ways to think about stress, your beliefs, and your responses to stress.

Reflective Writing

Individuals with panic disorder often feel they are in real imminent physical danger that is life threatening. Positive self-talk can be used to give the individual cognitive control over the situation and decrease the fear of losing control. Imagine yourself in a situation where you feel out of control and overwhelmed by anxiety. Write one negative thought and feeling about this experience. Write a positive self-talk response to help you cope with the previous negative thought or feeling. What resources do you have available to assist you and your clients with learning new coping techniques?

Thought	Response
I am going to die.	**I will get through this. I can handle this.**
I'm getting dizzy.	**This is only anxiety and it will pass.**
It is happening again.	**This is a symptom of anxiety. Some deep breathing will help.**

Feeling	Response
I'm afraid to go outside.	**I can go outside for a few minutes and come right back inside.**

Any positive response to the negative thought or feeling is acceptable. Exercise helps students realize how difficult it is to overcome negative thoughts without help. Students may identify that clients will need to attend some education groups to learn new techniques for coping.

References

Boyd, M. A. & Nihart, M. A. (1998). *Psychiatric nursing contemporary practice.* Chap. 17, Anxiety and related disorders, 478–509. Philadelphia: Lippincott.

Fishel, A. H. (1998). Nursing management of anxiety and panic. *Nursing Clinics of North America,* 33(1), 135–151.

Kaplan, A. (1998). Treating panic disorder and agoraphobia without pushing the panic button. *Psychiatric Times,* 15(10), *http://www.mhsource.com/psychiatrictimes.html*

CASE #8 MADELINE MAYFIELD

Learning Objectives

1. Identify assessment questions specific to generalized anxiety disorder.
2. Identify assessment data characteristic of generalized anxiety disorder.
3. Identify nursing interventions for clients with generalized anxiety disorder.
4. Identify educational interventions for clients on BuSpar.
5. Explore the implications of psychobiological research on the stigma of mental health and treatment.

- **Instructor may want to use cases 6, 7, and 8 together, assigning a small group of students to each case. A general class discussion regarding similarities and differences of the clients could follow.**

Sherrie Kennedy, R.N., is working in the crisis mental health clinic. As she returns from dinner, a new patient, Madeline Mayfield, walks in the clinic door. Without making eye contact with Sherrie, Madeline asks if someone can talk with her. She wants to know if she is going crazy.

Focus Question

1. What assessment questions would Sherrie ask?

   What is happening to make you concerned about your mental health? Do you have difficulty relaxing or falling asleep? Do you find yourself feeling anxious or tense about a variety of things every day? Do you get anxious about how you can get through the day? Do you find yourself worrying frequently about a number of different things? Do you think your reaction to situations that make you anxious is more intense than you would like it to be? The nurse should find out Madeline's psychiatric history and whether she is presently being seen by a psychiatrist.

Madeline is a 38-year-old real estate agent, married with children. Madeline reports that she worries about maintaining her status as the top real estate agent in her company, about being a good mother, and about getting older. In fact she reports worrying about everything. Madeline feels high strung, is easily irritated, and has difficulty concentrating. She feels muscle tension all over her body. As she talks she fidgets, shakes her leg constantly, makes no eye contact, and clears her voice frequently. "I know my fears are unjustified, but I can't seem to control them," Madeline states. Sherrie calls Madeline's physician and finds she has a history of generalized anxiety disorder.

Focus Questions

1. What objective and subjective data indicate Madeline is having generalized anxiety?
   - **Objective data—She fidgets when talking, shakes her leg constantly, makes no eye contact, and clears her voice frequently.**
   - **Subjective data—worries about everything, feels high strung, is easily irritated, reports difficulty concentrating, states feels muscle tension, and is aware that anxiety is out of proportion to the situation but cannot control anxious feelings.**
2. What interventions can Sherrie suggest to help Madeline deal with some of her anxiety?

   Reassure Madeline that her anxiety will decrease with treatment. Help Madeline identify behaviors that indicate the presence of anxiety, such as shaking her leg, clearing her voice frequently, avoiding eye contact, fidgeting, having muscle tension, and feeling out of control. (Madeline must identify that anxiety is present before she can take actions to decrease anxiety.) Next identify feelings related to anxiety—fear, guilt, anger, frustration. Try to connect the feeling with the situation since different anxiety situations may stimulate different feelings and behaviors. (This denotes a cause and effect relationship that contributes to anxiety.) List some possible ways to decrease anxiety and deal with the situation. Identify possible signs of muscle tension and try relaxation techniques such as deep breathing. Implement one intervention at a time to decrease anxiety. Discuss community health resources available for individuals with generalized anxiety disorders.

Madeline was just started on BuSpar, and she does not know anything about the drug. She doesn't like to take medication and is worried that she will get addicted to the medicine.

Focus Question

1. What can Sherrie tell Madeline about BuSpar that will be educational and reassure her that addiction will not be a problem?

   BuSpar is very effective for clients with generalized anxiety disorder because it targets symptoms of anxiety and related problems of difficulty concentrating, tension, insomnia, restlessness, irritability, and fatigue. It does not have the potential for creating physical or psychological dependence. The most frequently experienced side effects are dizziness, drowsiness (avoid driving until you get used to the drug), nausea (frequent small meals help), excitement (will disappear when drug is discontinued), and headache. Consult your physician if side effects are problematic. Do not use this drug if breast-feeding or pregnant. Avoid drinking alcohol while taking BuSpar.

Reflective Writing

After Madeline leaves, Sherrie thinks about her expressed concerns that she was crazy and did not want to take medication. How could Sherrie help clients understand the biological approach to management of mental illness and the importance of following the treatment regimen?

With advances in medical technology, researchers have been able to understand the brain's structure and function. Knowing how changes in neurotransmitters and their receptors are manifest with different mental health disorders has led to new treatments. Understanding there is a physiological cause for mental illness destroys the myths that evil spirits and demons create uncontrollable individuals and offers hope of a new treatment available for restoring one's ability to function in society. If Madeline understands she has a physical problem of excess or deficient neurotransmitters that can be corrected by medication, she may be more compliant in taking her medication.

References

Boyd, M. A. & Nihart, M. A. (1998). *Psychiatric nursing contemporary practice.* Chap. 17 Anxiety and related disorders, 509–512. Philadelphia: Lippincott.

Fishel, A. H. (1998). Nursing management of anxiety and panic. *Nursing Clinics of North America,* 33(1), 135–151.

CASE #9 MADISON MARCUM

Learning Objectives

1. Identify assessment questions appropriate for obsessive-compulsive disorders.
2. Interpret assessment data characteristic of obsessive-compulsive disorders.
3. Identify implications of ritualistic behaviors and the implications for nursing care.
4. Identify nursing interventions appropriate for ritualistic behaviors.
5. Develop patient outcome criteria for clients with obsessive-compulsive disorders.
6. Discuss personal feelings about how the influence of mental health stigma and one's personal perspectives impacts one's value of the mental health nursing role.

Sandy Parrot, R.N., is finishing up her charts at the crisis mental health center. It is 10:30 P.M. and a new patient walks in the crisis unit door. It is a young student, Madison Marcum, from the college. She is alone and neatly dressed, but when she signs in you notice her hands are dry and the skin is cracked. Madison has never been to the doctor before for mental problems, but her mother told her to go to the clinic before she went to bed tonight. Madison says, "I just can't seem to stop doing things over and over again."

Focus Questions

1. What assessment questions should Sandy ask?

   Do you ever feel out of control or anxious? What helps you feel less anxious? Do you find yourself frequently repeating certain activities even though you know you have performed this activity already? Does this happen every day? How much is this repetitive activity interfering with your life?

2. What might Sandy suspect regarding the dry and cracked hands and what action should she take?

   Madison may have a hand washing compulsion and needs to have her skin condition checked for breakdown and secondary infection. At this time, Sandy should encourage Madison to protect her skin by using hand cream after washing her hands.

Madison was 12 years old when she began practicing compulsive behaviors to handle her anxieties and fears. Her first ritual was making sure she closed the closet door four times and set the alarm three times before she went to bed. She is now 19 and repetitively washes her hands after using the bathroom. She also changes her clothes three times each morning and twice in the afternoon. Her rituals have begun to increase in numbers and she has been having difficulty getting to classes on time.

Focus Questions

1. How can Sandy help Madison get to class on time?

   Encourage Madison to set her alarm earlier in the day to allow her more time to complete her rituals before leaving for class. Having a dual alarm clock may be helpful as she can set it for different departure times during the day. Sandy may want to use rating scales to help identify symptoms and monitor improvement in daily functioning. Such scales may include Yale-Brown Obsessive-Compulsive Scale or the Maudsley Obsessive-Compulsive Inventory (Goodman, Price, & Rasmussen, 1989).

2. What is the primary gain of Madison's rituals?

   The performance of the ritual helps relieve anxiety and worry temporarily.

3. What would happen if Sandy asked Madison to stop the rituals and how can she help Madison at this time?

   Restricting performance of the rituals would only increase Madison's worry and possibly create severe anxiety. Initial intervention should focus on protection of the skin and observation for secondary infection. Sandy should listen to Madison's life stressors and show empathy for Madison's need to perform the rituals. Sandy can speak to the discomfort caused by the frequent hand washing and suggest relief by use of hand creams and washing for a shorter length of time.

4. What outcomes would Sandy plan with Madison that would demonstrate an improvement in her behaviors?

   Outcomes—Madison will:

   - **Decrease the frequency of hand washing or decrease the length of time the hands are washed.**
   - **Have no impairment of skin integrity or secondary infection.**
   - **Not be late for class.**
   - **Explore two alternative ways to cope when feeling out of control.**

Reflective Writing

Your best friend works in a pediatric intensive care unit. She frequently makes comments about how easy your job as a mental health nurse is and the merits of her job over yours. Last week she saved a child's life and asked you how you can continue to work with "those people." How do you feel about her opinion and what is a "real" nurse to you?

The student may express anger, hurt, and frustration that the friend thinks mental health nursing is easier than caring for individuals with medical-surgical conditions. Writing should reflect insight that the peer's statement reflects misunderstandings and misconceptions about mental illness and the specific challenges of mental-health nursing. The student may reflect that the "real" nurse gets beyond the stigma of mental health and understands that the patient with mental illness, like the medical-surgical patient, does not have control over or cause one's mental health problem. Hopefully

the student will reflect insight as to how the friend might be enlightened to respect the role of the mental health nurse without causing alienation. It is important that the student identify that mental health nursing is a valued role in the profession. The student may also indicate that the stigma of mental illness and the related treatment is as much a social problem as it is a professional problem. Therefore, change in other's views may not occur until the society view of mental illness changes. These changes often occur by nurses becoming more socially active in creating reform.

References

Boyd, M. A. & Nihart, M. A. (1998). *Psychiatric nursing contemporary practice.* Chap. 17, Anxiety and related disorders, 512–522. Philadelphia: Lippincott.

Goodman, W., Price, L., Rasmussen, S., et.al. (1989). The Yale-Brown obsessive compulsory scale (Y-BOS): Part I. Development, use and reliability. *Archives of General Psychiatry,* 46, 1006–1011.

Paisley, L. M. (January 27, 1998). Clarity and parity: Understanding the roles of the advanced practice psychiatric nurse. *Online Journal of Issues in Nursing.* Available online at: *http://www.nursingworld.org/ojin/tpc1_8.htm.*

Rachman, S. & Hodgson, R. (1980). *Obsessions and Compulsions.* New York: Prentice Hall.

CASE # 10 SUSAN SINGLETON

Learning Objectives

1. Interpret assessment data and determine the implications for managing nursing care for patients with manic disorder.
2. Identify priority of nursing interventions for patients with manic disorders.
3. Identify the nursing implications of Lithium treatment in manic depression.
4. Discuss self-management of health after discharge and supportive resources available.

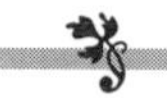

While working on the mental health unit, Jerrie Bedford, R.N., receives a call from the emergency room that there is a patient to be admitted to her unit, Susan Singleton, age 28, with an acute manic episode. The police were called to her apartment for a domestic disturbance. Susan was running around in the street and began to undress in the front yard. Her husband asked the police to take her to the hospital because she would not take her medicine and was out of control. He said Susan had not slept for two days and had eaten very little food. She has a history of bipolar disorder. She was assessed as having poor judgment and decreased attention span and concentration. The mental health unit has two available beds on the open unit, one private and one semi-private, and two available private beds on the closed secure unit.

Focus Questions

1. Where should Jerrie admit Susan? What information influenced this decision?

   Admit Susan to one of the beds on the closed secure unit because she needs a secure, safe environment with close supervision and limited stimulation.

2. What questions should Jerrie ask the ER nurse prior to Susan's transfer?

   What, if any, medications were given in the ER? Is there a husband or a family member available to provide the patient's history? What is the client's current status of activity, distractibility, and hostility?

3. What are the top priorities of care for Susan at this time? List nursing interventions that will meet those priorities.

   Rest and nutrition are high priorities of Susan's care at this time. Minimal stimulation in the environment will facilitate rest. Darken the room as much as possible. Finger foods should be available on the unit, such as vegetable tray, pieces of fruit in a cup, chicken strips, vienna sausages, or hot dogs. Susan would benefit from high protein and low calorie foods.

Susan has been taking Lithium at home, but her Lithium level is 0.1 mEq/L. She has an order for Valparoic acid (Depakote) 500 mg tid and Lithium 300 mg. b.i.d. On the unit Susan makes inappropriate sexual comments to all the males. She changes her clothes frequently and is often observed pacing the halls.

Focus Questions

1. Why did the physician order both Depakote and Lithium?

   Depakote will help get Susan's agitation under control while she is waiting for the Lithium to reach a therapeutic level, which may take two weeks.

2. What nursing action could Jerrie take if Susan gets agitated or demonstrates sexually inappropriate behavior when she is out of her room?

   Jerrie can use distraction and redirection to change Susan's behavior and prevent a hostile reaction.

Several days later, Jerrie finds hyperactive deep tendon reflexes, drowsiness, and vomiting when assessing Susan. Tomorrow is a group outing. Susan has attended group and received instructions regarding Lithium. Susan plans to go on the picnic and play volleyball. The weather forecast calls for a high temperature of 98 degrees with high humidity.

Focus Questions

1. What does the assessment data tell Jerrie about the Lithium level?

   Susan's Lithium level is too high.

2. What additional assessment data would confirm Jerrie's suspicions?

   Anorexia, c/o nausea, hand tremor, muscle twitching, ataxia, tinnitus, vertigo, and weakness would support the conclusion of a high Lithium level.

3. What are appropriate nursing actions considering Susan's assessment data?

   Alert Susan's physician and hold the Lithium for 24–48 hours.

4. How should Jerrie respond to Susan's plan for the picnic?

   Susan should plan to go on the outing but should not play volleyball in the heat and humidity. It could affect her Lithium levels.

5. What would be a priority concern for the bipolar client who is a rapid cycler and is taking Lithium?

   Susan is at high risk for suicide if she is a rapid cycler because of the frequent shift of moods from high to low.

Reflective Writing

Susan is leaving the medication group and you hear her telling another patient that she enjoys the highs of her illness and isn't too sure she wants to take medication. She is being discharged in two days. What could you do to improve Susan's chances of self-management of her health?

Meet with Susan and set personal goals for self-management. Provide her with appropriate reading information to explain bipolar disorder. Provide her with a list of local support group meeting locations and times. Encourage her to keep her follow-up appointments and explain the reason for blood monitoring. Help her identify a family member or a friend who will be her support system to remind her of meetings and monitor her medication administration. Give her a number to contact when she has questions about her health. Encourage her to talk with other individuals who have bipolar disorder and their family members. Make arangements for her aftercare treatment program.

References

Fortinash, K. M. & Holoday-Worret, P. A. (1996). *Psychiatric mental health nursing,* Chap. 12, Mood disorders: Depression and mania, 251–283. St. Louis: Mosby-Year Book, Inc.

Frisch, N. C. & Frisch, L. E. (1998). *Psychiatric mental health nursing: Understanding the client as well as the condition,* Chap. 13, The client experiencing mania, 267–291. Ibid. Psychopharmacology, 155–157. Albany, NY: Delmar.

Pollack, L. E. (1996). Inpatients with bipolar disorder: Their quest to understand. *Journal of Psychosocial Nursing, 34* (6),19–24.

CASE # 11 ANDREW AND ROWEENA ABBOTT

Learning Objectives

1. Identify assessment data characteristic of Alzheimer's disease and late life depression.
2. Modify communication strategies to meet the needs of the client with Alzheimer's disease.
3. Formulate nursing interventions to address self-care deficits of the client with Alzheimer's disease.
4. Apply the Progressively Lowered Stress Threshold (PLST) conceptual framework to the care of clients with Alzheimer's disease.
5. Identify strategies to address wandering behavior in a community care setting.
6. Analyze the suicide risk and lethality of an older adult.
7. Determine personal strengths and limitations in providing nursing care to suicidal clients and clients with Alzheimer's disease and related dementias.

Andrew Abbott, age 80, is the primary caregiver for his wife Roweena, age 78. Roweena was diagnosed with Alzheimer's disease three years ago. Mr. Abbott has just begun bringing his wife to the Adult Day Care Center (ADC) at Manorview, a continuing care retirement community. He tells you that the most problematic situations related to caring for his wife at the present time are: (1) episodes of incontinence, especially during the night; (2) increasingly unsteady gait and difficulty walking leading to falls; and (3) her continued behavior of following him from room to room in the home. He also stated that sometimes she doesn't know he is her husband. He is having difficulty getting her ready to come to the ADC because of difficulties she has with dressing. Today, she had her slip on over her dress. Mr. Abbott talked briefly (and tearfully) of his hopes for retirement life and how Rowena's disease had taken away their plans for later life.

Focus Questions

1. Given the above data, in what stage of Alzheimer's disease is Mrs. Abbott?

   Roweena is in the moderate to severe stage. In this stage the individual exhibits severe agnosia and advanced apraxia. Incontinence often occurs because the person cannot remember where the toilet is. In this stage the level of care is very demanding.

2. What strategies will be most useful in helping you communicate with Mrs. Abbott?

   Observe body language to determine receptiveness. Be sure you have her undivided attention. Begin each interaction by introducing yourself, explaining your role, and telling why you are there. Reduce all background noise and distractions. Match verbal and nonverbal messages—calm, low pitched voice, converse at eye level. Use concrete, common words; avoid generalizations and cliches. Reduce speed of speech. Use simple words and sentences; avoid conjunctions. Avoid logical discussions; focus on feelings being expressed. Avoid open-ended questions. Help with word finding by giving two alternative choices. Help when she gets off-track by restating the original topic as a question or by repeating the last words said. Give positive directions rather than telling her not to do something. Give one direction at a time and help start the activity if necessary. When asking a question, give the choice at the end of the question. Use smiling, relaxed demeanor.

3. What strategies would you suggest to Mr. Abbott that might help him with dressing Mrs. Abbott in the morning?

   Strategies: Divide task into single directions; provide directions calmly. Lay out clothes in order. Do not hurry Mrs. Abbott. Provide other cueing if necessary. Consider replacing buttons and zippers with velcro. Use slacks and skirts with elastic waists. Provide teaching about effective communication as in question 2.

Mrs. Abbott is initially attending Adult Day Care (ADC) four days a week, from 9:00 A.M. to 5:00 P.M. The ADC uses the Progressively Lowered Stress Threshold Model (PLST) as a theoretical framework for provision of care. You are responsible for supervising the ADC staff. During her first week, Mrs. Abbott tried to leave the building on two occasions, repeatedly saying she had to leave school because it was time for her to get home to do her chores. She is not eating well, and she has had two episodes of urinary incontinence.

Focus Questions

1. Develop a short-term goal and nursing interventions for Mrs. Abbott's diagnosis of *Self-care deficit related to cognitive impairment.* Consider eating as well as bowel and bladder function.

   Given the guiding theoretical framework of Hall and Buckwalter (1987), interventions should address controlling the following factors hypothesized to increase stress and anxiety: fatigue; physical stressors; demands to function beyond the person's capability; change of routine, caregiver, or environment; and overwhelming or competing stimuli.

   - **Short-Term Goal: Mrs. Abbott will follow step-by-step instructions for eating.**
   - **Interventions: Use one staff member consistently. Divide task into single directions. Provide other cueing if necessary (e.g., put fork in her hand, model eating). Offer**

finger foods if necessary. If necessary, provide only one food item at a time. Minimize other competing stimulation in dining room; if necessary have Mrs. Abbott eat in a small dining room with one other participant and staff member.

- **Short-Term Goal: Mrs. Abbott will remain continent during her time at the ADC.**
- **Interventions: Use one staff member consistently. Make certain there are labels (large signs and pictures) on bathroom doors and doors to other rooms. Accompany to bathroom at frequent intervals, in the early morning and after all meals and snacks. Segment task into single steps. Simplify clothing as previously described.**

2. Develop a short-term goal and nursing interventions for Mrs. Abbott's diagnosis of *Potential for injury related to wandering secondary to cognitive impairment.*

    - **Short-Term Goal: Client will wander only in protected area.**
    - **Interventions: Determine underlying need being met by wandering and attempt to meet need. Is Mrs. Abbott trying to find something? Is wandering meeting a need for tactile stimulation? Has Mrs. Abbott used physical activity as a means of reducing tension during her lifetime? Is wandering related to previous lifestyle/roles? Does she have to urinate, have a bowel movement? Involve Mrs. Abbott in physical activity using large motor movement. Reduce environmental cues for leaving the building. Remove any coats/coat racks from immediate area. Disguise doors with visual barriers. Assess for fatigue; provide rest periods. Use a symbol on Mrs. Abbott's nametag to identify her as a wanderer to staff and visitors.**

3. As Mrs. Abbott attempts to leave the building, she says, "I have to leave school. It's time for me to get home to do my chores." How would you respond to Mrs. Abbott's verbalization. Why would you respond this way?

    Guidelines for responding would include: Facing Mrs. Abbott and using touch if this does not seem threatening. Link the statement to Mrs. Abbott's feelings. Repeat specific words "time to do your chores" or the emotional need "you need to go home"; "you're worrried you won't finish your chores." Do not provide orientation to the present unless it is calming to Mrs. Abbott. Response should indicate awareness of importance of acknowledging Mrs. Abbott's feelings rather than pointing out her cognitive deficits by correcting her. Therapeutic responses might focus on speaking to her about school or her chores, while also acknowledging her desire to be at home. Discussing previous areas of competence can increase Mrs. Abbott's sense of mastery and self-esteem.

When discussing his situation, Mr. Abbott became tearful at times. He seemed especially sad when talking about his children. He indicated that they did not like to talk about his feelings and their feelings regarding their mother's illness, but they would only discuss practical concerns related to the situation. He also revealed his belief that he and his wife had lived longer than they should have. When discussing the tragic nature of Alzheimer's disease, he also stated, "They should just shoot us and get it over with." Several times Mr. Abbott asked, "When do you know it's time for a nursing home?"

Focus Questions

1. What assessment questions would you ask to determine if Mr. Abbott was depressed?

    Questions should focus on the following characteristics of later life depression:

    - **Memory deficits, difficulty concentrating, slowed thinking (these cognitive changes may be exaggerated; often the predominant symptom of depression in older adults).**

- **Anxiety and irritability.**
- **Focus on feeling "worried" or "down" or "empty," expressions of hopelessness and pessimism about the future.**
- **Changes in sleep patterns that may include insomnia, hypersomnia, frequent awakening, early morning awakening.**
- **Loss of appetite, weight loss, digestive system complaints.**
- **Discomfort/pain, loss of energy and fatigue, slowing of psychomotor functioning.**

2. It is important to determine Mr. Abbott's suicide risk. How would you do this?

The Sad Persons Scale can to used to evaluate major risk factors for suicide potential (Varcarolis, 1994).

S Sex

A Age

D Depression

P Previous attempts

E ETOH (alcohol)

R Rational thinking loss

S Social supports lacking

O Organized plan

N No spouse

S Sickness

One point is given for each factor. General guidelines for interpretation of scores are:

7–10 points	**Client needs to be hospitalized**
5–6 points	**Hospitalization should be strongly considered**
3–4 points	**Close follow-up; possible hospitalization**
0–2	**Home; follow-up care if necessary**

It is also important to assess for any nonverbal indicators of suicide intent, such as serious self-neglect, excessive use of alcohol or drugs and/or accumulation of prescription drugs, frequent physician visits, and behaviors such as giving possessions away.

If Mr. Abbott acknowledges suicidal ideation, it is important to determine if he has a plan. The nurse then needs to evaluate the suicide plan to determine the degree of suicide risk or lethality. Specificity of details, lethality of methods, and availability of means are considered when evaluating lethality. It is also important to determine if Mr. Abbott has ever started to act on a plan and under what circumstances he would act on his plan. (Robie, *et al.*, 1999)

3. How would you respond to Mr. Abbott's statements? Why would you respond this way?

It is important to make covert indications of suicide overt. Questions that would do this include:

- **Are you experiencing thoughts of suicide?**
- **How often and when do you experience the thoughts?**
- **How compelling are your thoughts?**

These questions should be asked in a dialogue such as:

"You said, 'they should just shoot us and get it over with.' It sounds like, for you, life is not worth living right now. Is that true?"

"Some people who feel that life is not worth living think about killing themselves. Are you thinking of killing yourself, Mr. Abbott?"

Reflective Writing

What are the most important characteristics and skills of the nurse caring for: (a) a suicidal client; (b) clients with Alzheimer's disease and their families? What are your strengths and areas for growth in this regard?

In order to work with suicidal clients effectively, the nurse must work through expected emotions and reactions to the client. These stages include shock and denial; recognition, which includes fear, anxiety, and helplessness; responsibility, which include feelings of being responsible, guilt, and anger; and the stage of individual choice, when the nurse realizes that the client is the only one who can ultimately choose life. Openness to emotions and supervision is crucial. Nurses have to exhibit warmth, openness, concern, and consistency. The nurse must be able to encourage realistic problem solving and also reaffirm the hope of the suicidal client. In order to be effective with clients with Alzheimer's disease, nurses need special training. Characteristics and skills include the ability to set realistic goals as well as the ability to find satisfaction in small accomplishments.

References

Hall, G. R. & Buckwalter, K. C. (1987). Progressively lowered stress threshold: A conceptual model for care of adults with Alzheimer's disease. *Archives of Psychiatric Nursing*, 1, 399–406.

Miller, C. A. (1995). *Nursing care of older adults: Theory and practice.* (2nd ed.). Philadelphia: J. B. Lippincott Co.

Rader, J, Doan, J., & Schwab, M. (1985). How to decrease wandering, a form of agenda behavior. *Geriatric Nursing*, 6, 196–199.

Robie, D, Edgemon-Hill, E., Phelps, B, Schmitz, C., & Laughlin, J. Suicide prevention protocol. *American Journal of Nursing*, 99(12), 53–57.

Varcarolis, E. M. (1994). *Foundations of psychiatric mental health nursing* (2nd ed.). Philadelphia: W. B. Saunders Co.

chapter **4**

Annotated Medical Surgical Cases

CASE #1 JACK TAYLOR

Learning Objectives

1. Discuss the pathophysiology for Type II diabetes.
2. Discuss appropriate teaching content for a newly diagnosed Type II diabetic.
3. Identify psychosocial needs of clients dealing with a need to alter their lifestyles.
4. Discuss ways the nurse might intervene with clients who are noncompliant.
5. Identify appropriate community resources for a client with Type II diabetes.

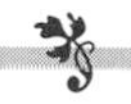

Jack Taylor is a 34-year-old male who came to the clinic with a complaint of a sinus infection. He had an episode of hematuria yesterday, so the clinic nurse checked his urine sample with a dipstick. Jack is 6 feet tall, 272 pounds, and his VS were T101.6°, P. 68, R. 18. The urine sample had the following results: Glucose ++, Protein +, Ketones trace, Blood trace, Specific gravity 1.020, Leukocytes none, and Nitrites none. The health care provider orders a fingerstick glucose and the clinic nurse reports a result of 274. The health care provider schedules Jack to return tomorrow for diabetic education and writes an order for home glucose monitoring equipment and for Augmentin 875/125 mg 1 tablet by mouth twice a day for 10 days.

Focus Questions

1. Discuss the pathophysiology of diabetes as applied to Jack.

   Jack has developed Type II diabetes. His pancreas is producing some insulin but the quantity is not sufficient to lower blood glucose levels. While insulin is assisting in transporting some glucose across membranes into muscle and fat cells, the additional glucose remains in the blood stream resulting in hyperglycemia. When blood glucose levels exceed the renal threshold of approximately 180 mg/dl, glucose is excreted in urine. The presence of insulin is sufficient to prevent the breakdown of most fats, thus the trace ketone finding. Type II diabetics rarely develop ketosis. Risk factors for Type II diabetes include family history, obesity, increasing age, and ethnicity. Type II diabetes has greater prevalence among Hispanic Americans, Native Americans, and African Americans. In reviewing Jack's information, he is obese.

2. What educational information should the nurse provide Jack today?

   Today the nurse should provide Jack with information about his prescribed antibiotic. Instructions include evenly spacing the doses across 24 hours; taking the medication on an empty stomach, either 1 hour before or 2 hours after a meal; taking with a full glass

of water; and reporting vomiting, diarrhea, rash, and continued or new symptoms of infection. If nausea is a problem for Jack, a few bites of crackers or bread may relieve this side effect. Additional instructions are to complete all ten days of medication and to drink plenty of water and other noncaloric fluids over the next several days. If he does not feel there has been any improvement in his infection after 4 to 5 days of antibiotic therapy, he should return to the office for further evaluation. The nurse must also provide information about his diet for the next day. As the health care provider has not identified a specific diet, Jack should be counseled to avoid concentrated sweets and choose protein, fruits, and vegetables instead.

3. Are there any questions that the nurse should ask Jack today to assist in preparing for tomorrow's educational intervention?

   The nurse should ask Jack what his immediate concerns are, what experiences he has had with diabetes (family members may be diabetics), what his usual dietary and exercise patterns are, what a typical day and week are like, and what his food preferences are.

4. What educational information should the nurse prepare for tomorrow's session?

   The nurse should prepare educational information about diet, exercise, use of a home glucose monitor, and how to record the monitor results. If possible, Jack should bring to the session the glucose monitor he will be using at home. The health care provider will order the diet appropriate for Jack. Written materials, diagrams, or charts will be useful to Jack at home.

Jack returns for his follow-up appointment. He has not eaten breakfast, so a fingerstick fasting glucose is performed. The result is 168. Jack is quite unhappy about this sudden diagnosis. He listens politely to the nurse's information but gives every indication he will do as he pleases. During the discussion, Jack reveals that he had a work-related accident four years ago that resulted in permanent disability. He has a weight lifting restriction of 10 pounds and cannot stand or walk for more than 20 minutes. His typical meal pattern is one meal a day for three or four days per week. He usually does not eat on the other days of the week. He is the family cook as he is home while his wife works. There are two children, ages 6 and 9, at home. Jack consumes a wide variety of foods, preferring to fry meats.

Focus Questions

1. What adjustments should the nurse make in the teaching plan?

   The nurse should focus on Jack's emotional reaction first. Provide Jack with some time to vent his emotions. Asking Jack about how he handled previous health problems will allow the nurse to reinforce positive coping strategies and explore negative coping strategies. In the therapeutic use of self, the nurse expresses optimism that Jack will learn to handle his diabetes just as he has successfully coped with previous health concerns.

2. What referrals are appropriate for Jack?

   Jack should be given a referral to a dietician to assist him in proper meal planning. A physical therapy referral may assist Jack to find some exercises that are within his physical capabilities. The nurse should explore with Jack whether he would like to participate in a diabetes educational group. A nearby hospital may offer such group opportunities.

3. What psychosocial needs might Jack have?

   The psychosocial needs Jack seems to be exhibiting are frustration/anger, resistance to changing his eating habits, and perhaps denial concerning his illness.

4. How will the nurse address his psychosocial needs?

   The nurse should use therapeutic communication skills to direct Jack toward taking control of his diabetes rather than allowing the diabetes to control him. Listening, reflecting, questioning, supporting would all be good techniques for communicating with Jack.

After 3 months, Jack returns for a follow-up appointment. His blood glucose monitoring log reveals fasting blood sugars of 155 to 210 and evening blood sugars of 220 to 286. He states that he has been watching what he eats and trying to eat more regularly. He is not exercising. His weight today is 255 pounds. The health care provider orders Glucophage 500 mg 1 tablet by mouth 3 times per day.

Focus Questions

1. How could the nurse obtain a more accurate picture of Jack's diet?

   Ask Jack to write down a 3-day recall of his intake. Asking Jack to record his intake for a week would provide even more information about his diet. The nurse assesses whether Jack's diet meets the prescribed diet and assists Jack in problem solving to improve his diet. Also, monitor the Hgb A1C to show diabetic control and adherence to prescribed regimen.

2. What educational information is appropriate to discuss with Jack today?

   Information about Glucophage is one topic that must be addressed today. Glucophage does not effect pancreatic insulin secretion; the actions are to increase the use of glucose by muscle and fat cells, decrease hepatic glucose production, and decrease intestinal absorption of glucose. Glucophage does not produce hypoglycemia. The doses should be taken with the morning and evening meals. Renal function tests will be ordered today and at least yearly during the time the client takes this medication. Jack should monitor his blood glucose at home as he is adjusting to this medication. Jack must continue diet and exercise treatments for best control of his blood sugars. Exercise must also be addressed today. Another offer of a referral to physical therapy would be appropriate in light of Jack's comment about not exercising. A discussion should also take place about the desired level of fasting blood sugars. This discussion could incorporate the complications that maintaining good control of blood sugar levels will help to prevent.

3. What psychosocial support can the nurse give Jack today?

   The nurse should ask Jack how he feels emotionally and physically, providing an opening for him to talk about the changes. The nurse should praise Jack for his weight loss and his improved eating pattern. Reinforcing that the changes Jack faced as a result of his diagnosis are indeed difficult and that he is being successful will encourage Jack to continue making changes.

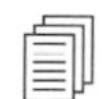

Reflective Writing

As a nurse, how will you work with clients who choose not to follow the advice of the health care provider?

There are two conflicting positions for the nurse in this case. Jack has a moral right to ignore the advice of the health care provider. The nurse must be assured that Jack understands that the choice he is making will lead to more physical complications than have occurred so far. The nurse may be in a position to assist Jack to sort through the emotions of this situation and then make informed choices about how to treat his

diabetes. The nurse is interested in helping Jack to take control of his health, and education is the best way for the nurse to intervene in this situation.

References

Abrams, A. C. (1998). *Clinical drug therapy: Rationales for nursing practice* (5th ed.). Philadelphia: Lippincott.

LeMone, P. & Burke, K. M. (1996). *Medical surgical nursing: Critical thinking in client care.* Menlo Park, Calif.: Addison-Wesley.

Phipps, W. J., Sands, J. K. & Marek, J. F. (1999). *Medical-surgical nursing: Concepts & clinical practice* (6th ed.). St. Louis: Mosby.

Ward-Collins, D. (1998). Noncompliant: Isn't there a better way to say it? *American Journal of Nursing,* 98(5), 27–31.

CASE #2 JOHN JACOBS

Learning Objectives

1. Relate risk factors to the pathophysiology of cerebral vascular accident (CVA).
2. Describe client teaching related to computed tomography (CT) scan and angiogram.
3. Discuss the nursing diagnoses common to the CVA patient.
4. Describe common medications used in management of clients with CVA.
5. Plan individualized discharge treatment for the CVA patient and family.

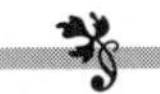

At 0645 John Jacobs, a 65-year-old white male, is admitted to Miami University Hospital. He was seen in the Emergency Department with the following symptoms: right side hemaparesis, homonymous hemianopia, and expressive aphasia. He is drowsy, his weight is 230 lbs. and he is 5ft. 11in. tall with BP 200/120. He has a history of cocaine abuse as a young adult. He is scheduled for a CT scan and cerebral angiogram prior to admission to the floor to rule out cerebral vascular accident (CVA). His wife accompanies him and states, "I found him unconscious on the floor in the bathroom."

Focus Questions

1. What are the risk factors in this case? Describe how they might contribute to the development of a cerebral vascular accident (CVA).
   - ***Age*—highest incidence of stroke is in people over 65; *gender*—more frequent in men**
   - ***Hypertension*—increased blood pressure damages blood vessels including the cerebral vessels**
   - ***Substance abuse*—increases risk of intracranial hemorrhage and decreases cerebral blood flow**
   - ***Obesity*—leads to hyperlipidemia and atherosclerosis, which obstructs cerebral vessels with plaque**
2. What other data would you want to collect related to possible risk factors?

   Family history of stroke; current medication—Is he taking medication for hypertension? Does he have any history of diabetes or heart disease such as arrhythmias, polycythemia, history of smoking, or gout? What about his lifestyle related to diet and exercise?

3. Describe what hemaparesis, homonymous hemianopia, and expressive aphasia will mean in relationship to nursing care.

   - ***Hemaparesis*—is weakness on one side of the body. Nursing goals would include maintaining and improving functional/ability related mobility. Interventions would include: (a) active and passive ROM for all extremities, (b) turning every 2 hours, (c) checking for Homan's sign to prevent thrombophebitis, (d) collaborating with physical therapy for rehabilitation, (e) assisting the client with activities of daily living as he improves—using the unaffected side for bathing, dressing, and eating, (f) instructing him to dress the affected extremities first, (g) collaborating with occupational therapy in use of assistive devices (special eating and dressing devices).**

   - ***Expressive aphasia*—is a motor speech problem in which the patient can understand what is being said, but can only respond in short phrases. Nursing goals for impaired communication are to meet his communication needs during all phases of care. Interventions would include: (a) accepting client's anger and frustration, (b) trying alternative methods of communication (writing on tablets, picture boards), (c) approaching and treating him as an adult, (d) not assuming he is hard of hearing, (e) allowing him time to respond, (f) being honest when you don't understand.**

   - ***Homonymous hemianopia*—loss of the same half of the visual field in each eye. Nursing care would involve teaching the client to scan his environment, and approach him and place objects within his field of vision.**

4. How should the nurse prepare John and his wife now for the CT scan and later for the angiogram?

   Both of these tests reveal the extent and specificity of the CVA. In both tests a consent form will need to be signed, an IV will be started, and dye may be used. The nurse must assess for any history of allergy to seafood (shell fish) or iodine as the dye used in these tests is iodine based. When the dye is injected, John may feel a warm sensation and have a metallic taste in his mouth. In the CT scan the patient's head will be positioned in a cradle and strapped across the forehead to keep his head immobilized. A CT scanner will revolve around the head, making a loud clicking noise. The CT test is painless and lasts 30–90 minutes. Someone will always be with them during the test. With the angiogram, the dye is inserted into a vessel in the arm or the femoral area. After this test the nurse will inspect the dressing at the insertion site and will monitor vital signs and radial/pedal pulses frequently.

John has had all of his tests completed. He has a blockage of the middle cerebral artery. He is started on Mannitol, Heparin, Dilantin, and Decadron.

Focus Questions

1. What are the nursing diagnoses for John?

   - **Altered cerebral tissue perfusion related to vessel occlusion.**
   - **Ineffective airway clearance related to the loss of cough reflex, loss of gag reflex, and cognitive impairment.**
   - **High risk for injury related to increased intercranial pressure (ICP).**
   - **Altered thought processes related to tissue injury or inflammation.**
   - **Ineffective breathing pattern related to damage or inflammation of respiratory centers of the brain.**

- **Altered nutrition: less than body requirements related to insufficient intake.**
- **Impaired physical ability related to paralysis or weakness.**
- **Anxiety related to actual risk to health status.**
- **Hopelessness related to deteriorating neurologic and physical functioning.**
- **Self-care deficit related to muscle weakness or paralysis.**
- **Ineffective family coping related to knowledge deficit or losses.**

2. What are the rationales for each of John's medications?

   Mannitol **is an osmotic diuretic used to take excessive fluid from the brain because of increased intracranial pressure.** ***Heparin*** **is an anticoagulant used to prevent extension of an existing blood clot and formation of new clots.** ***Dilantin*** **is an anticonvulsant drug used to prevent seizure because of irritation of brain from increased intracranial pressure.** ***Decadron*** **is used to decrease intracranial pressure by reducing inflammation.**

Day of discharge. Medications for discharge include: Dilantin 300 mg qd, Vasotec 10 mg qd, Ticlid 250 mg bid po, and Tylenol gr.X q4h prn for headache. Continue PT/OT 3x/week. His wife seems overwhelmed with the thought of taking John home. She is especially concerned about his dysphagia.

Focus Questions

1. How would the nurse explain the medications to John and his wife at discharge?

   Dilantin **prevents John from developing a seizure.** ***Vasotec*** **helps control his high blood pressure.** ***Ticlid*** **prevents the development of further strokes by preventing clot formation.** ***Tylenol*** **is an analgesic and anti-inflammatory drug for pain relief and reduction of fever. John should not take aspirin in conjunction with the Ticlid.**

2. What is dysphagia? Explain interventions the wife could use to help with his eating.

   Dysphagia means the patient has difficulty swallowing. Patients should not be overtired before eating; plan activities so that he has at least 30 minutes rest before eating. Place him in high Fowler's position. Stay with him during eating if aspiration has been an issue. Allow him twice as long to eat. Serve foods at room temperature. Semi-solid foods are tolerated best. Foods such as casseroles, custards, strained fruits and vegetables, and cooked cereals are moist enough not to crumble and dry enough not to form a bolus. Yogurt and cottage cheese are well tolerated. Avoid dry foods such as crackers or toast. Make sure he is placing food on unaffected side and be sure he clears his mouth after every bite. Avoid use of straws. Have suction at the bedside. (Gauwitz, 1995).

3. As a coordinator of care, how might the nurse plan for John's discharge?

   The need for discharge planning starts with the admission of the patient. Will he go to a rehabilitation center or straight home? How can he manage at home? What help is available to him in the home setting? What will be the expected outcome of rehab as far as mobility is concerned? It is important that someone make a home visit to evaluate the home and the needs of the patient (condition of the residence, i.e., will steps be involved in getting to the house? Is there a bedroom on the first floor? etc.). Prepare the patient and family while in the hospital by teaching medications and the use and side effects of each. Have the family involved with the various therapies and care of the patient. Have the family discuss with the dietitian what dietary needs may be involved with this patient and how to get adequate supplements if the patient is having difficulty with eating. If the home is not conducive to the patient returning there immediately, it may be necessary to collaborate with the social worker to have the patient have

more extensive rehabilitation. You may have to look at the financial capabilities of the family. Options you may offer to the wife would be seeking home care with home health aides or respite care to ease her responsibility.

Reflective Writing

Describe how you would feel if the person having the stroke were related to you.

This case has presented a catastrophic change to a family and causes many sudden role changes in all family members. It is important that the nurse takes the time to listen to all family members as each will see the problem differently. John may also have difficulty following the stroke with powerlessness related to the loss of mobility, social isolation, and self-esteem disturbances. The nurse should care for both John and his other family members.

References

Gauwitz, D. (1995). How to protect the dysphagic stroke patient. *American Journal of Nursing*, 95(8), 34–38.

Hayn, M. A. & Fisher, T. R. (1997). Stroke rehabilitation: Salvaging ability after the storm. *Nursing* 97. 27(3), 40–48.

Lemone, P. & Burke, K. (2000). *Medical surgical nursing: Critical thinking in client care.* 2nd edition. Upper Saddle River, N.J.: Prentice Hall.

Mower, D. M. (1997). Brain attack: Treating acute ischemic CVA, *Nursing 97*, 27(3), 34–39.

Sommers, M. S. (1994). *Concepts and Activities Medical-Surgical Nursing*. Springhouse, P.: Springhouse Publications.

CASE #3 GEORGE JONES

Learning Objectives

1. Assess data from several sources regarding Mr. Jones and his health needs.
2. Identify the pathophysiology of Parkinson's disease and hip fracture, and plan appropriate nursing interventions.
3. Individualize pre- and postoperative teaching for elderly clients.
4. Provide discharge planning for clients.

Mr. George Jones is a 78-year-old man with Parkinson's disease. Following a fall at home, he was admitted to the hospital with an intertrochanteric fracture of the right hip. Yesterday he had a internal fixation with a Jewett nail, and today is his first postoperative day.

Focus Questions

1. What assessment data would the nurse want to collect from the chart and the client?

   Assessment data: **age, family, religion, living arrangement. Who lives with him? Health history, cause of fracture, medication he has been taking; past level of activity, hobbies/how he uses time; how much pain, what pain medication and how often is he getting it; how leg is immobilized, fracture bedpan being used or not.**

2. What teaching should be done preoperatively and postoperatively for the client? How would the nurse individualize care for an elderly client?

   - ***Preoperative:*** **Explain what will happen in surgery and how he will feel on return from surgery; teach coughing and deep breathing; explain turning; explain pain medication and how it will be administered.**

- *Postoperative:* **Check to be sure patient still understands what was taught pre-operatively and that patient understands how to use patient controlled analgesia (PCA) and passive and active range of motion**
- *Individualized teaching for elderly clients:* **Nurse should speak up so as to be easily heard, not talk too fast, check that hearing aid is in place and turned on if client uses one, look at client when talking with him, not teach too much at one time (as client may tire), be sure if written instructions are provided, that they are in large print so he can easily read them.**

3. List nursing diagnoses for Mr. Jones.

Nursing diagnoses

- **pain related to surgical incision**
- **high risk for altered respiratory function related to anesthesia, immobility, and Parkinson's disease**
- **high risk for infection related to surgical incision**
- **fluid volume deficit related to decreased fluid intake preoperatively**
- **impaired mobility related to surgical pain, procedure, and Parkinson's disease**
- **altered bowel elimination related to Parkinson's disease**
- **bathing/grooming/dressing self-care deficit related to surgery and Parkinson's disease**

  (Faculty may want students to prioritize diagnoses.)

Postop day 3. The physical therapist has been working with Mr. Jones. The therapist has shown Mr. Jones some exercises and has ambulated him with the use of a walker. The therapist notes that Mr. Jones has the form of Parkinson's disease in which rigidity is the primary symptom. Mr. Jones' physician decides that another drug might aid Mr. Jones, so he orders Tasmar 100 mg tid, and reduces the Sinemet 25/100 to tid.

Focus Questions

1. What are the major symptoms of Parkinson's disease (PD)?

   Major symptoms of Parkinson's disease: tremors (involuntary shaking of extremities), rigidity (stiffness of muscles to movement), bradykinesia or akinesia (slowness or an absence of movement of muscles); others—impaired vision, dementia, soft voice, hand writing very small, drooling, stooped posture.

2. How may Parkinson's disease (PD) affect recovery from a hip fracture?

   PD may cause stiffness of movement, difficulty starting movement, tremor, difficulty in using walker, difficulty maintaining balance because of rigidity and tremor, possible difficulty in doing two tasks at same time, need sufficient time to carry out tasks, others may have difficulty understanding patient, constipation, fear of falling especially if a fall was the cause of the hip fracture.

3. What kinds of drugs are Tasmar and Sinemet, and what teaching should the nurse provide about these drugs?

Sinemet and Tasmar

Sinemet 25/100 **is a combination of Carbidopa 25 mg. and Levodopa 100 mg. Carbidopa decreases effect of Levodopa in peripheral area of body but not in the brain where it is**

converted to dopamine. Dopamine is the chemical that is decreased in the brain and the cause of Parkinson's disease. Possible side effects are: dyskinesia, muscle and eyelid twitching, orthostatic hypotension, agitation, hallucinations, nausea and vomiting, anorexia, blurred vision, diplopia.

Tasmar is a catechol-o-methyltransferase (COMT) inhibitor. COMT drugs are used as adjunct therapy for Sinemet. COMT drugs enhance the effect of levodopa/carbidopa therapy by blocking the enzyme that breaks down levodopa before levodopa can reach the brain. Side effects include orthostatic hypotension, dyskinesia, nausea, sleep disorders, diarrhea, excessive dreaming, muscle cramps, confusion.

Teach family that Sinemet supplies the chemical to the brain that is in short supply in Parkinson's disease, and Tasmar enhances the effect of Sinement. When taking Tasmar the patient usually requires less Sinemet. The side effects of both drugs are similar to the effect of Parkinson's disease, thus an increase in Parkinson's disease symptoms should be reported to the physcian. Also muscle and eyelid twitching is a sign of too much medicine and should be reported to the doctor. The patient should be told to come to a standing position slowly. Other possible symptoms to report to the physician would be vomiting, diarrhea that does not stop in a few days, and sleep problems.

Postop day 10. Mr. Jones is ready for discharge. He has spent the last 7 days on the long-term care unit of the hospital. While he was in the long-term care unit, he received physical and occupational therapy. He has developed his skill at walking with a walker and dressing himself. Mrs. Jones expresses some anxiety as to whether he is ready to go home and how they will manage.

Focus Questions

1. What does the nurse need to know about their home situation?

   Home situation: Assess the home: Are the bedroom, living room, and bathroom all on one floor? How many steps will the patient have to be able to climb to get to the bathroom/bedroom/house? Do the toilets have a raised seat? Are there bars around the toilet to aid the patient in getting up and down? How does the patient take a shower/bath? Are there bars around shower? If patient takes a bath, is there a bathtub seat for use now? Are there throw rugs in the house? Is it easy to get around in the house or is there a lot of clutter?

2. What discharge teaching do Mr. and Mrs. Jones need?

   Teaching for discharge: May need social services to assist client's family to obtain equipment, should get a raised toilet seat with handles, need handles or bars in tub or shower, rails on outside steps or a ramp, no throw rugs in the house, clear pathways throughout the house, need bedroom/toilet/living area on one level, teach and help patient return to demonstration of dressing self, wife needs to be taught how to assist client to do as much for self as possible, wife needs to be taught how to assist client in walking and bathing and exercises for hip strengthening, review information on drugs client is to take.

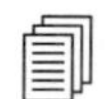

Reflective Writing

Mrs. Jones tells you that she often feels overwhelmed at the prognosis for Parkinson's disease and fears for their future. How do you feel about this comment and what would you do?

Assess what is making Mrs. Jones feel overwhelmed, and help to find solutions for this. Recommend that she contact local Parkinson's Disease Association (give her address and phone number), and encourage Mr. and Mrs. Jones to attend the Parkinson's disease support group.

References

Baker, S.; Grant, A. & Hudnicki, D. (1998). Parkinson's disease: A holistic approach. *American Journal of Nursing*, 98 (11), 48A–48H.

Carpenito, L. J. (1993). *Nursing diagnosis application to clinical practice.* (5th ed.) Philadelphia: J. B. Lippincott.

Chenitz, W. C., Stone J. T., & Salisburg, C. S. (eds.). (1991). *Clinical gerontological nursing.* Philadelphia: W. B. Saunders.

Ignatavicius, D. D., Workman, M. L., & Mishler, M. A. (1995). *Medical-surgical nursing.* Philadelphia: W. B. Saunders.

Spratto, G. R. & Woods, A. L. (1998). *Delmar's A–Z nurses drug reference—98.* Albany: Delmar.

CASE #4 WILLIAM MILLER

Learning Objectives

1. Apply assessment data and risk factors to the pathophysiology of a myocardial infarction (MI).
2. Plan nursing care to help prevent complications of an MI.
3. Apply the principles of pain management to a client with an MI.
4. Develop plans for discharge instructions.

Day 1, 0200. William Miller is a 51-year-old African American male admitted to the Coronary Care Unit for a Rule Out myocardial infarction (MI). William presented in the ER at 2400 with severe substernal chest pain radiating to the back, neck, and down the left arm. He received $MS0_4$ 4 mg IV at 2430, 2440, and 0100. He now reports his pain level as a 5/10, down from a 10/10 before pain medication. Admission interview notes a positive family history of cardiovascular disease with his mother dying of a stroke at age 62 and his father dying of a heart attack at age 58. He also has a history of hypertension, which has been effectively treated with Vasotec for the past 5 years. V.S. 158/90, P 100, R 24, temperature 99.8° oral. Height 5 ft. 8 in. weight 244 lbs. Cardiac monitor shows sinus tachycardia with occasional PVC. Cardiac enzymes were drawn in ER, and a 12 lead ECG was obtained. An automobile accident 8 days ago in which the client sustained a head injury eliminated him as a candidate for thrombolytic therapy.

Focus Questions

1. This client is presenting with what risk factors for an MI? What other assessment data must the nurse collect related to cardiovascular disease? What is the significance of his weight based on the updated 1998 weight recommendations?

   Coronary Heart Disease (CHD) is higher in men than in women. Risk of CHD increases with age. This client presents with a family history of heart disease, which is also a risk factor. High blood pressure is known to predispose an individual to the risk of developing CHD, and hypertension is higher in African Americans than Caucasians. His weight for his height also is a risk factor and points to the fact he probably leads a sedentary lifestyle. Lack of exercise has been noted as a risk factor for developing heart disease. Additional assessment data would include obtaining a thorough history that would investigate other risk factors for the development of CHD. Cigarette smoking, stress, history of hyperlipidemia, and diabetes mellitus have all been linked to the development of heart disease. Obtaining a history regarding the chest pain including onset, intensity, duration, and radiation would be important. According to the 1998 weight recommendations, at 5 ft. 8 in. and 244 lbs. he is considered significantly overweight.

2. What complications must the nurse prepare for when a client presents with a suspected MI?

   - **Dysrhythmias: Approximately 80% of individuals develop dysrhythmias after an MI because of the myocardial cells sensitivity to nerve impulses due to ischemia, electrolyte imbalances, and stimulation of the sympathetic nervous system. The heart rate can be increased, decreased or develop irregular beats. Lethal dysrhythmias (ventricular tachycardia or ventricular fibrillation) most often occur within the first 4 hours after the onset of pain. All clients with a suspected MI are closely monitored for the development of dysrhythmias.**
   - **Extension of the infarction: A client who has recurrent chest pain, ECG changes, and deterioration of condition may be experiencing an extension of the ischemia to the myocardium leading to further heart damage.**
   - **Heart Failure: A myocardial infarction results in some damage to the left ventricle. The larger the damaged area, the greater the risk the pumping action of the heart will be compromised.**
   - **Cardiogenic Shock: When the damage to the left ventricle is severe, the pumping action of the heart may be inadequate to meet the circulatory needs of the body. A state of circulatory failure develops. Cardiogenic shock has a high mortality rate.**
   - **Pericarditis: Inflammation of the pericardium can develop in 2–3 days after an MI. This can be a common complication causing cardiac compression and chest pain. Often a friction rub can be auscultated over the pericardium.**
   - **Ventricular aneurysm: The infarcted area of the myocardium may become thin and can bulge out during contractions. A ventricular aneurysm can cause congestive heart failure, dysrhythmias, angina, or ventricular rupture. Surgical excision of the aneurysm is necessary.**
   - **Thromboembolism: The dysrhythmias, congestive heart failure (CHF), and inactivity that can occur after an MI can place an individual at an increase risk for developing blood clots or a pulmonary embolism. Anticoagulants are often administered to prevent this occurrence.**
   - **Papillary muscle dysfunction: If the infarcted area of the myocardium is close to the papillary muscles, mitral regurgitation can occur. Mitral valve replacement may be necessary.**
   - **Dressler syndrome: Also called "Post MI Syndrome," Dressler's syndrome can develop 1–4 weeks after an MI and is characterized by pericarditis with effusion and fever. Corticosteroids are usually used to treat this condition.**

3. Discuss pain management in a client with chest pain. What nursing interventions should be initiated to control and prevent chest pain?

   It is essential that pain is managed promptly in an acute myocardial infarction since anxiety will increase oxygen consumption, which can cause further myocardial damage. Pain medication (usually Morphine Sulfate) is given via the IV route so it is readily assimilated. Morphine reduces pain, anxiety, and myocardial oxygen consumption, and it lowers the BP and the pulse. Re-medicate as allowed as long as vital signs remain stable. Intravenous nitroglycerin is often ordered for the management of chest pain. The infusion is started slowly, and vital signs, particularly BP, are monitored carefully. Infusion is titrated to control chest pain.

   Oxygen is generally administered via nasal cannula, which can help lessen chest pain by assuring the myocardium is adequately oxygenated. Elevating the head of the bed can foster adequate respiration. Activity is limited to decrease the need for increased cardiac output and increased oxygen consumption. Clear explanations with a calm, quiet environment can help limit client's anxiety, reducing oxygen consumption.

Day 2, 2000. William's ECG shows ST elevation, T inversion, and pathophysiologic Q wave in leads II and III and aVf consistent with an inferior wall MI. Cardiac enzymes CK, LDH, and AST are all elevated. CKMB bands elevated over 5%. Earlier in the day, William's occasional PVC's increased to over 10/min with occasional coupling noted. Lidocaine 100 mg bolus was given as well as a Lidocaine drip of 500 cc D5W with 2 gms. Lidocaine is now infusing at 2 mg/min. Monitor currently shows no further coupling and only an occasional PVC. Chest pain has continued to be a significant problem requiring MSO_4 4 mg q hour. William's O_2 has been increased to 4 L per min per cannula. An IV drip of Nitroglycerin (NTG) has been started and titrated to control chest pain.

Focus Questions

1. What are the risks to William related to his dysrhythmia? How does Lidocaine control PVCs? Discuss the possible adverse effects of Lidocaine and identify how the nurse can help prevent these adverse problems.

   Myocardial ischemia leads to an irritable myocardium, predisposing the client to abnormal beats and rhythms. Premature ventricular contractions (PVCs) are the most frequent arrhythmia seen after an MI. PVCs may proceed ventricular tachycardia or ventricular fibrillation, both of which can be fatal. Early treatment of PVCs that occur greater than 5 per minute or in groups of two (coupling) or more is essential.

   Lidocaine is the treatment of choice for PVCs as it controls PVCs by stabilizing the cardiac membrane and decreasing cardiac automaticity. Adverse effects can include confusion, convulsions, blurred vision, nausea, vomiting, hypotension, bradycardia, heart block, arrest, dyspnea, and respiratory depression.

   The nurse can help prevent these adverse side effects by carefully monitoring the Lidocaine infusion and placing the infusion on a pump to minimize the risk of overdose. Continuous cardiac monitoring is necessary to determine if the PR or QRS intervals are increasing. If these develop it can signal increasing heart block, which warrants decreasing the rate or discontinuing the Lidocaine. Monitor VS frequently for any changes in BP, pulse, or respirations. Assess for any central nervous system effects such as confusion or dizziness. When PVCs diminish or are no longer present, the infusion is gradually titrated off.

2. What can William's continued chest pain signify? What role does oxygen therapy and NTG IV play in pain control with MI clients?

   Continued chest pain may mean ongoing myocardial ischemia and the risk for further myocardial damage. Both oxygen therapy and NTG help control chest pain by assuring adequate oxygenation to the myocardium. Oxygen therapy increases oxygenation of the myocardium and prevents further tissue ischemia. NTG enhances collateral blood flow, causes dilation of the coronary arteries, and redistributes blood flow toward the subendocardium, all of which improves oxygenation.

William has had an uncomplicated course after his pain was controlled and no further dysrhythmias noted. He is to be discharged to home with cardiac rehabilitation follow-up.

Day of discharge:	**Discharge instructions include:**
Diet:	***2 gm Na, low fat, low cholesterol**
Activity:	***may walk up 1 flight of stairs**
	***no lifting, carrying, and pushing heavy objects**
	***begin cardiac outpatient Rehab Program tomorrow**

Appointment:	***Schedule Dr. appointment for 1 week**
Meds:	***Vasotec 5 mg qd**
	***ASA 5 gr qd**
	***Colace 100 mg qd**

William's wife pulls you aside after you have discussed these instructions and nervously inquires when they can resume sexual relations.

Focus Questions

1. How can the nurse assess if William and his wife understand the discharge instructions?

   They understand if: William and his wife are able to identify cardiac risk factors and can relate the discharge instructions to these risk factors. William and his wife can answer questions regarding the disease process and explain rationale for treatment. Both can explain what foods are included and which foods should be avoided on a low Na, low fat, and low cholesterol diet. Both can explain the purpose of each drug, their side effects, and what should be reported to the physician.

2. How can the nurse investigate if any other supportive services are necessary to follow through on these instructions?

   The nurse should ask specifically if Mr. or Mrs. Miller has any concerns about their ability to follow through on the instructions. Are there any financial concerns or knowledge deficits that could prevent follow through? Investigate how many flights of stairs are in their home. Where is the location of the bedroom? What arrangements have they made to get to the outpatient rehab program? Both the client and the wife should confirm that they understand the discharge instructions and intend to comply with the treatment regime.

3. What are the standard teaching instructions regarding sexual relations for a client recovering from an MI?

   The environment should be comfortable with a familiar partner. Use positions of comfort that cause less strain on the recovering cardiac client. The cardiac client should be well rested. Avoid environmental extremes such as rooms too cold or too hot. Avoid intercourse after a heavy meal, should wait 3–4 hours after meal. Client should avoid holding breath during intercourse since this can trigger the valsalva maneuver causing hypotension and reflex tachcardia leading to angina. Anal intercourse can induce a vasovagal response and should be avoided. Prophylactic use of NTG may be encouraged prior to sexual activity to prevent angina. The following should be reported: rapid heart beat and respirations lasting more than 15 minutes after activity, chest pain during or after intercourse, and extreme fatigue the next day.

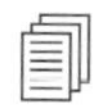

Reflective Writing

Sometimes it is necessary for the nurse to discuss intimate and personal matters such as sexual relations with a client and family. How comfortable are you in discussing such matters? Do you feel such discussions should be part of the nurse's role? How can you improve your comfort level with this topic?

Students can often decrease their anxiety regarding this topic by practicing interview skills on each other. Practicing ways to pose questions and explaining topics to each other can help in the development of some comfort level with this subject matter. It is important students learn to use words clients would understand and not be emb

rassed by the client's words. Both the client and the nurse will feel more comfortable in discussing sexual issues if they begin discussing less sensitive issues first. Once a trusting relationship has been established, the client will feel free to question the nurse as needed. It is important all clients and significant others are given an opportunity to have their questions about sexual issues answered.

References

Gerard, P. & Ringel, K. A. (1997). Nursing care of clients with disorders of cardiac function. In J. M. Black & E. Matassarin-Jacobs (eds.). *Medical-surgical nursing: Clinical management for continuity of care* (5th ed.) 1258–1270. Philadelphia: W. B. Saunders.

Griego, L. & House-Fancher, M. A. (1996). Nursing role in management: Coronary artery disease. In S. M. Lewis, I. C. Collier, & M. M. Heitkemper (Eds.). *Medical-surgical nursing: Assessment and management of clinical problems* (4th ed.) 907–929. St. Louis: Mosby.

Lemone, P. & Burke, K. M. (2000). *Medical surgical nursing: Critical thinking in client care.* (2nd ed.) 1030–1170. Upper Saddle River, NJ: Prentice Hall.

Mavroukakis, S.A. & Stine, A. (1998). Nursing management of adults with disorders of the coronary arteries, myocardium, or pericardium. In P. G. Beare & J. L. Myers (Eds.). *Adult Health Nursing* (3rd ed.) 579–597. St. Louis: Mosby.

CASE #5 JIM LAWSON

Learning Objectives

1. Apply assessment findings to the pathophysiology of chronic obstructive pulmonary disease (COPD).
2. Develop a teaching plan for a COPD client.
3. Recognize the complications that could develop from COPD.
4. Plan interventions to prevent or minimize the complications of COPD.

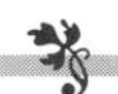

Day 1, 1330. Jim Lawson is a 64-year-old Caucasian male admitted to the hospital medical floor for a respiratory infection. Jim, a 2-pack-a-day smoker, has a history of chronic obstructive pulmonary disease (COPD). He awakened in the morning with increased shortness of breath and coughing with the production of green-brown sputum. Vital signs are BP 144/88, P 94, R 30, temperature 100.2° orally. Physician's orders include: ABG's stat, sputum for C & S then begin Ampicillin 500 mg IV q 6 hours, IV D_5W 100cc/hour, Theo Dur 1 bid, Albuterol 3 mg per nebulizer qid and prn acute dyspnea, O_2 1.5L/min.

Focus Questions

1. Relate this clinical data to the diagnosis of COPD. What other symptoms would the nurse expect the client to exhibit?

   Chronic obstructive pulmonary disease (COPD) includes any condition characterized by chronic obstruction to airflow during expiration. This leads to difficulty in emptying the lungs resulting in an increase in residual lung volume and air trapping. Jim has several risk factors for COPD. History of smoking is one of the leading risk factors. Men have an increased risk. Age is also a risk factor due to the decline in respiratory quality that occurs in normal aging. Increased exposure to causative agents as one ages has also been linked to the development of COPD as well as repeated respiratory infections. Mortality rates from COPD are higher in whites than nonwhites. Jim's presenting symptoms of SOB, coughing, and respiratory rate of 30 are consistent with the diagnosis of COPD.

Respiratory muscles become less efficient with the hyperinflation of the lungs. Jim's temperature elevation and productive green-brown sputum along with worsening SOB are all symptoms of a pulmonary infection. However, not all COPD clients will have a temperature elevation. Additional assessment data needed by the nurse includes a thorough history to determine when symptoms worsened. Activity intolerance and weight loss would point to a worsening of condition and has been linked to increased morbidity and mortality with COPD clients. Physical exam should include observation of the use of accessory muscles in breathing. Increased anterior posterior diameter of the chest is common in COPD because of the chronic air trapping. Color may be cyanotic due to poor gas exchange. Auscultation of the chest often reveals distant heart sounds with diminished breath sounds due to the air trapping. Crackles and other adventitious breath sounds are not uncommon, especially during an infection or productive sputum. Finger clubbing may be noted and results from conditions causing long term hypoxemia.

2. What are the benefits and risks of O_2 therapy in a client with COPD? Why was the O_2 therapy limited to 1.5 L/min?

   Over time, changes in the lungs of COPD clients leads to hypercapnea and respiratory acidosis. Normally the chemoreceptors in the medulla respond to hypercapnea by stimulating an increase in respiratory rate to help remove the excess CO_2. As COPD progresses the chemoreceptor response may diminish. In COPD clients, hypoxemia becomes the primary drive for breathing, not hypercapnea. This is referred to as the "hypoxic drive." Oxygen helps relieve shortness of breath and hypoxemia in COPD clients but must be used with caution. Low flow rates of 1–2 L/min. are recommended. Higher flow rates can depress the "hypoxic drive," which is the COPD client's only stimulus to breath.

3. What should be included in a teaching plan for a client with COPD?

   A teaching plan should include: Avoid smoke and other airway irritants. Avoid exposure to pollutants: occupational, household, and community. Avoid exposure to respiratory tract infections and receive annual flu vaccine. Avoid extremes in temperature and humidity especially hot/humid and cold/dry. Encourage fluid intake 2–3L/day, smaller, more frequent meals tolerated better. Report any increase in size of feet or ankles to physician (may indicate right-side heart failure). Avoid high altitudes because of their low oxygen levels. Teach about any home therapies needed, i.e., chest physiotherapy, oxygen therapy, nebulizers, medication, breathing exercises, relaxation exercises, dyspneic positions, etc.

Day 1, 2300. Jim puts on his call light in an acute episode of dyspnea. He is breathing rapidly and shallowly at 40/min. His color is dusky with circumoral cyanosis. He is frightened and diaphoretic, sitting upright in bed. You call for a stat nebulizer with Albuterol as you assist Jim to an orthopneic position.

Focus Questions

1. Describe positions a dyspneic client should assume to reduce the workload of breathing while standing, sitting, or in bed.

   - *Standing:* **A COPD client who becomes short of breath while walking should be taught to move to a wall. Client should rest against the wall with back and hips. Feet should be about 12 inches from the wall and shoulders should be relaxed and bent forward.**

   - *Sitting:* **Place pillows over a nightstand. Client should sit on the side of the bed and bend over the nightstand with arms folded resting on the pillows.**

If a person is sitting in a chair and does not have a nightstand, he should spread feet a shoulder width apart and lean forward with elbows resting on knees.

- ***In bed:*** **Assist client to a sitting position or raise head of bed. Using pillows and a nightstand, encourage client to bend over the nightstand with arms folded resting on the pillows.**

Each of these positions reduces the workload of breathing by removing the weight of the arms from the chest and allowing better chest expansion.

2. Describe the breathing exercises that should be included in Jim's teaching plan.

Pursed lip and diaphragmatic breathing techniques help reduce air trapping and minimizes fatigue. Clients should be taught and encouraged to practice these techniques so the client will automatically use these breathing techniques during episodes of dyspnea.

- ***Pursed lip breathing:*** **With mouth closed, inhale through the nose. Exhale slowly through pursed lips as if blowing out a candle. Exhalation should last twice as long as inhalation.**

- ***Diaphragmatic breathing:*** **Helps use the larger muscles of respiration to decrease the work of breathing. Have client place one hand on the chest and one on the abdomen. Encourage client to concentrate on pushing the hand on the abdomen outward during inhalation while keeping the chest hand still. Exhalation should be slow. The hand on the abdomen should move inward during exhalation and the chest hand should again remain still.**

3. What other actions should the nurse take with a client experiencing severe dyspnea?

A stat pulse oximeter reading would be necessary to determine the level of hypoxia. The nurse should assess the O_2 to make sure it is patent and set to the proper flow rate. Do not try to teach during an acute episode of dyspnea but reinforce any earlier teaching about breathing exercises and relaxation exercises. Client should be coached to begin pursed lip and abdominal breathing and practice whatever relaxation exercises that have been helpful in the past. Do not leave the client alone. A calm, confident manner from the nurse can help the client begin to gain control over his breathing. Sometimes it is helpful to allow a family member to help calm the client. The nurse needs to be prepared to notify the physician if the pulse oximeter reading is below the client's baseline or client remains unresponsive to these interventions.

4. How does nebulizer therapy assist a dyspneic client? Describe the actions of Albuterol. What are the possible complications of this treatment?

Nebulized medication is reduced to a fine spray that can be inhaled into a client's tracheobronchial tree. An advantage of this method of medication administration is that it is very fast acting with minimized systemic effects. Albuterol is a noncatecholamine bronchodilator. Albuterol relaxes bronchial smooth muscle, reduces airway resistance, and improves airflow. There are few complications of this treatment. Side effects of Albuterol include: tremors, insomnia, dizziness, headache, anxiety, restlessness, irritability, cardiac palpitations, tachycardia, angina, nausea, vomiting, and muscle cramps. A disadvantage of nebulizers is that the equipment unit can be a source of respiratory infection unless it is cleaned regularly.

Day 2, 0100. Jim's condition continues to deteriorate. He received little relief from the nebulizer therapy, dyspneic positions, or the nurse's coaching with his breathing exercises. The physician was notified, stat ABG's were ordered with the following results: pH 7.3, O_2 48, CO_2 55, HCO_3

30. The physician has asked the resident on call to intubate Jim and place him on a mechanical ventilator.

Focus Questions

1. Analyze these ABG's. What acid-base problem exists? Why are COPD clients at risk for this problem? What are the indicators in these ABG's that signify the need for intubation?

   These arterial blood gas results indicate Mr. Lawson is in respiratory acidosis. The pH of 7.3 = acidosis. The high CO_2 level of 55 points to the fact the problem is respiratory in nature. The HCO_3 is rising in an attempt to compensate for the acidotic state. COPD clients are at risk for respiratory acidosis due to the poor gas exchange that occurs in the damaged lungs.

   Indicators in the ABGs that signify the need for intubation: pH less than 7.35; $PaCO_2$ greater than 50; PaO_2 less than 50; all three of these indicators point to how poorly this client is exchanging gases. Without intervention, his pH and oxygen levels will continue to fall as his CO_2 rises.

2. What is the nurse's role in assisting with endotracheal intubation? What equipment must the nurse assemble?

   The nurse must be familiar with all emergency equipment and the crash cart. Most carts contain the supplies necessary for endotracheal intubation. Some hospital rooms routinely stock such supplies. It requires special training to perform endotracheal intubation. The nurse's role is usually to assist the physician by having all supplies assembled so the tube can be inserted quickly. The head of the bed in moved away from the wall and the head board removed so the physician has easy access to the client. Inserting an endotracheal tube may cause the client to vomit so it is necessary to have workable suction and tubing in the room. Oxygen equipment, tubing, and an ambubag are also needed. Other equipment includes: laryngoscope; endotracheal tube; stylet; 10 cc syringe; water-soluble lubricant, tape.

3. What are some of the possible complications of a mechanical ventilator? What are the risks of placing a COPD client on a ventilator?

   Complications of mechanical ventilation include: Pneumothorax because of the rupture of alveoli from high positive pressure. Increased intrathoracic pressure causing barotrauma to major vessels or organs in the thorax. This increased pressure may impede venous return leading to decreased cardiac output. The decreased venous return and blood pooling in the cerebral vessels can lead to increased intracranial pressure. The main risk of placing a client with COPD on a mechanical ventilator is that such individuals are often very difficult to eventually wean from the ventilator. COPD clients can become too accustomed to the mechanical support.

Reflective Writing

Jim's COPD developed, in part, because of his cigarette smoking of nearly 2 packs a day for 30 years. What if one of your nursing colleagues states, "It serves him right, he brought this on himself"? How do you feel about this comment? How would you respond to your colleague?

Regardless of one's personal attitude about smoking, it is important that nurses do not convey personal judgments to their clients. Even though the colleague said this to another nurse, her beliefs may well have been conveyed to the client as well. Remind your colleague that we know a lot more about the risks of smoking today than we did 30 years ago and we also understand the addictive qualities that have made it very difficult for some individuals to quit. Today, a smoker has many more intervention options to help them quit smoking. By remaining silent or agreeing you merely reinforce a judgmental stereotype and lose an opportunity to be a role model for caring and client advocacy.

References

Berry, J. K. & Larson, J. L. (1998). Nursing management of adults with lower airway disorders. In P. G. Beare & J. L. Myers (eds.). *Adult health nursing* (3rd ed.) 346–357. St. Louis: Mosby.

Cronin, S. N. (1997). Nursing care of clients with disorders of the lower airways and pulmonary vessels. In J. M. Black & E. Matassarin-Jacobs (Eds.). *Medical-surgical nursing: Clinical management for continuity of care* (5th ed.) 1111–1124. Philadelphia: W. B. Saunders.

Lemone, P. & Burke, K. M. (2000). *Medical surgical nursing: Critical thinking in client care* (2nd ed.) 1390–1505. Upper Saddle River, N.J.: Prentice Hall.

Weilitz, P.B. & Van Sciver, T. (1996). Nursing role in management of obstructive pulmonary diseases. In S. M. Lewis, I. C. Collier, & M. M. Heitkemper (Eds.). *Medical-surgical nursing: Assessment and management of clinical problems* (4th ed.) 706–729. St. Louis: Mosby.

CASE #6 MARY MARTIN

Learning Objectives

1. Relate cultural considerations with clients with End Stage Renal Disease (ESRD).
2. Plan and prioritize nursing care for ESRD.
3. Apply principles of fluid and electrolyte balance to clinical needs of renal clients.
4. Recognize and utilize resources for ESRD clients.

Day 1, 1000. Mary Martin a 62-year-old female of Native American decent is admitted to the hospital with increased fatigue, lethargy, and occasional confusion from chronic uremia secondary to End Stage Renal Disease (ESRD). Mary has a long history of diabetes mellitus resulting in permanent damage to her kidneys. Diagnostic tests ordered for Mary include: Renal scan and ultrasound, Hgb & Hct., BUN, serum creatinine, creatinine clearance, serum electrolytes, urinalysis, urine for C & S, fasting blood sugars, and fingerstick blood sugars AC & HS.

Focus Questions

1. Discuss the cultural/ethnic considerations of clients with ESRD. Which cultures have a higher incidence of ESRD?

   ESRD is more common among Native Americans and African Americans than among Caucasians. These groups also have a higher risk for hypertension and diabetes, which can lead to renal disease.

2. Identify the purpose of each diagnostic test ordered and why these tests would be needed with a diagnosis of ESRD.

   - **Renal Scan: Provides visualization of the urinary tract and can be used to detect infarctions, tumors, abscesses and other abnormalities in the kidneys.**
   - **Ultrasound: Determines the size of the kidneys. A reduction in size of the kidneys is often noted in chronic renal failure because of the destruction of the nephrons.**
   - **Hgb & Hct: Anemia is common in chronic renal failure because of decreased erythropoietin production by the kidneys leading to decreased erythropoiesis by the bone marrow.**
   - **BUN: Measures the amount of urea nitrogen in the blood. Urea is formed from protein metabolism and excreted exclusively by the kidneys. Blood levels of urea can be**

used to help determine the excretory function of the kidneys. Rising BUN levels can signal renal disease.

- Serum Creatinine: Creatinine is also excreted only by the kidneys and can be used as an indicator of kidney function. Elevated creatinine levels can indicate kidney disease. The BUN/creatinine levels are often reported as a ratio.
- Creatinine Clearance: This test is a measure of the glomerular filtration rate (the number of milliliters of filtrate made by kidneys per min). Both urine and serum creatinine levels are assessed, then the clearance rate is calculated. This requires a 24 hour urine specimen. A decrease in creatinine clearance is seen in renal disease.
- Serum Electrolytes: Blood levels of electrolytes help to determine if there is a balance between dietary intake and renal excretion of common electrolytes. Sodium, potassium, chloride, phosphorus, calcium, and carbon dioxide are common electrolytes evaluated. Elevation or deficit of these electrolytes can point to kidney dsyfunction.
- Urinalysis: This is a routine assessment test of the urine that notes appearance, color, odor; pH, and specific gravity measurements; presence of glucose, blood, protein, and ketones. Urine sediment is examined to detect casts, cells, crystals, and bacteria. Specific gravity may be decreased in a client with kidney dysfunction. Proteinuria and hematuria can also be sensitive indicators of kidney disease. An increase in casts can indicate renal problems, and bacteria in the urine indicates a urinary tract infection.
- Urine for C & S: A sterile urine specimen is collected and assessed for culture and sensitivity. A positive culture indicates an infection. The sensitivity will determine which antibiotics are effective against the organism. Repeated or severe urinary tract or kidney infections can lead to permanent kidney damage.
- Fasting blood sugars and fingersticks: Serum glucose is helpful in diagnosing and monitoring metabolic diseases particularly diabetes mellitus. A diagnosis of diabetes mellitus places an individual at increased risk over time for developing kidney disease.

3. Develop and prioritize five nursing diagnoses for Mary and three interventions for each diagnosis.

   a. Fluid volume excess related to inability of kidney to excrete fluid as manifested by edema. Nursing interventions:

      - Restrict fluid and sodium intake
      - Weigh daily
      - Teach about low sodium diets and ways to restrict fluids
      - Monitor intake and output
      - Provide skin care especially to edematous areas
      - Monitor blood pressure
      - Assess for worsening fluid volume excess; crackles in lungs, dyspnea, jugular vein distention, etc.

   b. Impaired skin integrity related to excess fluid as manifested by edema. Nursing interventions:

      - Monitor skin closely
      - Provide skin care especially to edematous areas
      - Apply ointments and creams for itching and dry skin
      - Keep nails trimmed to eliminate skin damage from scratching

c. **Altered thought processes related to effects of uremic toxins on the CNS as manifested by confusion. Nursing interventions:**
   - **Assess level of consciousness and mental status**
   - **Provide reassurance and explanations for the changing mental status**
   - **Keep periods of teaching brief and to the point**
   - **Provide a quiet, restful environment**

d. **Altered nutrition: less than body requirements, related to restricted intake of nutrients as manifested by loss of appetite. Nursing interventions:**
   - **Offer small, frequent meals**
   - **Provide oral hygiene**
   - **Involve the patient in planning and choosing food and fluid**
   - **Keep protein and phosphate within prescribed levels**
   - **Provide sugar-free hard candy or gum to help improve taste and decrease thirst**
   - **Encourage to suck on ice cubes to minimize thirst with little fluid**

e. **Activity intolerance related to anemia secondary to kidney disease as manifested by fatigue and lethargy. Nursing interventions:**
   - **Help patient plan activities to avoid fatigue**
   - **Assess patients tolerance to activities**
   - **Provide rest periods**
   - **Administer iron and erythropoietin as ordered**
   - **Monitor Hgb and Hct levels**

Day 3, 1100. Mary's renal status has continued to deteriorate. Creatinine clearance is 6 ml per minute and Mary is showing evidence of fluid intoxication despite conservative measures to restrict fluid. BP 160/96, weight has increased by 5 lbs. since admission, 2+ pitting edema noted in her ankles and feet, fine crackles are present bilaterally in bases of lungs on auscultation, jugular vein distention is evident. Mary's doctor has prepared her for the possibility of hemodialysis.

Focus Questions

1. What are included in conservative nursing measures to prevent fluid volume excess in clients with renal disease?

   Conservative management is attempted before maintenance on dialysis. The amount of fluids allowed depends on the client's daily urine output. Usually 500–600 ml in addition to the amount equal to the urine output is allowed. This allotment is spread throughout the 24-hour period to avoid thirst. Protein, sodium, potassium, and phosphate are also restricted.

2. Explain why Mary's symptoms may develop in a client with ESRD.

   As chronic renal failure progresses, it results in a systemic disease involving every body organ. Mary's symptoms are symptoms of fluid volume excess due to the kidney's inability to concentrate and excrete urine. This extra circulating fluid volume leads to increased BP, weight gain, edema, jugular vein distention, and fluid in the lungs.

3. Compare and contrast peritoneal dialysis and hemodialysis. What are the advantages and disadvantages of each?

   - **Dialysis is a technique in which substances move across a semipermeable membrane from the blood into a dialysis solution.**
   - **Dialysis is used to remove waste products and correct fluid and electrolyte imbalances.**
   - **In peritoneal dialysis (PD) the peritoneal membrane serves as the semipermeable membrane. A catheter is inserted through the anterior abdominal wall. The dialysis solution is infused into the peritoneum and remains in the peritoneum for approximately 30 minutes to several hours before it is drained out. Client's can perform PD at home. Usually at least four exchanges are required each day. Automated and manual PD systems are available. Advantages: PD is less complicated and requires less training than hemodialysis. PD is portable, has fewer dietary restrictions, and causes less cardiovascular stress. It is also a good dialysis method for individuals with poor vascular access. Disadvantages/complications include: risk of infection at the catheter site, peritonitis, abdominal pain, hernias, lower back pain, pulmonary complications, bleeding, lipid and carbohydrate abnormalities, and loss of ultrafiltration.**
   - **In hemodialysis a high blood flow is required. Vascular access for hemodialysis can be otained by an external cannula/shunt, internal arteriovenous fistula, or a looped graft in the forearm. Two needles are placed in the fistula or graft, arterial blood is removed from the client and sent to a dialyzer, which has a series of membranes through which the blood flows removing waste products. Blood is returned to the client via the venous line. Hemodialysis can be performed at home but is more complicated, and most clients choose to go to a community center for 3–4 hours 3 times a week. Advantages: Hemodialysis allows for rapid removal of fluids, lowers serum triglycerides, and is effective in the removal of potassium. Disadvantages/complications: Disequilibrium syndrome occurs because of the rapid change in the composition of the extracellular fluid. Other complications include hypotension, muscle cramps, loss of blood, hepatitis, and sepsis.**

Discharge day. Mary had an internal arteriovenous fistula surgically created two days ago. Mary will receive hemodialysis through a temporary access percutaneous cannula in her right subclavian until the fistula is ready for use. The nurse schedules Mary for hemodialysis at the outpatient dialysis center three times per week. She is scheduled for a doctor's appointment in one week at which time she will have serum electrolytes and a CBC drawn. The dietitian has met with Mary and instructed her on fluid, sodium, and potassium restriction and a low protein, 2,000 calorie diabetic diet. Mary lives alone on a fixed income. She expresses concern regarding her ability to get to the dialysis center three times per week and her financial capability to afford hemodialysis.

Focus Questions

1. Considering discharge planning, what other areas should the nurse investigate with Mary?

   Mary should understand she is at an increased risk for fractures related to alterations in absorption of calcium, excretion of phosphate, and altered vitamin D metabolism. Encourage activity that will help osteoblast activity. Fluid and nutrition restrictions may make her prone for constipation. Activity will help increase bowel peristalsis. Avoid over-the-counter laxatives since they can lead to hypermagnesemia. Make sure Mary understands she is at an increased risk for infection because of her renal disease and her recently created fistula. Advise her to avoid crowds and people with infections. Observe for any local

signs of infection at the fistula site, such as warmth, redness, swelling, soreness, or drainage. Report any fever or chills. Encourage good personal hygiene. Assess her understanding of the therapeutic regime. Does she understand the importance of frequent monitoring of blood levels, ongoing dialysis, dietary restrictions, keeping track of intake and output, weight, and BP? She should know to report a weight gain of more than 2 pounds, any shortness of breath, confusion, lethargy, and increasing fatigue or weakness. Assess her ability to cope with her disease and these restrictions. She lives alone, but what other support systems does she have, such as church, neighbors, or social groups?

2. What are some of the options the nurse might explore with Mary regarding transportation and financial resources?

   Provide information on community services available. Provide information on support groups. Provide the address and phone number of the National Kidney Foundation. Discuss the ESRD Medicare Program and refer Mary to the hospital social worker to help Mary with this and other financial and transportation information.

3. How has the ESRD Medicare Program assisted individuals with renal disease? How can the nurse help Mary access this resource?

   The incidence of ESRD has increased over the years. Dialysis is often the only viable treatment due to the lack of sufficient numbers of organ donors. Because of this program, almost every client with ESRD is offered dialysis, regardless of age. This program covers nearly 80% of the cost of dialysis once the client has been on dialysis approximately three months. The nurse's referral to the hospital social worker will ensure that all avenues of economic support will be investigated.

Reflective Writing

If Mary does not do well on hemodialysis, renal transplantation may be her only other option. Considering the scarcity of donor organs, Mary will be placed on a waiting list with many others. Recently, there has been public debate about donor organs being given to someone who may have damaged their organs through drug abuse or chronic alcoholism. How do you feel about this matter? What are some of the ethical issues that must be considered in such a debate?

Our national organ procurement system is set up to be neutral about the client except in the areas of biologic and psychologic that are relevant to the transplantation. No person on the list is more important than another. The current system assures only the best matched client will receive the transplant. Medical necessity, prognosis, and need are the standards for organ transplantation. There are many ethical issues involved if the health professional's opinion of the client's worth were to be taken into account. What would be the criteria set for transplantation and who would have the authority to decide? Blaming clients for their medical conditions is contrary to the professional detachment owed all clients. Any belief that the system of organ procurement is not fair could negatively impact the pool of available organs since organ donation is voluntary in this country.

References

Johnson-Brennan, K. C. (1998). Nursing management of adults with renal disorders. In P. G. Beare & J. L. Myers (Eds.). *Adult health nursing* (3rd ed.) 811–832. St. Louis: Mosby.

Lemone, P. & Burke, K. M. (2000). *Medical surgical nursing: Critical thinking in client care.* (2nd ed.) 948–1011. Upper Saddle River, N.J.: Prentice Hall.

Matassarin-Jacobs, E. (1997). Nursing care of clients with renal disorders. In J. M. Black & E. Matassarin-Jacobs (eds.). *Medical-surgical nursing: Clinical management of continuity of care* (5th ed.) 1258–1270. Philadelphia: W. B. Saunders.

McCarley, T. & Lewis, S. (1996). Nursing role in management: Acute and chronic renal failure. In S.M. Lewis, I. C. Collier, & M. M. Heitkemper (eds.). *Medical-surgical nursing: Assessment and management of clinical problems* (4th ed.) 1379–1409. St. Louis: Mosby.

Roark, D. (2000). Overhauling the organ donation system. *American Journal of Nursing, 100*(6), 45–48.

CASE #7 MARY BREWER

Learning Objectives

1. Differentiate between characteristics of benign versus malignant breast lumps.
2. List risk factors associated with breast cancer.
3. Discuss differences between diagnostic and screening mammograms.
4. Describe characteristics of tumors with a less aggressive metastatic potential.
5. Discuss side effects of chemotherapy (CMF).
6. Discuss appropriate nursing interventions for clients experiencing chemotherapy post-mastectomy.

Mary Brewer is a 36-year-old overweight white, married female who works as a receptionist in the dentist's office where you have an appointment. Knowing you are a nurse who works with cancer patients, Mary confides that she had found a small lump in the upper outer quadrant in her right breast. The lump is hard, moveable, and sore. She says no one in her family has had breast cancer.

Focus Question

1. What information suggests that the lump may be benign versus malignant?
   - **The greatest risk for breast cancer is being female.**
   - **Seventy percent of breast cancer occurs in women over 50 years old.**
   - **Obesity poses a slight increase in risk for breast cancer but usually more so for postmenopausal women.**
   - **The upper outer quadrant of the breast is the most frequent site for primary breast adenocarcinomas.**
   - **Benign breast lumps tend to be smooth, firm, moveable, may be painful, and may change characteristics with hormonal changes; malignant tumors more often are hard, irregular, may be fixed, and are usually not painful; however, any lump manually manipulated over time may become tender or sore.**
   - **Only 20% of women with breast cancer have a familial history of breast cancer.**
   - **Approximately 70% of women who are diagnosed with breast cancer have no known risk factors.**
   - **Most breast lumps (80%) are benign.**

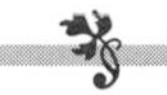

Since you know cancer cannot be diagnosed without further interventions, you recommend to Mary that she consult with her physician. Mary states she plans to go to the breast screening unit in the mall later that afternoon.

Focus Question

1. Why would you suggest that she needs a diagnostic mammogram and not a screening mammogram?

The screening mammogram is for the purpose of detecting a malignancy before there are any obvious signs or symptoms of a lesion. Diagnostic mammograms provide multiple views as needed and provides more specific details when a thickening or a lesion has been detected.

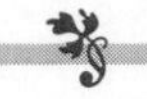

Mary is to be seen in the ambulatory oncology clinic in which you practice. She has had a right modified radical mastectomy for a Stage II infiltrating ductal adenocarcinoma. The lymph nodes were negative, but the tumor mass measured 3.0 cm. The tumor was determined to be estrogen receptor/progesterone receptor positive. The flow cytology revealed the cells were diploid and had a lower S-phase calculation. Histologically, the tumor was classified as a Grade I or as being well-differentiated.

Focus Question

1. There is no one parameter that is predictive of recurrence, but Mary has factors that indicate a less aggressive metastatic potential. What are they?
   - **Axillary lymph node—negative status;**
   - **No known metastasis (per Stage II definition);**
   - **Diploid (tumor cells with normal amount of DNA) vs. aneuploid (tumor cells with abnormal amount of DNA);**
   - **Lower S-phase calculation;**
   - **Well-differentiated cells (suggests less aggressive characteristic);**
   - **ER/PR positive status predicts a better response to hormone manipulation (by controlling the environment through additive or ablative therapy in reducing the amount of female hormones, any remaining clinically undetected malignant cells are less likely to be stimulated to proliferate).**

Mary is to begin adjuvant chemotherapy in a couple of weeks. She is to receive CMF (Cytoxan, Methotrexate, and 5-Fluorouracil). She has had a venous access port implanted.

Focus Question

1. What are the major side effects of CMF?

   Myelosuppression, gastrointestinal tract disturbances, hair loss, hemorrhagic cystitis

Mary had been divorced for four years and remarried eight months ago. She has a six- year-old son from her first marriage and had a spontaneous miscarriage three month ago. She is anxious and cries easily. When you ask what she fears the most, she answers, "My hair falling out."

Focus Question

1. What interventions/teaching may be appropriate?
   - **Use of therapeutic communication skills/listening.**
   - **Determine what coping mechanisms have worked for her in the past and how these strategies can be integrated in this situation.**
   - **Explain that (a) gradual thinning of hair over 6–8 months of treatments may occur and that hair begins to grow back within a month of ending therapy, (b) hair usually regrows approximately 1/4 inch/month, (c) a sample of hair can be cut from under-**

layers of hair before chemotherapy begins so that the color of the wig can be better matched to her own color of hair if needed, (d) shopping for a wig prior to chemotherapy better enables selection of a wig more comparable with her own hair and style (although she may not want to purchase the wig until one is actually needed since not all patients experience significant hair loss).

- **Refer to "Look Good . . . Feel Better," an American Cancer Society program to address ways of maintaining grooming and appearance while undergoing treatments for cancer.**
- **Explore need for fertility counseling since chemotherapy, especially alkylating agents of which Cytoxan is one, can cause ovarian failure, irregular menses, hot flashes, and night sweats.**
- **Arrange social service consult to identify and intercede in evolving psycho-social needs of this new family in medical crisis.**
- **Refer to appropriate support services such as community mastectomy hydrotherapy exercise program, "I Can Cope," and other support groups.**
- ***Teaching needs include:* (a) How chemotherapy works; (b) schedule for treatments and what to expect when she comes to the clinic; (c) specific side effects of CMF to report, e.g., symptoms of bladder infection (Cytoxan can cause hemorrhagic cystitis; teach to take oral doses in the morning, to drink 1–2 liters fluids every day, and to void every 1–2 hours), dry or sore places in the mouth (possible precursors to stomatitis), importance of follow-up labs to detect leukopenia and other abnormal labs related to chemotherapy treatment; (d) side effects that will be reported to Mary by health care providers, e.g., leukopenia (so she can know to avoid crowds especially at that time, how to recognize signs and symptoms of occult infection, and to receive colony stimulating factors if ordered); (e) possible ovarian failure, irregular menses, hot flashes and night sweats, and implications for family planning; (f) teach client or appropriate other to flush port or schedule for flushing port as recommended by manufacturer or policy (usually flush every 4–6 weeks when not being used); (g) review precautions to be taken with right upper extremity as result of axillary node dissection re: localized immunosuppression and impaired lymphatic drainage leading to lymphedema; (h) need for dental exam with repair of any dental caries and maintenance of oral health prior to initiation of chemotherapy; (i) nutrition needs during treatment, e.g., maintaining nourishment when alteration of appetite and/or ability to eat occurs, controlling amount of weight gain associated with chemotherapy.**

Reflective Writing

Why do you think women avoid self-breast examination, gynecological visits, and mammograms despite the widespread media coverage of the benefits of early detection and cure?

In responding to this question, students could bring out theory related to the health belief model, discussing components such as perceived susceptibility and seriousness of the disease. Students might also discuss coping strategies of denial, locus of control, and developmental issues related to risk taking, as well as psychological defense mechanisms such as rationalization.

References

Corbett, J. V. (1996). *Laboratory tests & diagnostic procedures with nursing diagnoses* (4th ed.). Stamford, Conn.: Appleton & Lange.

Groenwald, S.L., Frogge, M. H., Goodman, M., & Yarbro, C. H. (1998). *Comprehensive cancer nursing review* (4th ed.). Boston: Jones and Bartlett Publishers.

Hoskins, C. & Haber, J. (2000). Adjusting to breast cancer. *American Journal of Nursing. 100*(4), 26–31.

Itano, J. K. & Taoka, K. N. (1998). *Core curriculum for oncology nursing* (3rd ed.). Philadelphia: W. B. Saunders Company.

Kuhn, M. (1998). *Pharmacotherapeutics: A nursing process approach* (4th ed.). Philadelphia: F. A. Davis Company.

LeMone, P. & Burke, K. (1996). *Medical-surgical nursing: Critical thinking in client care.* Menlo Park, Calif.: Addison-Wesley.

McCance, K. L. & Huether, S. E. (1990). Pathophysiology: The biologic basis for disease in adults and children. St. Louis: Mosby.

Petersen, M. & Fieler, V. (2000). Breast cancer. *American Journal of Nursing*, supp. 9–12.

Sommers, S. & Johnson, S. (1997). *Davis's manual of nursing therapeutics for diseases and disorder*. Philadelphia: F.A. Davis Co.

CASE #8 JOE FROST

Learning Objectives

1. Identify data collection that leads to a need for a more comprehensive and in-depth assessment.
2. Recognize inherent safety factors and what information is necessary in caring for clients with multiple problems.
3. Assimilate lab data to facilitate problem identification and to monitor for complications and track progress.
4. Develop a teaching plan for the complex needs of a client with multiple problems.

Joe Frost is a 76-year-old black widowed male. He is scheduled for outpatient inguinal herniorrhaphy. During your intake assessment prior to his elective procedure, you notice that Mr. Frost winces when he changes positions as when he climbed onto the examination table. Upon questioning, you learn that he has had constant dull mid-back pain for about a week. He denies having fallen or injuring himself. The pain is initiated or aggravated with movement, straining, coughing, sneezing, and sitting, and it is radicular. Mr. Frost also appears somewhat unsteady as he stands to walk to the exam table. He acknowledges he is "a little weak in my legs" and he "feels a little light-headed at times." His speech is slightly thick, which he attributes to his mouth being dry. His history includes a diagnosis of prostate cancer and hypertension. The cancer had been diagnosed ten years ago and treated with Leuprolide acetate (Lupron) injections every three months. He takes Hytrin 1 mg/hs and Demadex 40 mg every morning. His vital signs are: T—97.8° (o), AP—92, R—16, BP 116/80 (left arm/sitting). Mr. Frost lives alone in a second-floor apartment. He has meals on wheels delivered three days a week.

Focus Question

1. What further assessment would you conduct?
   - **Check orthostatic blood pressure to assess for possible volume depletion (most accurate method to clinically assess for volume depletion). Volume depletion may result from (1) being NPO for surgery, (2) possible chronic less-than-required oral fluid intake that sometimes occurs with elderly persons because of deterioration of the thirst center, and (3) possible increased urinary output R/T diuretic therapy resulting in hypovolemia; assess heart rate as part of the effect of postural changes; compare heart rate with record; heart rate may be rapid due to hypovolemia or from pain or because of anxiety;**
   - **Check muscle strength by (1) having Mr. Frost squeeze your two fingers as firmly as possible with each hand, and (2) having him resist plantar flexion of his feet. Compare results of both sides (hemiplegia may indicate spinal cord compression, which is an oncology emergency to be reported immediately, but hemiplegia and thickened speech may suggest a cerebrovascular mishap);**
   - **Assess for spinal cord compression (SCC) as a cause for motor weakness in Mr. Frost's legs. Gently tap down his vertebrae with the knuckle of your index finger to**

illicit pain response, which may indicate metastasis to the vertebra(e). (Back pain is the first symptom of SCC in 96% of patients). Assess for loss of sensation for light touch, pain, and temperature. Check coordination by having Mr. Frost tap your hand as quickly as possible with the ball of each foot or having him place the heel of one foot on the shin of the opposite leg and sliding the heel down the shin. (Sexual impotence may be another early sign of SCC. However, the Lupron may have already rendered him to be impotent.)

You discover that Mr. Frost does exhibit postural hypotension indicating volume depletion. From a sitting position to standing for two minutes, his blood pressure in the same arm dropped to 104/72 and his heart rate increased to 102. But he also cried out abruptly in response to your tapping his T-8 and T-9 vertebrae. On a scale of 1–10 with "1" being no pain to "10" being unbearable pain, Mr. Frost rates his pain at a "6" with "4" being tolerable. He does exhibit muscle weakness, especially of his left lower extremity.

Focus Question

1. What are the issues that need rapid intervention?
   - **Patient safety by keeping him quiet and in a comfortable position; if there is a spinal cord compression (SCC), the vertebra can collapse and cause paraplegia.**
   - **Caution to not make rapid position changes or to ambulate alone since orthostatic hypotension can cause dizziness, placing him at high risk for falls.**
   - **Volume replacement; note pre-admission test results for altered electrolytes as (1) hypokalemia from nonpotassium sparing diuretic therapy contributing to rapid heart rate, (2) hypercalcemia if there is metastasis, and (3) possible falsely elevated lab values due to dehydration, e.g., BUN, serum creatinine, serum albumin, specific gravity of urine.**
   - **Initiate pain management when patient's self-report of pain is not required to guide medical diagnosis,**
   - **Test(s) to diagnose SCC.**
   - **Handle gently; log roll if necessary to turn patient in bed.**

You collaborated with the anesthesiologist and the neurosurgeon who ordered: bed rest with bathroom privileges and 1,000 cc. NaCl with 30 mEq KCL per IV infusion at 150 cc/hour (potassium level was 3.1 mEq/L and calcium was 11.4 mg/dl). Also ordered were Ibuprofen 200 mg po and a magnetic resonance imaging (MRI) stat. (The MRI is becoming the primary test to diagnose and localize spinal metastasis; other tests could include spinal films, bone scan, CT scan, and myelogram.) The elective surgery was postponed. Metastatic tumor causing SCC at T-9 was diagnosed per the MRI. The urologist ordered Decadron 20 mg IVP stat with 10 mg po q6h for controlling the edema and pain. It was decided that debulking or spinal stabilization were not indicated, and a radiation oncologist was consulted. Radiation therapy at 3,000 cGy fractionated over five weeks was initiated. Mr. Frost was admitted for 23-hour observation.

Focus Question

1. What monitoring and plan of care would you provide?
   - **Provide for continued safety since identifying Mr. Frost as high risk for falls due to (1) motor weakness from SCC and electrolyte imbalances, and (2) potential altered mental status from hypercalcemia if high level not just reflection of his dehydration;**

- **Provide pain assessment and management;**
- **Monitor vital signs and orthostatic blood pressure changes to assess improved hydration; also assess mucous membranes and speech for improved hydration;**
- **Monitor apical heart rate for irregularities that may cue myocardial irritability related to hypokalemia; perform ECG monitoring as ordered;**
- **Avoid circulatory overload;**
- **Monitor follow-up labs;**
- **Teach: (1) reportable signs and symptoms of SCC; (2) making position changes slowly; (3) care of radiation site; (4) increasing oral fluid intake; (5) medication actions, side effects, precautions, and schedule; (6) importance of compliance with lab and medical follow-up for managing electrolytes; (7) supporting inguinal hernia and reportable signs and symptoms related to possible strangulation;**
- **Obtain social service consult for discharge preparation, i.e., home evaluation for accessibility and safety, transportation for radiation treatments, assurance that schedule for Meals on Wheels is optimal, and to search out other support services available;**
- **Assess Mr. Frost's ability to ambulate to bathroom; if deficit observed, collaborate with physician regarding physical therapy evaluation and home health care needs.**

Reflective Writing

What's the importance of a holistic assessment in the care of clients rather than assessing based on their medical diagnosis?

Students in reflecting on Mr. Frost could note his diagnosis for inguinal hernia and only focus on preop and postop assessment for this surgery. In this case they would have missed his metastatic prostate cancer and hypertension, as well as his home situation. It is important to give total client care, and that necessitates a holistic approach.

References

Corbett, J. V. (1996). *Laboratory tests & diagnostic procedures with nursing diagnoses.* (4th ed.). Stamford, Conn.: Appleton & Lange.

Groenwald, S. L., Frogge, M. H., Goodman, M., & Yarbro, C. H. (1998). *Comprehensive cancer nursing review* (4th ed.). Boston: Jones and Bartlett Publishers.

Itano, J. K. & Taoka, K. N. (1998). *Core curriculum for oncology nursing* (3rd ed.). Philadelphia: W. B. Saunders Company.

Kuhn, M. (1998). *Pharmacotherapeutics: A nursing process approach* (4th ed.). Philadelphia: F. A. Davis Company.

McCance, K. L. & Huether, S. E. (1990). *Pathophysiology: The biologic basis for disease in adults and children.* St. Louis: Mosby.

CASE #9 TY EVANS

Learning Objectives

1. Identify questions to be probed based on initial and progressive nursing assessment of the client.
2. Synthesize data from multiple sources to determine nursing problems and interventions.
3. Recognize the home health nurse's role as coordinator of care.
4. Document specific assessments with accuracy and clarity.

Ty Evans is a 73-year-old black married male living with his spouse. You are making your first home care visit with Mr. Evans since his regular nurse is on vacation. He weighs 185 lbs. and is 6 ft. 3 in. He has lost 10 pounds in the past 6 weeks. He had a central venous port implanted for previous chemotherapy administration for colon cancer, but the port is not currently being used. His apical heart rate is now 110 BPM, irregular and thready, with BP 110/60. His respirations are 25/minute, which he says is his usual respiratory pattern. He denies dyspnea but admits he uses three pillows under his head to sleep. The chart indicates medical diagnoses of COPD and CVA with right hemiparesis. Medications listed are as follows: Theodur 450 mg bid po, Furosemide 40 mg bid po, Proventil 4 puffs q4h INH, Lanoxin 0.25 mg qd po, Surfak 240 mg qd po.

Focus Question

1. What questions do you have?

   - **There is no medical diagnosis to support order for Lanoxin. Is there a diagnosed cardiac problem?**
   - **What is his digoxin level since he has an irregular tachycardia?**
   - **Since he is taking Lasix, does he have hypokalemia, which is the most common cause for digitalis toxicity? This toxicity could be a possible explanation for the irregular tachycardia. Does he have signs and symptoms of digitalis toxicity, e.g., mentation changes, irritability, nausea, rapid heart rate, visual changes such as white, yellow, or green spots or halos around objects?**
   - **What was the interpretation of his most recent electrocardiogram since atrial fibrillation (AF) is irregular and is not uncommon in elderly persons? If he does have AF, he is experiencing uncontrolled ventricular response, which needs intervention.**
   - **Does he have signs and symptoms of hypovolemia, which could account for tachycardia as a compensatory mechanism? Hypovolemia could result from a lack of intake because of nausea, the loss of fluid through loose stools, the positive action of diuretic therapy, and the increased perfusion of the renal system as a result of vasodilation from Theodur. The most reliable tool to assess hypovolemia is to perform orthostatic blood pressure checks.**
   - **What is his skin turgor and status of his mucous membranes? What is the quality of his peripheral pulse? (If he is hypovolemic and requires intravenous fluids, remember to use the port!)**
   - **Mr. Evans' systolic blood pressure is low for a man his size; what is his baseline systolic pressure?**
   - **What is recorded as his usual respiratory pattern? What are his breath sounds?**
   - **What are the possible reasons for the weight loss? Does he have edema, a possible sign of malnourishment from lack of oncotic pressure because of lack of protein in the venous blood? Is a pre-albumin test indicated? (Pre-albumin reflects albumin level within last twelve hours versus the albumin test, which reflects the level over the past thirty days.) Does Mr. Evans need a dietitian consult? Does he need weekly weights? Are supplements, particularly those for pulmonary patients, indicated? Can Mr. Evans afford supplements? With his history of CVA, does he have dysphagia and need a speech therapy consult to evaluate swallowing?**
   - **What is the maintenance flushing schedule for the port?**

You learn that Mr. Evans' last ECG two weeks ago noted "Atrial fibrillation with controlled ventricular response." He has not had a digoxin level drawn for two months. He states that he was in the hospital a year ago for congestion in his heart. His respirations are recorded as being 20–27/minute and that he frequently has sonorous wheezes on expiration in the right bronchovesicular area with crackles in the right middle lobe, which you confirm through auscultation during your assessment. The home health aid has left a note from the day before for the nurse: "Patient is flushed, has loose stools, and says he's nauseated."

Focus Question

1. What questions do you have now?

   - **What is/are the cause(s) for the nausea? Is it a symptom of digitalis toxicity? Is it a side effect of Theodur toxicity (should take Theodur after meals or food and with eight ounces of water to minimize gastrointestinal disturbances)? Could the nausea be emanating from bowel problem as evidenced by loose stools (most garden-variety nausea caused by upset bowel)?**

   - **How many loose stools did patient have? Is he continuing to experience loose stools? Is Mr. Evans still taking Surfak? When was the patient's last "normal" stool? What is his evacuation pattern? Could he be impacted? Are there associated signs or symptoms of bowel distress? Are there abnormal bowel sounds? What does palpation/percussion of abdomen reveal? Is his liver enlarged? Since early metastasis of GI malignancies are often evidenced in the liver, is the size or consistency of the liver changed if palpated? Is jaundice apparent in icterus of the sclera? Are there any recent labs on liver enzymes? Is he febrile and simply has a GI virus? Has there been any dietary change? What is the color, consistency, and amount of stool? Is there blood or mucus evident? Is there indication for checking occult blood in stool? Has the patient taken a laxative lately? Synthesis of vitamin K may be impaired with diarrhea, so need to observe for signs/symptoms of bleeding.**

   - **Is Mr. Evans hypokalemic? Potassium can be lost through loose stools and diuretic effects. Is an order needed for a lab draw for potassium level? Does Mr. Evans and his wife know to increase potassium-rich foods such as avocado, bananas, cantaloupe, dates, figs, molasses, orange juice, potatoes, prunes, some salt substitutes, soybeans, and tomato juice?**

   - **Do the adventitious breath sounds clear with cough?**

   - **It would be expected that with a diagnosis of COPD that Mr. Evans would be in a compensated respiratory acidosis state. However, diuretic therapy can cause metabolic alkalosis with hypocalcemia resulting. (The measurement of calcium in the serum in alkalosis would not be lower but less calcium is in an ionized state.) A positive Chvostek's and/or Trousseau's sign would be significant reportable sign(s) in that inadequate amounts of ionized calcium may alter the inotropic state of the heart. Because Lanoxin and Lasix are ordered and there is a self-reported suggestion of a history of CHF, Mr. Evans may be at risk for CHF if the myocardial contractility is compromised.**

   - **What is causing the patient to be flushed? Is he febrile? Is the environmental temperature high? Is the flushing a response to the Theodur affecting the beta-2 receptors causing vasodilation? If his COPD is related to emphysema, flushing may be a sign of respiratory acidosis seen in the "pink puffer" appearance of the emphysematous patient. Flushing can be a subjective observation, and it can be transient.**

As you conduct your assessment, you discover a sacral pressure ulcer. The latest entry in the nurses' documentation states: "Stage III pressure ulcer on sacral area is healing and is now a Stage II. Wife demonstrated wound cleansing with NaCl solution and application of Duoderm.

Wound is 3 cm × 3 cm × 2 mm with no tunneling, intact skin around edges dark red and blanches well, no exudate, pink granulation with thin layer of gray film noted. c/o local soreness. Wife verbalizes knowledge of and compliance with turning patient at least q2h."

Focus Question

1. What is wrong with this documentation?

   Reverse staging of pressure ulcers in not appropriate. It is important to show progress so a Stage III remains a Stage III and cannot become a Stage II as it heals. Instead it can be stated that the ulcer is a healing Stage III and then describe those observations that demonstrate the wound has improved.

Reflective Writing

As an experienced acute care nurse, what things will you have to take into consideration if you decide to become a home heath nurse? In other words, how do you compare the role of the nurse in each area?

Students should identify that the same nursing process is used in caring for patients regardless of the setting. As a home health nurse, you are the bridge between the patient and the health care system, more so than the client who is hospitalized and seen daily by a variety of health care professionals. Therefore the nurse must be able to identify potential problems as well as treat actual ones. Because the environments are different, the nurse must realize that she is a guest in the client's home and being a partner in the client's care is even more important.

References

Corbett, J. V. (1996). *Laboratory tests & diagnostic procedures with nursing diagnoses* (4th ed.). Stamford, Conn.: Appleton & Lange.

Groenwald, S. L., Frogge, M. H., Goodman, M., & Yarbro, C. H. (1998). *Comprehensive cancer nursing review* (4th ed.). Boston: Jones and Bartlett Publishers.

Itano, J. K. & Taoka, K. N. (1998). *Core curriculum for oncology nursing* (3rd ed.). Philadelphia: W. B. Saunders Company.

Kuhn, M. (1998). *Pharmacotherapeutics: A nursing process approach* (4th ed.). Philadelphia: F. A. Davis Company.

McCance, K. L. & Huether, S. E. (1990). *Pathophysiology: The biologic basis for disease in adults and children.* St. Louis: Mosby.

CASE #10 C.J. BARNES

Learning Objectives

1. Interpret client data using discipline specific language.
2. Discuss signs and symptoms of heart failure, also referred to as congestive heart failure (CHF).
3. Relate pathophysiology to assessment data.
4. Analyze assessment data.
5. Implement clinical judgment through clinical decision making.
6. Describe nursing and collaborative interventions for CHF.
7. Develop a plan of care for client experiencing acute CHF.

8. Identify educational interventions related to CHF.
9. Identify evaluative criteria related to collaborative interventions.

1300. C. J. Barnes, a 50-year-old professor, is 5 hours post-laproscopic cholecystectomy. He is alert, oriented, with physical assessment within normal limits including active bowel sounds, soft slightly tender abdomen. He is sipping on clear liquids and conversant with his wife. The nurse is performing the final assessment and providing discharge client education. C. J. states he feels a little tired because of all the excitement about going home and feeling so good after surgery. While checking his vital signs for the discharge form, the nurse notices that his pulse is 110/ minute and irregular compared to the 86 to 90/minute regular pulse, which he had been having since surgery. C. J. states it is just his excitement, he feels great, and his wife is waiting in the car at the client discharge area for him.

Focus Questions

1. What should the nurse do?

   The nurse should delay discharge, reassess the client and inform the physician ASAP of the change in condition. Reassessment should include repeating the vital signs, auscultate apical pulse, auscultate breath sounds, assess peripheral pulses, assess for JVD (jugular vein distention), orthostatic hypotension, auscultatory gap, respiratory rhythm and effort, level of orientation, and peripheral edema. The nurse also needs to calculate intake and output for the past 24 hours. The nurse should also notify Mr. Barnes wife of the delayed discharge.

2. What should the nurse say to C. J.?

   Appropriate verbal and nonverbal communications are important. C. J. needs to be educated on the importance of evaluating his fatigue and change in vital signs. The nurse should reassure C. J. that all effort is being used to consult with his physician in a timely manner so as to minimize the delay in discharge. It is important to demonstrate respect for the client and his wife.

3. Is there any significance in an irregular pulse? If yes, then describe.

   An irregular pulse is a significant change in a client's condition. An irregular pulse is usually associated with cardiac dysrhythmia and reduced cardiac output.

1400. You inform the physician of the irregular pulse and other assessment finding. The physician requests a STAT ECG and chest x-ray, and cancels the prior written discharge order. The ECG shows atrial fibrillation with a ventricular rate of 118, with QRS and ST configurations suggesting an old anterior wall MI (myocardial infarction). C. J. continues to rest in semi-Fowler's position in bed. His wife has returned to his bedside. Upon auscultation you note that C. J. has fine crackles in both bases, an occasional dry nonproductive cough, and hiccoughs, and he denies difficulty in breathing. As you turn to leave the room, you observe C. J. getting out of bed and walking toward the restroom. He is holding onto the bed rails as he walks. His wife looks frightened and asks him if he is all right. He stops, holds onto the footboard stating, "I don't know. I feel sort of weak." He appears slightly tachypneic.

Focus Questions

1. Should the nurse continue to exit the room? If not, then what should the nurse say and do?

   The nurse should immediately assist C. J. to sit at the bedside. The nurse should assess C. J. for orthostatic hypotension, initiate prn oxygen if ordered, and ensure he is in a

safe position. Then obtain a urinal or BSC (bedside commode) for him to use and educate both C. J. and his wife that he should only get out of bed with assistance and initiate a turning schedule.

2. Why does C. J. have the crackles and cough at rest and tachypnea with walking?

   In left heart failure, there is increased pulmonary vascular pressure usually due to decreased left ventricle cardiac output. This leads to increased pulmonary capillary oncotic pressure resulting in alveolar and interstitial infiltrates. The infiltrates can stimulate cough and bronchial constriction leading to wheezes. Crackles are sign of alveolar infiltrates. Infiltrates compromise oxygenation leading to hypoxia as evidenced by dyspnea, tachypnea, fatigue, and altered cognitive function. Clients can also develop altered renal function, angina and poor peripheral perfusion.

3. Identify independent nursing interventions for this client.

Monitor BP qh until stable	**Record intake and output**	**Report decreased urine output**
Monitor cardiac rate and rhythm	**Notify physician immediately of dysrhythmia**	**Assess and note heart sounds**
Palpate peripheral pulses	**Assess breath sounds**	**Assess cognitive function**
If intracardiac catheter is present, monitor pressures and cardiac output	**Monitor SaO_2 and notify physician if decreased**	**Assess for leg tenderness, redness, edema, homan sign**
Encourage rest	**Assess for impaired skin**	**Provide skin pressure relief or reduction**
Elevate legs if edema present	**Encourage/assist with range of motion**	**Educate client and significant other**
Assess response to medications, withhold and notify physician	**Assess for cyanosis (indicates 5gm+ blood lack oxygen)**	**Assess for JVD**
Assist client to reduce stress	**Weigh client daily**	**Limit intake to 2,000cc/24hr**
Assess activity tolerance	**Assist with ADL as needed**	**Refer to Cardiac Education RN**
Recommend Home Health RN visit post discharge	**Assess nutrition status**	**Assess skin turgor**

4. Identify collaborative nursing interventions for this client.

Monitor electrolytes	**Administer oxygen**	**Administer medications**
Monitor medication serum levels	**Monitor chest x-ray results**	**Monitor coagulation, liver, renal studies**

5. What medications and lab tests would commonly be prescribed for this client?

   - **Medications: Digoxin, diuretic, oxygen, and Heparin infusion. Potassium, if using potassium wasting diuretic**
   - **Lab tests: APTT (also PT & INR if long term anticoagulation planned); electrolytes, BUN, creatinine, AST, LDH, digoxin level**

Reflective Writing

Your patient is to be discharged today. You recognize signs of a major complication and report it to the third-year resident on call. The resident instructs you to discharge the patient. What should you do?

Document your assessment data and the call to the resident as well as his or her instructions. Notify your immediate supervisor of your concerns and follow the hospital's chain of command. Be sure to document all of your attempts to advocate for the client. The attending physician will need to be called.

References

Doenges, M., Moorhouse, M., & Geissler, A. (2000). *Nursing care plans: Guidelines for individualizing patient care,* 5th ed. Philadelphia: F. A. Davis.

Ignatavicius, D., Workman, M., & Mishler, M. (1999). *Medical-surgical nursing across the health care continuum,* 3rd ed., Philadelphia: W. B. Saunders Company.

Swearingen, P. & Keen, J., eds. (1995). *Manual of critical care nursing,* 3rd ed. St. Louis: Mosby.

CASE #11 CARMEN COSTA

Learning Objectives

1. Identify assessment data related to complications of postoperative patients.
2. Interpret assessment data characteristic of postoperative patients.
3. Identify nursing interventions related to complications of postoperative patients.
4. Identify collaborative management interventions related to postoperative patients.

Carmen Costa is a 67-year-old female with IDDM admitted on Sunday for severe abdominal discomfort. On admission her vital signs were: BP 116/80, heart rate 86, respirations 20, temperature 98.4°. Her blood sugar (BS) was 115 and her initial lab work was WNL. Carmen's x-rays revealed an abdominal mass, and she was scheduled for an exploratory laparotomy on Monday. During surgery Carmen was diagnosed with a cancerous tumor. The tumor was removed, and Carmen was taken to a medical/surgical unit. Postoperatively Carmen had an IV of 1,000ml D_5W infusing at 50ml/hr, an NG to intermittent suction, a Foley draining clear amber urine, and a midline abdominal dressing that was dry/intact (D/I). Nurse Nancy is assigned to care for Carmen on her first POD. Carmen is alert/oriented and her color is gray/pale. Her morning accucheck is 210 and she receives 8 units of regular insulin. Carmen's NG is draining brown/green mucous, her abdominal dressing is D/I, and she has an IV of D_5W at 50ml/hr. Carmen has very limited conversation this morning but states, "I'm very tired and sick to my stomach."

Focus Questions

1. What collaborative management and postoperative teaching strategies are needed for Carmen and why? (Discuss postoperative management and types of medications she might need.)

Collaborative Management/Teaching Strategies:

A. Monitor and manage clinical status for postoperative patient

- **Maintain adequate ventilation/oxygenation—apply O_2, cough and deep breathing techniques, use of incentive spirometer, early ambulation, elevate HOB greater than**

30 degrees, reposition patient q2h. ***Rationale*: Aids in aerating alveoli that may be underinflated with the patient's postoperative breathing patterns, improves distribution of ventilation and perfusion of the lungs, helps mobilize secretions that could impair ventilation/perfusion of the lungs**

- **Assess pain level. *Rationale:* Geriatric patients may be less likely to complain of pain because they may be less able to differentiate different degrees of pain. Postoperative pain decreases lung function, increases O_2 consumption, and depletes the patient's energy level.**
- **Provide pain relief. Pharmacological (analgesics). Nonpharmacological measures: change position—*Rationale:* eliminates formation of gas from abdominal surgery; relaxation and imaging strategies—*Rationale:* relieves muscle tension; straighten linens—*Rationale:* provides comfort**
- **Assess for abdominal distention/nausea/flatus/bowel movement. Check NG for accurate placement and drainage (type and amount)—*Rationale:* decrease or lack of drainage could indicate an obstruction in flow of gastric secretions and could cause the patient abdominal distention and discomfort. Limit or restrain from P.O intake until peristalsis returns. Decrease fear and anxiety—*Rationale:* relaxes smooth muscle contraction.**
- **Provide supportive care. Involvement of: pastoral care, social worker, family/support system, nurses, and physicians. *Rationale:* Provides comfort and reassurance to the patient. The needs of each patient are unique. Interventions by an experienced nurse, minister, social worker, or physician may be needed to relieve anxiety.**

B. Pharmacotherapeutics

- **Antiemetics—drugs used to prevent or relieve nausea/vomiting**
- **Analgesics—drugs used to relieve pain, administration of narcotic analgesic is integral part of nursing care for postoperative patients**
- **IV therapy—maintains body's H_2O and electrolyte balance and distribution. The response to surgery and anesthesia causes conservation of fluids and salt by the kidneys related to sympathetic stimulation, ADH secretion, and activation of the renin-angiotension system. Extracellular fluid volume decreases as a result of inadequate fluid replacement postoperative. (0.9% NaCl, 0.45% NaCl, or lactated ringers restore fluid volume; D_5W results in intracellular expansion not an increase in intravascular volume)**

**** With all the collaborative measures listed, the nurse needs to remember: nausea and vomiting may develop from medications, gastric distention, surgical manipulation, pain, or psychological factors. Assessment of all these areas is important in determining the cause and appropriate treatment.**

2. Prioritize a list of nursing diagnosis appropriate for Carmen.

- **Impaired gas exchange related to drug effects/incisional pain (gray/pale coloration)**
- **Alteration in comfort: nausea/vomiting related to movement in postoperative period, anxiety, ineffective action of antiemetic (complaint of nausea and "sick to my stomach")**
- **Pain, acute related to surgical incision, positioning (very limited conversation this morning)**
- **Anxiety, risk for related to possible change in health status, pain, strange environment (very limited conversation this morning)**
- **Risk for fluid volume deficit related to insufficient IV fluids (IV solution of D_5W instead of 0.9 NaCl/0.45 NaCl/or LR)**

The physician ordered Carmen to be OOB tid starting today. At 1000 Nancy gives Carmen a complete bed bath and then decides to ambulate her to the chair per order while she changes her sheets. While sitting at the bedside Carmen states, "I don't feel very well." After waiting 30 seconds, Nancy decides to get Carmen in the chair. While in the chair her color becomes more pale and her skin is diaphoretic. Her BP is 88/64, and her abdominal dressing has a 3x3 area of sanguinous drainage.

Focus Questions

1. What could be happening to Carmen in relation to the introduction of this new data?

   Carmen could be experiencing:

   - **orthostatic hypotension**
   - **hypovolemia related to blood loss or decreased fluid volume.**

2. What data supports this/these conclusions?

   - **Orthostatic hypotension is a common complication in the postoperative period. It occurs either from a change in body position or from fluid volume deficit. The manifestation of orthostatic hypotension in postoperative patients is assessed by taking the BP when the patient is supine. Then when the patient stands or sets the BP is taken immediately. A drop in systolic BP greater than 15mmHg or a heart rate greater than 15 bpm difference from onset of activity is indicative of orthostatic hypotension. Carmen's initial BP was 116/80. Upon dangling at the bedside, it changed to 88/64, a difference in systolic BP of 28mmHg.**

   - **Adequate circulation is important in the postoperative period. Pallor can indicate decreased circulation to the skin. Vasoconstriction may occur because of cold temperatures or because of a decrease blood volume due to blood loss. Assessment of the nail beds for capillary refill or change in vital signs (significant drop in systolic BP) could be an indication of hemorrhage or circulatory failure. Also, the patient could become anxious or restless with skin that is cold, moist, or cyanotic. Hemorrhage most likely occurs within 48 hours after surgery and can be caused by slipping of sutures or dislodging of a clot or reestablishment of blood flow. Hypovolemia is a deficit in fluid/blood volume that also affects the circulatory system. Hypovolemia is caused by an inadequate IV fluid administration or loss of blood/fluids from wounds or drains. The manifestation of blood loss in postoperative patients is: postural hypotension, tachycardia, tachypnea, decreased urinary output, cool clammy skin, and a change in the level of consciousness. Carmen's assessment findings for fluid volume deficit included: significant changes in systolic BP, pale diaphoretic skin, and new sanguinous drainage on the wound dressing with position change.**

3. What nursing interventions should Nancy implement at this time?

   a. **The nursing intervention for orthostatic hypotension is to have the patient dangle before standing and ambulating for the first time after surgery. Dangling is done to assess the patient's tolerance to activity. Have the patient change position gradually and avoid standing upright for more than 3 minutes. This will help reduce the risk of blood pooling in the lower extremities. When a patient stands, approximately 500–700ml of blood shifts from the thoracic cavity to the pelvic region and the lower extremities. This change in fluid shift (blood volume) is completed in 2–3 minutes with a drop in arterial pressure. To avoid these changes from occurring, the nurse should reinforce the following preoperative and postoperative measure:**

   - **leg exercises to promote venous return and reduce the risk of vagal stimulation**
   - **taking slow, deep breaths with activity to promote a calming effect, to promote venous return, and reduce the risk of vagal stimulation**

- **while standing have the patient wiggle his or her toes and contract their leg muscles to promote venous return to the heart**
- **have nurse assist in position changes until the patient no longer experiences signs and symptoms of fluid volume deficit/orthostatic hypotension**
- **provide continuous assessment of heart rate, BP, and level of consciousness in the postoperative period**

b. To assess for hemorrhage from the wound, careful assessment in BP changes, wound dressing, and drainage systems are essential in the postoperative period. If changes in vital signs, color, skin temperature, level of consciousness, or wound dressing/drains are assessed, the surgeon should be notified immediately.

The second POD Carmen has ambulated to the chair 3 times, her BP remains approximately 94/56 all day, BS 200's with each accucheck, and her abdominal dressing remains dry and intact (D/I). By 1630 that evening, Carmen complains of nausea. At 1700 her sensorium began changing and her pulse oximeter was 88% with O_2 at 2L/nasal cannula. At 1830, the family found the patient dangling at the bedside, restless and trying to gag herself to vomit. Her NG was draining dark brown/black aspirate, her accucheck was 232, P 133 and irregular. At 1845 Carmen was found thrashing in bed. Her daughter ran to get the nurse. At 1850, Nancy found Carmen unconscious with Cheyne-Stokes respirations, P 67, BP 60 systolic. ABG's were drawn at 1908 with the results: pH 7.13, HCO_3 19.8, O_2 sat 18.4%, $PaCO_2$, 59.5, PaO_2 18.8. At 1910: P 107, BP 40 palpable.

Lab values from first POD:		Lab values at 1908, second POD:	
RBC	4.3	RBC	3.29
Hgb	11.5	Hgb	6.8
Hct	28.8	Hct	23.3
K	4.35	K	6.9
Na	134	Na	134.4
CO_2	26.1	CO_2	12.7
Glucose	354	Glucose	383
BUN	5	BUN	8
Cr	0.8	Cr	1.1

1915 ABG's were repeated. The results were: pH 7.12, $PaCO_2$ 24.5, HCO_3 8.1, PaO_2 80.9, O_2 Sat 92.3 %.

Focus Questions

1. What could be happening in this scenario?

   - **Acute gastric dilatation: can mimic signs of shock**

   S&S: restless, rapid weak pulse, decreased BP, vomiting
   Other S&S of gastric dilatation, not seen with shock: gastric distention, decreased or absent drainage from NG, weight gain, increased abdominal girth

   - **Postoperative shock—one of the most common complications after surgery.**

   Causes include: respiratory acidosis, narcotics, postoperative pain, abdominal distention, surgery with high abdominal incision causes pain with ventilation, hemorrhage, hypovolemic state, pulmonary emboli. The most common cause is hemorrhage. S&S of hemorrhage: postural hypotension, decreased urinary output, tachycardia, cool, clammy skin, tachypnea, decreased level of consciousness. The second most common cause is hypovolemic shock, not specific to hemorrhage. Subjective signs and symptoms include: feeling sick, weak, cold, nausea, dizziness, shortness of breath, and

confusion. Objective signs and symptoms: decreased BP (systolic and diastolic), decreased cardiac output, decreased urinary output, increased respirations, alterations in heart rate, dyspnea, and altered sensorium.

- **Pulmonary embolism—arising from immobility and venous stasis. S&S: sudden shortness of breath, tachypnea, tachycardia, anxiety. End result is a respiratory arrest if left untreated.**
- **Metabolic acidosis—caused by tissue breakdown from shock, malnutrition and lactic release; also can be caused from diabetic ketoacidosis. S&S: Kussmaul respirations, restless, HCO_3 less than 24mEq/L, pH less than 7.35, when attempting to have respiratory compensation: $PaCO_2$ less than 35mmHg.**

2. What data supports your conclusion(s)?
   - **Data pertaining to Carmen that supports gastric dilatation: restless, vomiting, rapid pulse, decreased BP**
   - **Data pertaining to Carmen that supports hypovolemic shock: states "feel sick", decreased BP, weak, increased respirations, cold, alteration in heart rate, nausea, confused, short of breath**
   - **Data pertaining to Carmen that supports hemorrhage: postural hypotension, cool, clammy skin, increased heart rate, decreased level of consciousness, tachypnea, decreased Hgb, ABG—metabolic acidosis, decreased Hct, decreased RBC**
   - **Data pertaining to Carmen that supports pulmonary embolism: sudden shortness of breath, anxiety, tachycardia, experienced a respiratory arrest**
   - **Data pertaining to Carmen that supports metabolic acidosis:**
     1. **pH less than 7.35 (7.12)**
     2. **HCO_3 less than 24mEq/L (8.1)**
     3. **$PaCO_2$ less than 35mmHg (24.5)**

   The probable conclusion would be that Carmen developed hypovolemic shock secondary to a hemorrhagic event. This change in condition caused her to have an acid-base imbalance of metabolic acidosis.

3. What collaborative management strategies need to be initiated to manage shock, respiratory, and cardiac changes and blood sugar? What other disciplines need to be involved?

Coordinated efforts with other disciplines:

- **Immediate action would be to notify the physician/surgeon of the current changes.**
- **Notify respiratory therapy for possible intubation and need for changes in O_2 management.**
- **Notify other staff nurses for assistance.**
- **Notify pastoral care service to facilitate family concerns/needs.**

Collaborative Management Strategies:

- **Hypovolemic shock**
  1. **blood administration/plasma expanders: albumin, PRBC, fresh frozen plasma**
  2. **vasoconstrictors: Dopamine, Levophed**
  3. **IV fluid administration: 0.45 NaCl or 0.9 NaCl should be initiated to increase intravascular volume**

4. place the patient in modified trendelenburg position (elevate the foot of bed 30–45%); promotes venous return to the heart
5. monitor continual changes in vital signs

   * The above treatment strategies are used to correct the low blood volume that is causing changes in Carmen's level of consciousness, decreased Hgb, Hct, RBC, BP, and fluctuations in her heart rate and rhythm.

- Respiratory/Cardiac:
  1. monitor changes in cardiac status: obtain a 12 lead ECG
  2. have a crash cart available for intubation and possible code status
  3. apply a 100% O_2 mask
  4. reassess ABG:

     —1st set were drawn from a venous puncture (PaO_2 18.8)

     —2nd set were drawn from an arterial puncture (PaO_2 80.9)

     —the ABG results indicate the patient is in metabolic acidosis (pH 7.12 HCO_3 8.1)

  *Treatment would include giving HCO_3 IV to correct the HCO_3 level.

- Blood Sugar:
  1. increases when:
     a. body is under stress
     b. DKA
     c. infective process

  * Can be corrected by giving insulin or removing the cause.

Reflective Writing

Write a reaction to how this situation could have been prevented from the nurse/patient/family's viewpoint.

This situation could have been eliminated or the severity of the situation reduced. The major issues of concern, in this situation, deal with communication and assessment. The patient could or should have been more descriptive and less vague in describing her feelings. Carmen frequently described her symptoms using words such as "sick to my stomach, I'm tired, I don't feel very well." These phrases do not lend accurate data for analyzing changes in conditions by the health care team. To better facilitate the needs of the patient, the nurse could have used therapeutic communication techniques to achieve more accurate data. The nurse could have used broad, open-ended questions or asked the patient to describe her feelings based on the pain scale 0–10. These measures would have elicited more detailed information from Carmen. The family's involvement is always important. When the patient was responding with vague statements, the nurse could have utilized the family for feedback on how Carmen responded or reacted in similar situations. This could have facilitated a better, more effective delivery of care for Carmen. The nurses should have responded more quickly to the change in Carmen's sensorium. At 1700, when Carmen's sensorium changed, the physician should have been notified for an evaluation of her current status. A person's level of consciousness is the first change frequently seen when there are physical changes occurring in the body. By not responding at 1700 to this change, Carmen's condition continued to deteriorate to a near death/death status. Health care requires prompt and accurate assess-

ment of our patients with involvement from the patients, their families or support systems, and the health care team. In this situation, the patient's health was jeopardized due to ineffective communication and a slow response to the needs of Carmen.

References

Beare, P. & Myers, J. (1998). *Adult health nursing* (3rd ed.). St. Louis: Mosby.

Black, J. & Matassarin-Jacobs, E. (1997). *Medical-surgical nursing: Clinical management for continuity of care* (5th ed.). Philadelphia: W. B. Saunders.

Burrell, C., Gerlach, M., & Pless, B. (1997). *Adult nursing: Acute and community care* (2nd ed.). Stamford, Conn.: Appleton & Lange.

LeFever Kee, J. (1998). *Laboratory & diagnostic tests with nursing implications* (4th ed.). Stamford, Conn.: Appleton & Lange.

Lewis, S., Heitkamper, M., & Dorksen, S. (2000). *Medical surgical nursing assessment and management of clinical problems* (5th ed.). St. Louis: Mosby.

Phipps, W., Sands, J., & Marek, J., (1999). *Medical surgical nursing: Concepts & clinical practice* (6th ed.). St. Louis: Mosby.

CASE # 12 MARY ELLEN MENKE

Learning Objectives

1. Discuss the pathophysiology related to rheumatoid arthritis.
2. Describe effects and side effects of the following drugs used in treatment of rheumatoid arthritis: Prednisone, Naprosyn, and Methotrexate.
3. Analyze the data for the client experiencing hemorrhage and determine the nurse's immediate interventions.
4. Describe the teaching needs of the client with rheumatoid arthritis.
5. Discuss resources that the client could use to care for herself and her mother.
6. Discuss discrimination in hiring practices of nurses with chronic illness.

Mary Ellen Menke is a 20-year-old single client with a history of rheumatoid arthritis. She lives with her mother who has metastatic cancer, and Mary Ellen is the primary caregiver. Lately she has been complaining of joint pain and weakness, which she attributes to the lifting and care giving of her mother. Her hands and feet are swollen and tender, and currently she has painful knees and hips. She has a marked swan neck deformity of the right index finger and mild ulnar deviation. Her current medications include Prednisone 5 mg bid po, Naprosyn 375 mg. bid po, and Methotrexate 7.5 mg weekly.

Focus Questions

1. Correlate the symptoms that Mary Ellen exhibits and explain in "lay terms" what arthritis is and what lifestyle modifications are indicated.

   Rheumatoid arthritis is an autoimmune disorder in which the body defenses attack its own tissues. Mary Ellen has weakness and painful and swollen joints as well as joint deformity and deviation. Patient experiences systemic signs of fatigue, weight loss, anorexia, fever, rheumatoid nodules, and anemia. Pain and stiffness are characteristic signs with red, hot, swollen joints that are limited in range of motion. Treatment modalities include rest and exercise, medications, and surgery. When coping with a chronic, debilitating disease, patients must alter their role performances because fatigue, pain, and the crippling effects of arthritis can interfere with the client's roles as spouse, caretaker, or career role.

2. What are the actions and side effects associated with her medications?

   ***Prednisone* is an anti-inflammatory steroid with side effects of fluid retention, depression, hypertension, nausea and anorexia, decreased wound healing, peptic ulceration, muscle wasting, hyperglycemia, and moon face. *Naprosyn*—management of mild to severe pain inhibits prostaglandins and suppresses inflammation. Headache, drowsiness, nausea, constipation, GI bleeding, and hepatitis are possible side effects. *Methotrexate*—small dosages are used in the treatment of immunosuppression of rheumatoid arthritis; side effects are stomatitis, anorexia, nausea, vomiting, hepatotoxicity, anemia, leukopenia, thrombocytopenia, and nephropathy.**

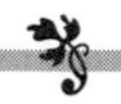

Mary Ellen was brought to the emergency room by a neighbor. She has had two episodes of syncope and is complaining of weakness. Vital signs are BP 130/75, P 100, R 28, T 100°. When asked if she has had any other symptoms, she reports right epigastric pain. While the nurse is away admitting another patient, Mary Ellen goes to the bathroom. When the nurse enters the room, she hears a loud thud followed by a cry for help. The nurse finds Mary Ellen on the floor in the bathroom. She denies being hurt and says, "I just got so dizzy. I think I hit my head." The nurse notes a black liquid stool in the toilet. After helping Mary Ellen back to bed, Mary Ellen exclaims, "I am going to be sick." She immediately vomits a large amount of bright red emesis into the bath basin that is sitting on the bedside table. Her vital signs are now: BP 80/40, P 120, R 32, T 100.4°. Her skin is cool, clammy, and pale. The nurse notes that Mary Ellen seems confused about where she is.

Focus Questions

1. What does the data indicate is happening? Why do you think this episode occurred?

   Mary Ellen is likely hemorrhaging; confusion could be related to decreased blood volume and shock or head injury from her fall; stools indicate bleeding as well as bright red vomitus, rapid pulse rate, and lowered blood pressure. The episode could have occurred because of the side effects of her medications, which caused a gastrointestinal GI bleeding.

2. What immediate interventions are necessary and what should the nurse anticipate happening next?

   The nurse should get Mary Ellen back to bed; initiate neurological assessment, raise HOB 15 degrees in case of head injury, but also raise feet to move blood to vital organs. Start an IV; call the phycian with current VS and report episode; anticipate the physician will order type and cross match for possible blood transfusion, H & H, prepare normal saline for possible gastric lavage (iced is no longer recommended because of risk of hypothermia and danger of severe vasoconstriction and ischemia of the gastric mucosa) (Lemone & Burke, 2000). Anticipate skull films to rule out skull fracture or other head trauma. Be sure to clarify appropriate client position with the physician. *Faculty may want to discuss pros and cons of positioning for this client with both a hemorrhage and a possible head injury.

Four days later Mary Ellen is stable on a medical unit. She has improved dramatically from the complication of a bleeding ulcer and is to be discharged in the morning. She shows the nurse a copper bracelet a friend brought to help control her disease. She states, "My friend thinks this bracelet will cure my arthritis, what do you think?"

Focus Questions

1. What teaching needs related to the management of rheumatoid arthritis should be discussed with Mary Ellen prior to discharge? How should the nurse respond to her question?

Teach about the disease and the importance of taking and understanding effects and side effects of medications, balancing rest and exercise, and nonpharmacological ways to manage pain, such as application of heat or cold, visualization or distraction, and relaxation; the importance of proper nutrition and weight control; strategies for managing altered role performance such as Mary Ellen getting help with her mother and coping with body image disturbances by talking about them or joining support groups such as the Arthritis Foundation. Quackery is a common problem in promising a cure for chronic illness and pain. Copper bracelets are not known to have any effect on the patient's pain or arthritis. Caution patients about this unethical practice that is expensive and ineffective.

2. What resources could the nurse help Mary Ellen connect with to assist her in managing her disease as well as assisting with problems with her mother?

   Home Health Aide services could be utilized to help with Mary Ellen's mother; respite care and care giver support groups in the community could help her cope. The American Cancer Society offers education and support as well. The Arthritis Foundation offers many programs to assist clients with arthritis, such as aquatic programs and support groups.

Reflective Writing

You are a nurse manager on a medical unit. You are currently hiring a staff nurse. There are two applicants equally qualified for the position. One of the candidates alludes to the fact that she has rheumatoid arthritis. Your supervisor tells you to hire the other candidate because people with rheumatoid arthritis are always sick and will not be able to pull their own weight on the unit. How do you feel about her suggestion? What are the ethical and legal implications?

You might feel that your supervisor's thinking could be true, yet it would be illegal to discriminate in such a way. You might secretly feel that way too because working on the unit is hard enough when you are well and strong. Both you and your supervisor are making generalizations about all arthritis clients. It would be illegal and unethical to judge a candidate in such a way, but disabled applicants are discriminated against every day. It would be necessary to challenge your own thinking about these discriminatory practices, as well as educate yourself regarding the Americans with Disabilities Act.

References

Mahat, G. (1998). Rheumatoid arthritis. *American Journal of Nursing*, 98(12), 42–43.

Lemone, P. & Burke, K. (2000). *Medical surgical nursing: Critical thinking in client care.* 2nd ed. Upper Saddle River, N.J.: Prentice Hall.

CASE #13 COLLEEN MURRAY

Learning Objectives

1. Apply assessment findings to pathophysiology of Inflammatory Bowel Disease.
2. Apply the symptom analysis process.
3. Apply Gordon's Functional Health Pattern as a process for assessment.
4. Apply clinical judgment to make clinical decisions and prioritize interventions.
5. Identify safety interventions for assisting client up to the chair.
6. Develop an individualized discharge plan.
7. Identify educational interventions for a client with altered bowel elimination.

8. Understand the roles and responsibilities of the RN and unlicensed assistive personnel (UAP)
9. Identify interventions for the Self Concept Functional Health Pattern.

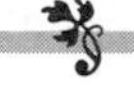

Day 1, 1000. Colleen is a 26-year-old unmarried secretary. She is being admitted to the hospital with LLQ pain and history of watery bowel movements containing bright red blood occurring every 2–3 hours for 30 hours. She has a four-year history of Inflammatory Bowel Disease, has been hospitalized once (at time of diagnosis), and is not taking any medications except Metamucil prn. She lives alone and is in the process of moving from an apartment into a house. Colleen's boyfriend informed the Emergency Department (ED) nurse that Colleen is worried about her finances. She has no income if she is off of work. Her insurance covers 70% of hospital expenses and some doctors' bills, but it does not cover prescriptions or doctor's office visits. Sam is the nurse on the medical unit assigned to do Colleen's admission assessment and develop an individualized plan of care. The ED nurse called the following report: BP 100/68, P 110 regular, R 18, T 100.4° F, hemoglobin 9.8 gm, hematocrit 29%, potassium 2.8, BUN 24 mg/dl, IV D_5W at 125 cc/hr. into L forearm, 2 bloody BMs during the past 4 hours in the ED, has not voided in the ED, height 5 ft. 6 in., weight 115 lbs., Na 142, Cl 98, creatinine 0.08 mg/dl. Admitting orders left by the gastroenterologist and general surgeon: Admit to medical unit, NPO except ice chips, IV fluid of D_5RL at 150 cc/hr., up in chair qid, plan for esophagastroduodenoscopy (EGD) and colonoscopy today at 1400; if begins vomiting insert NG tube and connect to low intermittent suction, irrigate NG tube prn.

Focus Questions

1. What additional assessment data need to be obtained regarding the elimination functional health pattern?
   - **What may have started this diarrhea?**
   - **What interventions helped to resolve any past episodes of diarrhea?**
   - **Has anything increased or decreased the diarrhea? Have you had any discomfort during the past 30 hours? Are you having any discomfort now? Describe.**
   - **Abdominal assessment: bowel sounds, distention, tenderness, flatulence, soft/firm.**
   - **Assess perineal and anal area for signs of skin irritation.**
   - **Assess recent physiologic stress such as bacterial or viral infection, altered eating pattern, long distance travel.**
   - **Assess change in usual diet: Within 48 hours to the onset of the red BM's, had she eaten spicy food or eaten at a restaurant? Obtain a 24-hour dietary history, noting significant increase in bulk-forming foods or fluids.**
   - **Assess recent significant increase in physical activity.**
   - **What was the volume for each BM she has had over the past 2 days?**
   - **When was the last time she took the Metamucil?**
   - **Describe her normal bowel pattern and characteristics of stool.**
2. Develop two priority nursing diagnoses and plan of care for Colleen. Indicate independent and collaborative interventions, rationale, and evaluative criteria.

   Priority #1: Diarrhea R/T inflammation, irritation or malabsorption as evidenced by bright red blood and watery bowel movements every 2–3 hours

   Desired Outcome: Client will return to more normal stool consistency

INDEPENDENT NURSING INTERVENTIONS

Intervention	Rationale	Evaluative Criteria
Observe & record stool characteristics	Assess severity of illness	Stool returns to client's normal characteristics
Observe & record precipitating factors	Help differentiate individual triggers & needs	Verify triggering effect
Promote bedrest, provide bedside commode	Rest will decrease intestinal motility and metabolic rate	Decreased frequency of BMs
Remove stool promptly, provide room deodorizer	Control odor & promote positive self-concept	Client will not be anxious with visitors in the room
Identify foods/fluids that precipitate diarrhea	Avoid intestinal irritants to promote healing & prevent future illness	Client able to identify irritants & avoids irritants.
When intake permitted, start with small amounts of clear liquids, avoid cold fluids	Promotes intestinal rest, minimal intestinal motility to prevent diarrhea	Intake resumed without cramping or frequent liquid BMs
Provide opportunities to discuss concerns & feeling R/T disease	Promote understanding of illness & effective coping	Client verbalizes concerns & feelings

COLLABORATIVE INTERVENTIONS

Intervention	Rationale	Evaluative Criteria
Administer medications appropriately if ordered	Promote healing	Desired & undesired effects of medications are assessed before & after administration & recorded
Prepare client for diagnostic studies & surgery (EGD, colonoscopy)	Client understands purpose of procedures & potential outcomes. Physician will be able to visualize intestines and prevent injury	Client verbalizes purpose, potential outcomes, & post-procedure follow-up

Priority #2: Risk for fluid volume deficit R/T diarrhea as evidenced by liquid BMs every 2–3 hr for 30 hours

Desired Outcome: Client will attain and maintain fluid balance

INDEPENDENT NURSING INTERVENTIONS

Intervention	Rationale	Evaluative Criteria
Monitor & record intake & output, including diaphoresis & urine specific gravity	Assess hydration level, renal & bowel function	Intake will equal or exceed output by maximum of 500cc/24 hr. Urine output will exceed 30cc/hr. yellow color. Normal specific gravity
Assess BP, P, T (cardiac output, SVR if appropriate)	Indicates response to fluid balance	Values are within normal limits

Assess skin turgor, moisture level of skin & mucous membranes, capillary refill	Indicates hydration level	Skin elastic, warm and dry, moist mucous membranes, capillary refill less than 3 seconds
Weigh daily	Indicates fluid balance & nutritional status	Weight gain correlates with other signs of improved hydration & nutrition.
Monitor & report bleeding, stool for guiac daily	Blood in stool should stop, indicating healing, altered nutrition intake & digestion can alter coagulation & increase risk for hemorrhage	No signs of bleeding or skin ecchymosis. Negative guiac
Assess skeletal muscle strength & peripheral pulses. Assess for cardiac dysrhythmias	Electrolyte imbalance may result from excess output causing weakness & increased excitability	Normal muscle tone, Normal sinus rhythm, peripheral pulses strong & regular

COLLABORATIVE INTERVENTIONS

Intervention	Rationale	Evaluative Criteria
Administer parenteral fluids, blood transfusions	Replace lost fluids and cells	Serum Hct and Hgb at safe level, urine output yellow, greater than 30cc/hr. Electrolytes at normal level
Monitor laboratory studies: potassium, sodium, chloride, magnesium, ABGs, Hgb, HCT	Indicates electrolyte & acid-base balance and effectiveness of interventions	Values in normal range
Administer medications	Promote healing & symptom control	Desired & undesired effects of medications are assessed before & after administration & recorded

3. Identify a discharge plan based on known data and the usual management of clients with this disease.

Intervention	Rationale	Evaluative Criteria
Assess resources & client ability to shop for &prepare meals	May have poor activity tolerance R/T fluid, electrolyte, blood, nutritional status	Client able to shop for and prepare meals without difficulty and still have energy to eat the meal.
Consult social service	To arrange home health aid, meals on wheels & financial consultation for hospital bill	Client's living area is clean, safe, has healthy meals, able to pay home and hospital bills

Educate client on home medications (prescriptions)	**Promote knowledge, understanding and healing**	**Client fills prescriptions, takes medications as prescribed, knows what to report to physician**
Educate client on disease process, precipitating factors, need for follow-up and related health promotion activities	**Promote rapid healing & prevent recurrence. Promote healthy lifestyle**	**Normal BMs. Activity tolerance, verbalized understanding of disease, precipitating factors, satisfying health promotion activities. Makes & keeps follow-up appointment. No recurrence in one year.**
Identify support groups and method of communication (local meetings, phone calls, Internet sites)	**Client's values, resources, time, self-concept influence accessing support groups. Support groups assist clients to cope effectively**	**Client verbalizes and demonstrates effective coping**

4. What should Sam do to promote safety and ensure that the client is up in the chair as prescribed?

   Assess for orthostatic hypotension. Document and maintain bed rest until free of orthostatic hypotension. Have chair within 2 feet of bed, assist client to wear nonslip footwear, have nurse call system within easy grasp, educate client on use of call system and symptoms to report. Begin at 15 minutes and gradually increase time in chair as tolerated. Plan for urgent restroom need. If client is weak, assist transfer with gait/transfer belt. If eating, then assist client into chair for meals.

5. If Sam has an unlicensed assistive personnel (UAP) as a team member, what client care tasks of Colleen might he delegate to the UAP and how should he determine this?

   - **Determine agency protocol and UAP competencies**
   - **Monitor and record vital signs except in relation to blood transfusion, assist to and from BSC and chair, assist with bath, dressing, oral and hair care, back rub, monitor and record oral intake and output, administer enema if ordered as procedure prep, assist with nutrition as appropriate, report to Sam urgently observations such as pink/red/black BM, vomiting, dizziness, or confusion**

6. What are the responsibilities of Sam in preparing Colleen for the EGD and colonoscopy?

   Assess for and notify physician of allergies or undesirable responses to sedation medications. Assess client's knowledge and understanding of the procedure and expected outcomes. Ask client to sign and Sam can witness client signing the Informed Consent for the procedures. (Responsibilities may be different dependent on agency. Sam's signature indicates witnessing client signing form only.) If client does not understand the procedures, then document this concern, inform physician, and delay having client sign form (Urbanski, 1997). Usually client is given a preparation to cleanse the bowel, but with Colleen's condition, this may not be needed. Maintain NPO to keep bowel clear and prevent nausea and vomiting with the sedation used during the procedures. Ensure client has secure and correct identification bracelet. Tape rings onto fingers. Some agencies require clients to remove and give all jewelry to significant other, and then nurse or UAP must record what jewelry was given to whom.

During the admission assessment and interview, Colleen informs Sam that the bleeding had started 4 days earlier after she used an enema to relieve constipation. Colleen complains of a dry mouth, thirst, and hunger and requests something to eat and drink. Sam assists her to sit in a chair, provides her with a cup of ice chips, and explains that the physician does not want her to eat anything except ice chips. Suddenly Colleen complains of severe nausea and has an emesis of 100cc of mucous and bright red blood.

Focus Questions

1. What should Sam do within the first 5 minutes after the emesis?

   Assess BP, P, R, level of consciousness, risk for aspiration, continued nausea, and safety to assist Colleen back to bed. If BP decreased and or P increased, then call for assistance to assist Colleen back to bed. Provide oral care. Stop ice chips (initiate NPO). Check orders for possible NG tube.

2. What should Sam do within the first 30 minutes?

   Assess breath sounds. Assist back to bed. Assess abdomen for pain or tenderness, distention, bowel sounds, firmness. Educate Colleen on NG tube purpose and insertion. Insert NG tube verifying correct placement per agency procedure. Connect to low intermittent suction. Assess NG output over 5 minutes. Inform physician of bloody emesis, continued nausea, vital signs, assessment data, NG output, NPO status, and Colleen's reported use of enema for constipation. Be prepared to inform physician of current lab values and intake and output totals.

3. What periodic assessments should be done? State timing.

   Assess BP, P, R, and level of consciousness every 15 minutes for 1 hour, then hourly ×2, then q4h. Assess breath sounds, comfort level, abdomen, urine, and NG output hourly ×3, then q4h.

The physician is informed of the hematemesis and the client's condition. The physician leaves the following orders: STAT hemoglobin (Hbg) and hematocrit (HCT), type and screen for 2 units of packed red cells (PRC), transfuse 2 units of PRC if Hbg is less than 8.4, obtain surgical consent for exploratory laparotomy and possible colostomy or ileostomy, surgery to immediately follow the EGD and colonoscopy.

Focus Questions

1. What information should be given to Colleen regarding the lab work?

   She should be informed of the tests ordered and that a lab technician would arrive in 15 minutes to draw the blood. She should be informed of the purpose of the tests and the order for transfusion.

2. When informed of the possible colostomy, Colleen cries stating she would "rather die than become so disfigured!" How might Sam respond?

   "You sound very upset about the possibility of a colostomy."

   "Tell me what you know about a colostomy." Sam needs to promote Colleen's verbalization of her feelings.

Colleen returns from surgery with an ileostomy. The ileostomy is draining 200 cc of green liquid every 3 hours. Colleen calls Sam to her bedside and requests Sam to immediately check her abdomen as it "feels wet." Sam finds the pouch leaking, loosened from the skin, and full. Colleen closed her eyes when Sam lifted the linens to examine her.

Focus Questions

1. How should Sam respond to Colleen closing her eyes during the exam?

   Sam should share the observation that Colleen closed her eyes while her abdomen was being examined. Then continue to explore Colleen's fears and feelings about her abdomen and the ileostomy. Sam will need to help Colleen to accept and cope effectively with the change in her body image. Colleen will need to be able to look at the ileostomy and then touch it.

2. Describe nutritional needs and potential problems of clients with an ileostomy.

   - **Risk for fluid and electrolyte imbalance because of high volume output.**
   - **Need to eat balanced meals plus 2,000–3,000 cc of fluid per day. Avoid high fiber food because it could further increase intestinal motility and thus output.**
   - **Promote healthy abdominal skin by emptying the pouch about 1 hour after eating. Avoid allowing the pouch to be more than three-fourths full so as to prevent leakage and premature loosening of the pouching appliance. Use and maintain an appropriate pouching system to prevent skin irritation and minimize expenses.**

3. What are the critical concepts Colleen needs to know prior to discharge from the hospital?

   - **Progress in psychosocial adjustment to living with an ileostomy.**
   - **Expected effluent volume, frequency, and characteristics. Signs and symptoms to report to physician.**
   - **Procedure for emptying the pouch.**
   - **Procedure for changing the pouching system.**
   - **Methods to prevent leakage while sleeping.**
   - **Appropriate method to care for incision line.**
   - **The name and phone number of a resource person such as Enterostomal RN to call for concerns and questions.**
   - **How and where to obtain supplies. Method of paying for supplies; amount insurance will cover.**

Reflective Writing

How might a nurse help you if you were faced with the situation Colleen is experiencing—young, unmarried, and with an ileostomy? What could the nurse do to help Colleen's boyfriend deal with helping Colleen to cope with this body image change?

Colleen needs time to talk about her fears, feelings, sexuality, and perception of altered body image. It is important that the nurse be able to gently encourage her to explore her feelings. The nurse should demonstrate acceptance and respect for Colleen. It may be helpful to tell Colleen that other young people are living normal lifestyles with an ileostomy. With Colleen's permission the nurse can explain the appearance and function of the ileostomy and Colleen's concerns. The boyfriend needs to be aware of his response to Colleen's change in body function and appearance. He needs to be accepting of Colleen and coping effectively in order to try to help Colleen. Her boyfriend may know Colleen's strengths and usual coping strategies. With this information the nurse can develop a plan to help Colleen cope.

References

Doenges, M., Moorhouse, M., & Geissler, A. (2000). *Nursing care plans: Guidelines for individualizing patient care*, 5th ed. Philadelphia: F.A. Davis.

Ignatavicius, D., Workman, M. & Mishler, M., (1999). *Medical-surgical nursing across the health care continuum*, 3rd ed., Philadelphia: W. B. Saunders Company.

Kozier, B., Erb, G., Berman, A., & Burke, K. (2000). *Fundamentals of nursing: Concepts, process, and practice*, 6th ed. Upper Saddle River, N.J.: Prentice Hall.

Simpson, K. (1997) Unlicensed assistive personnel: What nurses need to know. *Lifelines* 1, (3) 26–31.

Urbanski, P. (1997) Getting the go-ahead: Helping patients understand informed consent. *Lifelines* 1(3), 45–48.

CASE# 14 MARTY DICKERSON

Learning Objectives

1. Identify pertinent assessment data for a client experiencing multiple trauma.
2. Identify pertinent diagnostic tests for a client experiencing multiple trauma.
3. List nursing diagnoses and independent nursing interventions for a client with multiple trauma.
4. Identify goals of care in the post-anesthesia care unit (PACU) including critical assessment data.
5. Prioritize nursing diagnosis and interventions and describe discharge planning for a client following abdominal surgery.

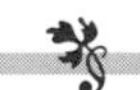

Marty Dickinson is a 35-year-old married father of two. He is driving home from work on the interstate at 65 mph when a car crosses the median and strikes his vehicle head-on. Marty, not wearing a seat belt, is thrown forward against the steering wheel. The front of the car is crushed, the steering wheel traps his torso, and the dashboard traps his lower extremities. Extrication takes 45 minutes; he is then flown to a Level I Trauma Center. He has two IV lines in place with #14 angiocath and is immobilized on a backboard with a cervical collar. His knees are flexed. The flight nurse notes that he has severe abdominal pain and is unable to lay with his legs flat. Vital signs during the flight are BP 90/60, P 120, R 36, oxygen saturation 88%. Supplemental oxygen is administered at 15 L/m via non-rebreather facemask. Other obvious injuries include contusions and edema in both knees. Distal pulses in the lower extremities are present.

Focus Questions

1. What should Marty's initial physical assessment include? Identify specific problems you are looking for and immediate actions.

- **Airway with Cervical Spine Immobilization**
  - **Open and maintain an open airway, use adjuncts as necessary.**
  - **Maintain cervical spine immobilization**
  - **Look for signs of airway obstruction in the mouth, oropharynx, and throat as manifested by dyspnea, diminished breath sounds with respiratory effort, hoarseness or stridor, dysphagia, and/or drooling.**
  - **Does patient need an airway created: intubation, cricothyrotomy, or tracheostomy?**

- Breathing
  - **Look, listen, and feel.**
  - **Is the patient breathing?**
  - **Is breathing effective or is assistance necessary with a bag-valve-mask or mechanical ventilation?**
  - **What is oxygen saturation level, blood gases, end-tidal carbon dioxide monitoring?**
  - **Place high flow oxygen (i.e., non-rebreather mask at 15–20 L/m; positive pressure ventilation).**
  - **If breathing is inadequate, consider presence of chest trauma including pneumothorax/tension pneumothorax, hemothorax, and ruptured diaphragm, open or sucking chest wound, flail chest segment. These will need immediate correction to improve breathing.**
- Circulation
  - **Presence of apical, symmetrical carotid, femoral, and distal extremity pulses.**
  - **Brisk capillary refill less than 2 sec.**
  - **Blood pressure greater than 100 systolic.**
  - **Cardiac rate and rhythm: regular and between 60–100.**
  - **Skin color and temperature, including inspection of mucous membranes.**
  - **Bleeding controlled.**
  - **Alterations indicate possible hypovolemia immediate fluid replacement. #14–16 angiocath (2)**
  - **Start with crystalloid solutions (normal saline or lactated ringers' solution) until blood products available.**
- Disability
  - **Maintain cervical spine immobilization.**
  - **Quick neuroexamination for LOC/ behavior and motor function.**
  - **Glasgow Coma Scale**
  - **PMS (pulse, movement, sensation)**
  - **If possible identify presence of alcohol or drugs.**

2. Assessment secondary survey is completed. Which diagnostic tests should be obtained immediately?

- Laboratory

  Urine/complete urinalysis or dipstick
  Complete blood count
  Chemistry profile include amylase, BUN
  Arterial blood gases
  Type and cross match for blood products

- Radiology

  Cervical spine (cross table films to clear spine are always first)
  KUB/abdominal CT
  Pelvis
  Chest
  Lower extremities

- *Other*

  EKG
  Peritoneal lavage

3. In addition to actual assessments being completed, what additional information regarding the mechanism of injuries and the accident is important to your data collection? Where would that information be obtained?

   - **Description of the incident**
   - **Description and/or pictures of the vehicles involved including speed, area of impact, condition of passenger compartment, use of seat belts, deployment of airbags, star patterns on windows, condition of steering wheel, dashboard**
   - **Need for extrication, and/or self-extrication**
   - **Condition of other persons involved (a fatality from any vehicle involved increases the risk for all persons involved)**
   - **Run report from responding fire and rescue units**
   - **Report from flight crew**

4. Identify and prioritize nursing diagnoses, with independent nursing interventions for Marty.

Nursing Diagnoses	• **Ineffective breathing patterns** • **Impaired gas exchange** • **Decreased cardiac output** • **Fluid volume deficit** • **Altered tissue perfusion**
Independent Interventions	• **Open and/or maintain patent airway, while keeping cervical spine immobilized until cleared by x-ray** • **Assist with ventilatory support maintain respiratory rate between 12 and 20, oxygen saturation greater than 92%,** • **PaO_2 greater than 60mmHG** • **Administer and monitor fluid volume replacement** • **Monitor hemodynamic status** • **Insert Foley catheter and nasogastric tube** • **Reassess Glasgow coma scale (GCS)** • **Provide care and treatment of other injuries** • **Tetanus booster if open wounds** • **Emotional support and explanations to Marty and family** • **Preparation for emergency laparotomy**

Despite fluid resuscitation, Marty's hemodynamic status continues to deteriorate and he is transferred to the OR for an exploratory laparotomy. Marty is transferred in stable condition to the post-anesthesia care unit (PACU) following a laparotomy with repairs to lacerations of the spleen and mesenteric vasculature. The urinary tract was free of injury. There is no repair needed to the knees.

Focus Questions

1. The goals of care in the PACU are to identify actual and potential problems that may occur as a result of anesthetic administration and surgical intervention and to intervene appropriately. What critical assessments are required? Include specifics for each identified area.

Respiratory	• **Airway patency** • **Secretions** • **Airway adjuncts** • **Breathing pattern, quality, type, rate** • **Breath sounds** • **Oxygen saturation**
Cardiovascular	• **Heart sounds** • **Blood pressure** • **Heart rate, rhythm, quality** • **EKG** • **Distal extremity pulse and capillary refill**
Neurological	• **Level of consciousness** • **Response to touch, pain** • **Gag reflex** • **Pain level**
Surgical site	• **Dressing dry and intact** • **Location and number of drains** • **Presence of bleeding and/or drainage**
Renal	• **Urine color** • **Intake and output**

2. What are the criteria that indicate the patient is stable and eligible for discharge from the PACU?

Patient is awake or at preoperative baseline, vital signs are stable, no excessive drainage or bleeding, respirations spontaneous and greater than 10, oxygen saturation greater than 90%, temperature greater than 96°F.

Marty is transferred to the medical surgical unit in stable condition. He is awake and continues to have oxygen by mask. His surgical site is a midline incision closed with staples and covered with a dry sterile dressing (DSD). His family is waiting on the unit. Assessment findings on arrival:

VS:	**T: 100.1°, BP: 100/70, P: 102, R: 24**
Airway:	**Patent, breath sounds present bilaterally**
Circulation:	**Skin cool, pale, good capillary refill, radial and pedal pulses present**
Neurological:	**Awake, responds to questions, denies pain, received $MS0_4$ in PACU**
	Moves all extremities on command
	Pupils are equal and responsive to light
Renal:	**Foley catheter in place draining amber urine**
Surgical site:	**Abdominal incision with DSD, dry and intact, no drainage noted**
	Jackson Pratt (JP) drain bulb from stab wound in LUQ
	Abdomen is soft without tenderness except around the incision site
Other:	**IV fluids lactated ringers at 150/hr; infusing into right forearm with #16 angiocath**
	NG: to suction, no drainage

Focus Question

1. Prioritize nursing diagnoses for Marty related to the patient following abdominal surgery. Identify appropriate nursing interventions for diagnoses.

Ineffective Breathing	• **Maintain patent airway** • **Cough and deep breathing, splint incision** • **Turn and position, ambulate as soon as possible** • **Monitor for signs or symptoms of atelectasis and pulmonary embolism**
Fluid Volume Deficit	• **Monitor vital signs** • **Maintain appropriate IV fluids and oral fluids as soon as possible** • **Monitor surgical site for drainage and hemorrhage** • **Monitor GI and urinary status** • **Record I and O**
Pain, acute	• **Provide comfort measures: turn and position, ambulate** • **Keep bed linens straightened** • **Mouth care as needed** • **Cool cloths, or heat as permitted** • **Massage** • **Relaxation and imaging or other distraction measures** • **Pain medication as needed, especially before procedures before activity** • **Encourage if available, use of patient controlled analgesia**
Impaired skin integrity **Risk for infection**	• **Sterile or optimal aseptic wound care** • **Good nutrition as permitted** • **Maintain optimal fluid intake** • **Ambulate when permitted**
Risk for altered elimination	• **Promote optimal urinary tract elimination** • **Note urine in drainage bag for color, consistency, odor, and amount** • **Monitor I and O** • **Promote return of peristalsis, noting presence of bowel sounds and flatus** • **Encourage ambulation** • **Encourage fluid intake** • **Assess for abdominal pain, distention, tenderness not associated with incision**

Marty is being discharged after an unremarkable postoperative course. His Foley catheter, IV, and NG tube were removed previously. Today his staples were replaced with steri-strips, and the JP was removed. He is to follow-up with his surgeon in 5 days. His diet is now as tolerated. He ambulates without assistance.

Focus Questions

1. What information would assist the health care team in planning for Marty's discharge?

   Occupation, education, family status—and dynamics, home environment (physical), daily routine, diet, substance use (tobacco, alcohol, drugs), chronic medical problems (patient and/or family), transportation resources, financial resources

2. What discharge instructions should Marty receive?

   Activity, prescriptions, wound care and signs of infection, nutrition and fluid needs, management of any elimination problem, complications related to surgery and action to take, follow-up care

Reflective Writing

How would you implement a trauma prevention educational program to reduce the incidence of injuries similar to Marty's? Include some age-related strategies.

- **Awareness of causative factors for traumatic injuries and fatalities from motor vehicle crashes**
- **Use of safety devices such as helmets, seatbelts, age appropriate child restraints, and other supplemental and passive restraint devices**
- **Reduction of alcohol and other substances that impair judgment**
- **Implications of driver age and inexperience especially in adverse weather conditions**
- **Awareness of how distractions such as shaving or makeup application, hairstyling, newspaper reading, adjusting sound systems, etc. can result in loss of vehicle control and/or driver concentration**

References

Kidd, P. & Wagner, K. (1997). *High acuity nursing*, 2nd ed. Stamford, Conn.: Appleton & Lange.

O'Keefe, M., et al. (1998). *Brady's emergency care*, 8th ed. Upper Saddle River, N.J.: Prentice Hall, Inc.

CASE # 15 TOMMY BENNETT

Learning Objectives

1. Discuss the clinical manifestations of tuberculosis (TB).
2. Discuss the pathophysiology of TB.
3. List nursing diagnoses and interventions for a client with TB.
4. Describe diagnostic tests commonly used to diagnose TB.
5. Identify drugs commonly used in treatement.
6. Discuss areas of importance in discharge planning for clients with TB.
7. Reflect on feelings related to homelessness.

0900. January 21 in a Northeastern inner-city. The police bring a 40-year-old male, Tommy Bennett, to the emergency room for possible frostbite to his toes bilaterally. He was found living below a bridge in a cardboard box in a homeless area with many other individuals. He is 5 ft. 10 in. tall and weighs 145 lbs. He reports fatigue, weight loss of 20 pounds over the last month despite no change in his usual nutrition, loss of appetite, chills, and night sweats. The nurse immediately places him in isolation in a negative airflow room.

Focus Questions

1. Determine from the current clinical data why the nurse placed the client in a negative airflow isolation room. (Use the following questions to guide your discussion.)
   a. In addition to the frostbite, considering the client's lifestyle and clinical data, for what major health problem is he most at risk and why?
   b. What clinical and lifestyle data will assist you on your decision?
   c. What other populations are also at risk for this major health problem and why?

   a. *Tuberculosis*

   Currently, tuberculosis primarily affects racial and ethnic minorities as well as the poor and homeless. These populations are more likely to use emergency departments rather than primary care physicians and typically do not practice primary, secondary, or tertiary levels of prevention.

   b. Tommy Bennett fits the profile for people who are at the greatest risk for contracting TB. He is homeless and lives in an area with many other individuals.

   Tommy Bennett's clinical manifestations suggestive of TB are:

   - **Weight loss of 20 pounds over the last month despite no change in his usual nutrition**
   - **Anorexia**
   - **Night sweats**

   Additional clinical manifestations of TB are:

   - **Low-grade afternoon fever**
   - **Initially a dry cough that becomes productive**
   - **Purulent and/or blood tinged sputum**

   c. Poor urban areas have seen an increased incidence of tuberculosis because of homelessness, malnutrition, and poor living conditions. These people are difficult to reach for primary, secondary, and tertiary preventive practices. Prolonged contact with infected persons increases the risk of exposure. A less-than-optimal immune system increases the susceptibility of the host. At-risk populations include:

   - **People in close contact with someone who has active TB**
   - **People without adequate health care. Young adults between 15–44 years of age frequently fall into this category.**
   - **People living in overcrowded, substandard housing**
   - **Overcrowded institutions such as: hospitals, homeless shelters, drug treatment enters, prisons, and residential facilities**
   - **Native Americans and Alaskan natives, non-Hispanic blacks, and Asian/Pacific islanders**
   - **Older adults and people with AIDS**
   - **Injection drug users and alcoholics**

1100. Tommy is admitted to a negative flow isolation room on a medical surgical unit for treatment of frostbite and to rule out active pulmonary tuberculosis (TB).

Focus Questions

1. Relate Tommy's current manifestations to the pathophysiology of active pulmonary TB.

   TB is a communicable disease caused by the bacterium *Mycobacterium tuberculosis.* It is spread from person to person through the inhalation of airborne particles (droplet nuclei) containing M. tuberculosis. These particles become airborne when an infected person forcefully exhales, coughs, sneezes, speaks, or sings. These infectious particles can remain suspended in the air and inhaled by someone sharing the same air. TB infection may occur when droplet nuclei are inhaled and then move down the trachea into the lungs until they reach the alveoli. However, the majority of infected people will not develop the disease. Alveolar inflammation and cellular reaction produces a small white, firm primary tubercle or *Ghon* focus. The center of the tubercle becomes necrotic and the liquefied material is expectorated, producing a cavity in the parenchyma, which is visible on a chest x-ray. If the immune system is adequate, scar tissue develops around the tubercle, encapsulating the bacilli. These calcified lesions are visible on an X-ray. A dormant form of TB can last for years. Reactivation can occur if the person becomes immunocompromised. Clinical manifestations of active pulmonary TB are often insidious and are initially nonspecific.

2. What additional screening methods, laboratory and diagnostic tests would the nurse expect to be ordered for this client? Describe each test and what constitutes significant findings.

Tuberculin test

Within 3–10 weeks after exposure to TB, a cellular or delayed hypersensitivity to the bacillus develops. An intradermal injection of a small amount of purified protein derivative (PPD) will activate this response after the hypersensitivity to the bacillus develops. Significant findings 48–72 hours after the test include:

- **greater than 15 mm induration is a positive response**
- **10–15 mm induration is a positive response for people who are in the high risk categoty**
- **5–9 mm induration is a positive response for people who: Are in close contact with someone with active TB, have an abnormal chest x-ray, and have HIV.**

Sputum Tests for the presence of the bacillus

Three consecutive early morning sputum specimens are sent for acid-fast and bacilli smear and culture.

Chest X-ray for the presence of dense lesions and possible cavity formation

Fiberoptic Bronchoscopy and Bronchial Washing **to obtain cultures from the client who is unable to produce a sputum specimen**

3. Discuss the pharmacological and surgical interventions to prevent and treat TB.

   - *Pharmacology*

   A newly diagnosed client is started on a combination of three antitubercular drugs, Isoniazid (INH), Rifampin, and Pyrazinamide, which are administered orally, daily, for the first two months. Four additional months with INH and Rifampin daily or weekly is prescribed. HIV infected TB clients are prescribed a combination of the three drugs for nine months.

   - *Surgery*

   A portion of the lung may be resected where the disease is localized or cavitation occurs and when the bacillus is resistant to the medications.

4. Describe prophylactic treatment for newly diagnosed clients and with noncompliant clients.

   Clients whose skin test converts from negative to positive without evidence of active pulmonary TB as defined through negative chest x-rays or sputum specimens or who have no other risk factors will be placed on single-dose drug therapy of INH for 6–9 months. When compliance is a problem, medications are administered under direct supervision twice weekly.

5. Apply the principle related to the spread of droplet nuclei to develop nursing interventions to prevent the spread of infection during Tommy's hospitalization, and when he is discharged.

   Because of the emergence of drug-resistance tuberculosis in large cities and HIV positive people, nursing care needs to focus on infection control and compliance with the treatment regime. Tuberculosis is spread by microscopic airborne droplets and thus requires respiratory precautions to prevent the spread of infection. While Tommy is in the hospital, respiratory precautions will include:

   - **Placing the client in a private room with negative airflow. Negative airflow control prevents air within the room from circulating into the hallway or other rooms. Air within these rooms is diluted with at least six fresh air exchanges per hour.**
   - **Maintaining universal precautions**
   - **Initiating tuberculosis isolation techniques, which includes personal protective devices such as the Occupational Safety and Health Administration (OSHA) required HEPA-filtered respirators to prevent occupational exposure to tuberculosis.**
   - **Placing a mask on the client when transporting to other areas of the hospital**
   - **Informing all personnel having contact with the client**
   - **Instructing visitors to mask prior to entering the client's room**

Tommy is discharged seven days after admission. He was diagnosed with active pulmonary TB. Discharge instructions related to his TB are written as follows: home health nurse to administer INH, Rifampin and Pyrazinamide twice weekly for the next two months. Chest x-ray and sputum specimens monthly for the next three months, avoid crowds and close physical contact, use respiratory precautions for the next two weeks.

Focus Questions

1. Plan the discharge for Tommy using each of the following focus areas: referral, client teaching, prevention of infection, and monitoring of drug toxicity and side effects.

   a. Referral

   - **Shelter placement or other housing and easily accessed and ongoing health care follow-up.**
   - **Public Health Department for management and follow-up.**

   b. Client teaching

   Teach the client how to collect sputum specimens and the importance of compliance with the treatment for the entire course of the regimen.

c. **Prevention of spread of infection**

Teach the client to:

- **Always cough and expectorate into tissues**
- **Properly dispose of tissues by placing them in a closed bag**
- **Wear a mask if unable to control respiratory secretions**

d. **Monitoring of drug toxicity/side effects**

- ***Isoniazid (INH, Laniazid, Nydrazid, Isotamine, Teebaconin)* adverse reactions are numbness and tingling of the extremities, hepatotoxicity that is diagnosed with abnormal liver function studies and scleral jaundice, and hypersensitivity reactions such a rash, anemia, bruising, and bleeding.**
- ***Rifampin (Rifadin, Rimactane, RoFact)* is low in toxicity but can produce hepatitis and occasionally renal failure.**
- ***Pyrazinamide (Tebrazid)* can cause liver toxicity**

Other anti-tuberculosis drugs include:

- ***Ethambutol Hydrochloride (Myambutol)* principal toxic effect is optic neuritis**
- ***Streptomycin* is ototoxic and toxic to the kidneys**

2. Prioritize a list of Nursing Diagnoses with three nursing interventions for each diagnosis.

Knowledge deficit related to medications, management of the disease, and prevention of the spread of infection.

- **Assess Tommy's knowledge about the disease process and medications.**
- **Assess Tommy's ability to learn, and his developmental level and interest in learning.**
- **Teach Tommy about tuberculosis, respiratory isolation, purpose, dosage, and side effects of his medications.**

Risk for infection related to spreading tuberculosis to others

- **Teach Tommy about measures to prevent the spread of the infection.**
- **Teach Tommy how to collect sputum specimens.**
- **Teach Tommy about the importance of compliance with the therapeutic treatment.**

Risk for noncompliance related to lack of resources

- **Refer to Social Services for follow-up.**
- **Develop a relationship of trust that will facilitate open discussion with Tommy about his disease.**
- **Institute a treatment program that best fits his lifestyle.**

Reflective Writing

If you were the home health nurse visiting Tommy in his box shelter under the bridge, how would you feel about providing his follow-up care in this environment? How might your personal feelings impact the nursing care you give Tommy?

Homelessness can evoke many feelings including disgust, pity, and ambivalence. It is important to first get in touch with your feelings about homeless people. Awareness is crucial in establishing a therapeutic relationship with your client so that you do not project these feelings when relating to them.

References

Smeltzer, S. & Bare, B. (1996). *Brunner and Suddarth's textbook of medical surgical nursing,* 8th Ed. Philadelphia: Lippincott.

LeMone, P. & Burke, K. (2000). *Medical surgical nursing: Critical thinking in client care,* 2nd Ed. Menlo Park, Calif.: Addison-Wesley.

Hermey, C. (1995). *Nursing management of tuberculosis: Instructor's resource booklet for Mosby's medical-surgical nursing video series.* Philadelphia: Mosby-Year Book, Inc.

CASE # 16 HUANG MEI LAN, RICHARD TANNER, JANE HOUSE, TIMOTHY MURPHY, AND STEVE CRON

Learning Objectives

1. Differentiate between the five types of shock including assessment, nursing diagnoses, pharmacologic, and therapeutic nursing interventions.
2. Reflect on how to handle a parent who wants to be with their child during resuscitation in the emergency department.

***The instructor may wish to assign each student group a different client. Similarities and differences of various types of shock could be discussed by the whole class.**

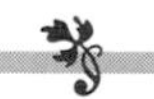

Client 1 Huang Mei Lan is a 43-year-old unmarried female who lives alone in a major West Coast city. Three years ago she was diagnosed with breast cancer and underwent a mastectomy of the affected breast and follow-up chemotherapy. Last month, Ms. Lan experienced a recurrence of cancer in at the lymph glands of the affected side. Surgery to remove the glands was performed and chemotherapy started. Ms. Lan has a central line, a urinary catheter, and a surgical incision. The nurse enters Ms. Lan's room and find her huddled in the middle of the bed, shivering violently.

Client 2 Richard Tanner, a 49-year-old truck driver, was admitted earlier this morning through the ER for chest pain. He was admitted to the CCU for r/o myocardial infarction (MI). He has no prior history of cardiac problems, however, he has been treated for the past 5 years for a total cholesterol of 285 (HDL 35, LDL 212). He was prescribed Mevacor, which he doesn't take regularly. He was recently diagnosed with hypertension with his normal BP 160/96 for which he doesn't take medication. He is overweight and exercises little. His father died of an MI at the age 50. The nurse enters his room and finds him lethargic and dyspneic.

Client 3 Jane House, 20 years old, was admitted to the ER following an MVA (motor vehicle accident) earlier in the day. She was an unrestrained passenger in an automobile that was T-boned by another motor vehicle on her side of the car. She was pinned in the wreckage for 30 minutes and an emergency transport helicopter brought her to the ER. She suffered a partially severed leg, chest contusion, possible fractured pelvis, open head wound, and fractured jaw. She has lost several units of blood. She has been in post-anesthesia care unit (PACU) for the past hour following surgery to reattach her leg and close her head wound. Her vital signs have been stable. The nurse enters the room to find Jane's NG draining copious amounts of sanguineous fluid.

Client 4 Timothy Murphy, 30 years old, was admitted to ICU earlier today from ER following a diving injury. He and his friends were swinging from a rope into a creek below when his head struck the bottom of the creek resulting in a cervical fracture and paralysis from his neck down. He has been alert and oriented, but his vital signs have been labile. He was placed on a ventilator on CMV at 12 BPM. His neck is immobilized in a cervical collar. The nurse enters the room because the ventilator alarms are going off.

Client 5 Steve Cron is a 76-year-old same-day surgery patient admitted to the unit a few minutes ago from PACU following left hip hemi-arthroplasty. The nurse started his second dose of Ancef IV five minutes ago. He calls the nurses's station and complains of itching and shortness of breath. The nurse arrives in his room and finds him extremely restless, anxious, and gasping.

Focus Questions

1. Relate each client's current manifestations to the pathophysiology of shock to determine what type of shock the client could be experiencing.

   Shock is a response of the body to illness or injury. It begins as a compensatory response to changes in the delivery or use of oxygen by tissues. Unless the conditions precipitating the response are treated, shock rapidly becomes a critical condition. As shock progresses, multisystem organ failure follows and death may result. Shock is triggered by a sustained drop in blood pressure.

Client 1, Huang Mei Lan

Septic Shock, warm phase (early phase)—**Begins with septicemia (presence of pathogens and toxins in the blood). As pathogens are destroyed, their ruptured cell membranes allow endotoxins to leak into the plasma. The endotoxins disrupt the vascular system, coagulation mechanism, and immune system and trigger an immune and inflammatory response. If untreated, it progresses from the warm phase (early phase) when cardiac output is high and systemic vascular resistance is low to the cold (late phase) resulting in expansion hypovolemia. Hypovolemia and intravascular coagulation lead to anerobic metabolism, lactic acidosis, and cellular death.**

Client 2, Richard Tanner

Cardiogenic shock—**Is caused by loss of critical contractile function of the heart and results in inadequate cardiac output and tissue perfusion. The most common cause is left ventricular myocardial infarction (MI) resulting in 40% or greater ventricular damage. Other causes that are also related to an MI are papillary muscle rupture, free wall rupture, and ventricular septral rupture. Cardiogenic shock often develops several hours after the onset of MI symptoms, after the client is admitted to the hospital.**

Client 3, Jane House

Hypovolemic shock—**Is the result of inadequate circulating blood volume. It is classified as either depletion or expansion and involves both intracellular and extracellular compartments. The most common cause of depletion hypovolemia is sudden blood loss and severe dehydration. Injuries such as burns cause significant fluid shifts from the intravascular space to the interstitial space resulting in expansion hypovolemia. Shock if untreated results in hypotension, electrolyte and acid-base imbalances, and organ failure from hypoperfusion.**

Client 4, Timothy Murphy

Neurogenic (vasogenic) shock—**Results from loss or disruption of the sympathetic nervous system, which causes peripheral vasodilitation and decreased tissue perfusion. The most common cause of neurogenic shock is a spinal cord injury above T6.**

Client 5, Steve Cron

Anaphylactic shock—**Results from a widespread, life threatening hypersensitive reaction to a specific allergen. It causes vasodilitation, capillary permeability, bronchoconstriction, coronary vasoconstriction, and cutaneous reactions, which result in hypovolemia and impaired tissue perfusion.**

2. Apply principles of collaborative care for clients experiencing shock to determine what the nurse's initial response should be and why.

The major focus of emergency care of the client is maintaining or restoring a level of tissue perfusion to sustain life. Assessment is always the initial action in the nursing process.

- **Obtain vital signs and an initial physical assessment**
- **Maintain a patent airway**
- **Initiate oxygen administration**
- **Obtain an IV access**

Additional interventions are specific to the type of shock

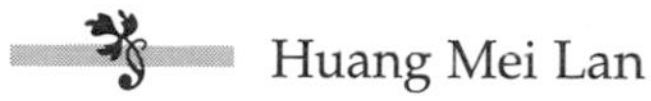

Huang Mei Lan	Her vital signs are: T 104°, P 110, R 30, BP 106/66 Skin—hot, dry, flushed with poor turgor Alert and oriented, restless, and anxious
Richard Tanner	His vital signs are: T 99.2°, P 110, rapid, thready EKG sinus tachycardia with frequent premature ventricular contractions (PVC's) R 30, labored, crackles, wheezing BP 106/66 Skin—pale, cyanotic, cold, and moist
Jane House	Her vital signs are: T 98° P 120, rapid, thready R 30 BP 80/60 Skin-cool, pale, moist, with dependent edema
Timothy Murphy	His vital signs are: T 99.6° P 60 and bounding, BP 82/60 R 28, he is bucking the ventilator Skin—warm and dry Anxious, extremely restless
Steve Cron	His vital signs are: T 100° P 130, and irregular R 40, dyspneic, stridor, wheezing BP 60 with a doppler Skin—warm, generalized edema Anxious, extremely restless

Focus Questions

Answer all the following questions for each client.

1. With this additional data, do you agree with your original interpretation of the kind of shock the client is experiencing? Why or why not?

Huang Mei Lan: Yes—All her symptoms correlate with warm (early phase) septic shock. She is experiencing vasodilation, which results in weakness and warm and flushed skin. Her high fever and chills are caused from septicemia. Here tachycardia and tachypnea indicate that her heart and lungs are compensating for the decreased tissue perfusion sufficiently to maintain a BP of 106/66.

Richard Tanner: Yes—Richard's temperature is within normal limits, his pulse is rapid, indicating that his heart is attempting to compensate for the decreased tissue perfusion through tachycardia, but his pulse is thready because of pump failure. His EKG arrhythmias indicate potential myocardial damage from his MI resulting in a disruption of the normal cardiac conduction system. He is experiencing tachypnea, labored respirations with crackles, and wheezing, which is indicative of congestive heart failure and pulmonary enema as a result of pump failure. Pale, cyanotic, cold, and moist skin are the result of vasoconstriction and the body's attempt to shunt blood to the vital organs. His BP of 106/66 indicates decompensation. Despite all of the body's compensatory efforts, his heart damage is so severe that it is unable to meet the body's metabolic demands.

Jane House: Yes—Considering the initial observation of her loss of several units of blood and her NG draining copious amounts of sanguineous fluid and her current rapid and thready pulse of 120, she is in hypovolemic shock from excessive blood loss. Her tachycardia and tachypnea indicate that her heart and lungs are attempting to compensate. The sympathetic nervous system response of vasoconstriction causes the pale and moist skin. The loss of cellular integrity results in dependent edema. Despite all the compensatory efforts, her thready pulse and BP of 80/60 indicate that the hypovolemia is so severe that her body is unable to meet its metabolic demands and is decompensating.

Timothy Murphy: Yes—Bradycardia occurs early in neurogenic shock. In the early stages, the extremities are warm and pink from venous pooling. Timothy's BP of 82/60 reflects decreasing stroke volume as a result of vasodilation. His anxiety and restlessness are related to hypoxia. Although he is on a ventilator, he is bucking the ventilator, which can cause inadequate oxygenation.

Steve Cron: Yes—Steve received his second IV dose of Ancef, a cephalosporin, a few minutes ago. Anaphylactic shock does not occur with the first exposure to an allergen. Anaphylaxis begins and progresses rapidly. Steve's hypersensitive reaction to this drug released large amounts of histamine and vasoactive amines throughout the circulatory system causing capillary permeability and massive vasodilation. The capillary permeability and vasodilation cause his profound hypotension of a BP of 60 with a doppler and warm skin with generalized edema. His initial symptom of pruritis is consistent with an allergic reaction. Dyspnea, restlessness, anxiety, respiratory rate of 40, stridor, and wheezing are signs of hypoxia related to the bronchoconstriction associated with anaphylaxis. Steve's temperature elevation is most probably related to the normal inflammatory response triggered by his surgery.

2. Now, based on new data, what type of shock is the client experiencing?

   Huang Mei Lan—Septic Shock

   Richard Tanner—Cardiogenic Shock

   Jane House—Hypovolemic Shock

   Timothy Murphy—Neurogenic (vasogenic) Shock

   Steve Cron—Anaphylactic Shock

3. What stage of shock (if applicable)?

   Shock advances through four stages: initial, compensatory, progressive, and irreversible.

Huang Mei Lan, Compensatory. Characterized by her: hypotention, poor skin turgor, increased respirations, rapid pulse, restlessness, and anxiety.

Richard Tanner, Progressive. Characterized by his: hypotension, cardiac dyarrhythmias; pale, cyanotic, cold and moist skin; rapid and thready pulse; and tachypnea.

Jane House, Progressive. Characterized by her: fluid loss of 35%–50% (1,800–2,500 cc); rapid, thready pulse; tachypnea; hypotension; and cool, pale, moist skin with dependent edema.

Timothy Murphy, Progressive. Characterized by his hypotension.

Steve Cron, Progressive. Characterized by his: severe hypotension, tachypnea, and generalized edema.

4. What would be the expected laboratory tests for each client?

   There are no routine laboratory tests to determine shock. Tests are used to assist the identification of the type of shock and assessing the client's response to shock.

   - **Tests to evaluate the effects of shock and the effectiveness of the body's compensatory mechanisms:**

     Arterial Blood Gasses (ABGs)—Determine oxygen, carbon dioxide, and pH levels. Declining compensatory mechanisms result in acidosis (declining pH levels), hypoxia (declining $Pa0_2$), and increasing carbon dioxide ($PaCO_2$).

     Serum Electrolytes—Measure the severity and progression of shock. As the stages of shock progress, glucose and sodium levels decrease, and potassium levels increase.

     Blood Urea Nitrogen (BUN), Serum Creatinine Levels, and Urine Specific Gravity and Osmolality—Measure renal function. As renal perfusion decreases, renal function is reduced. The BUN, creatinine, urine specific gravity, and osmolality increase.

   - **Tests specific to these clients:**

     Huang Mei Lan

     Tests used to evaluate infections:

     White blood count with differential—The total white count is increased in septic shock. Elevated neutrophils indicate acute infection, elevated monocytes indicate bacterial infection, and elevated esinophils indicate an allergic response.

     Blood, urine, wound, central line, and sputum cultures—Determine the source of the infection and the causative organisms.

     Richard Tanner

     Serum cardiac enzymes—Are elevated in cardiogenic shock: lactic dehyrogenase (LDH), creatine phosphokinase (CPK), and serum glutamic-oxaloacetic transaminase (SGOT).

     Jane House

     Blood hemoglobin and hematocrit—Changes in hematocrit concentrations occur in hypovolemic shock. Hypovolemic shock caused by hemorrhage results in lower than normal hemoglobin and hematocrit concentrations. Hypovolemic shock caused by intravascular fluid loss results in higher than normal hemoglobin and hematocrit levels.

     Tests to determine the extent of injury or damage or to locate the site of internal hemorrhage-X-rays, computerized tomography (CT) scans, magnetic resonance imaging (MRI), endoscopy, and echocardiograms.

     Timothy Murphy

     Tests to evaluate the effects of shock and the effectiveness of the body's compensatory mechanisms: ABGs, Serum Electrolytes, Blood Urea Nitrogen (BUN), Serum Creatinine Levels, and Urine Specific Gravity, and Osmolality

     Steve Cron

     Tests to evaluate the effects of shock and the effectiveness of the body's compensatory mechanisms: ABGs, Serum Electrolytes, Blood Urea Nitrogen (BUN), Serum Creatinine Levels, and Urine Specific Gravity, and Osmolality

5. Apply principles of collaborative care for clients experiencing shock to determine what are, in general and specific to each client, the expected medical/pharmaceutical treatments/interventions.

Standard management for all classifications of shock

The focus on nursing care for the client in shock is assessing and monitoring tissue perfusion and meeting the psychosocial needs of the client and his or her family. Assessment begins with a history and a physical assessment. A history of the client's presenting problem will provide clues in determining causative factors and the type of shock. Assessments specific to all classifications of shock are:

- **Vital signs**
- **Level of consciousness (LOC)**
- **Skin turgor, temperature, moisture or dryness, and color**
- **I & O**
- **Hourly urine output and urine color**
- **Peripheral pulses**
- **Hemodynamic monitoring of arterial, pulmonary artery, and central venous pressures**
- **Bowel sounds and abdominal distention**

Regardless of the classification of shock, the following interventions are initiated as soon the condition is diagnosed:

- **Establishing and maintaining a patent airway and adequate oxygenation with oxygen therapy by mask, nasal cannula, or endotracheal entubation**
- **Obtaining intravenous access through two large-bore peripheral lines or a central line**
- **Inserting a Foley catheter in order to monitor hourly urinary output**
- **Maintaining bed rest**

Specific care for each client

Huang Mei Lan

Initiate the standard management interventions. Obtain the appropriate laboratory tests as stated in focus question number 4. Considering her most recent assessment data the nurse should:

- **Administering an IV colloid solution (plasma expander) to maintain an adequate B/P**
- **Administering IV broad-spectrum antibiotics until the portal of entry and the organism are determined to treat the septicemia**
- **Reducing her body temperature with the administration of antipyretics such as acetaminophen and hypothermia blankets to reduce oxygen demands**

Richard Tanner

Initiate the standard management interventions. Obtain the appropriate laboratory tests as stated in focus question 4. Considering his most recent assessment data, the nurse should:

- **Administer a narcotic analgesic such as morphine sulfate IV to minimize sympathetic nervous system response and increase coronary tissue perfusion**

- Monitor EKG for arrhythmias
- Administer antiarrhythmic agents, cardioversion, or pacing as needed
- Correct any acid-base or electrolyte imbalances that could affect cardiac functioning
- Cautiously administer IV fluids, titrate according to left ventricular end diastolic pressures (LVEDP) to maximize cardiac output
- Administer IV inotropic drugs to increase cardiac output and maintain an adequate BP
- Administer vasodilators and mechanical support devices to decrease the workload of the left ventricle
- Initiate percutaneous translumenal coronary angioplasty, thrombolytic therapy, stent placement, and rotoblade therapy to expedite revascularization of the heart
- Maintain supine or semi-Fowler's position to decrease the workload of the left ventricle

Jane House

Initiate the standard management interventions. Obtain the appropriate laboratory tests as stated in focus question 4. Considering her most recent assessment data the nurse should:

- Apply military antishock trousers (MAST) while being transported to the ER to maintain arterial pressure
- Maintain supine position with legs elevated to increase venous return
- Administer IV colloid solutions (plasma expanders) and crystalloid solutions until blood or blood products arrive, to increase the amount of hemoglobin, increase vascular volume, and replace deficient substances such as platelets and clotting factors
- Administer IV inotropic drugs to increase cardiac output and improve tissue perfusion
- Administer IV vasopressors to improve systolic BP
- Administer pain medications
- Administer a tetanus immunization if she is unable to remember when her last tetanus immunization was given

Timothy Murphy

Initiate the standard management interventions. Obtain the appropriate laboratory tests as stated in focus question 4. Considering his most recent assessment data, the nurse should:

- Elevate the head of the bed 20–30 degrees considering his head and neck injury
- Maintain immobility of the spinal column
- Administer an IV colloid solution (plasma expander) to obtain an adequate BP
- Administer IV adrenergic (sympathomimetic) agents with both vasoconstrictors and inotropes to increase systemic blood pressure and increase the force and rate of myocardial contraction
- Administer a sedative or muscle relaxant to reduce Timothy's bucking the ventilator and improve oxygenation

Steve Cron

Initiate the standard management interventions. Obtain the appropriate laboratory tests as stated in focus question 4. Considering his most recent assessment data, the nurse should:

- **Immediately discontinue the Ancef**
- **Establish a patent airway through insertion of an endotracheal tube and initiating mechanical ventilation**
- **Admister IV Epinephrine**
- **Administer an IV colloid solution (plasma expander) to obtain an adequate BP**
- **Administer IV adrenergic (sympathomimetic) agents with both vasoconstrictors and inotropes to increase systemic blood pressure and increase the force and rate of myocardial contraction**

The appropriate medical/pharmaceutical interventions have been implemented for the respective clients.

Focus Questions

1. Discuss nursing implications for treatments and medications prescribed for these clients in shock.

   Nursing management of clients with shock center around:

   - **Hypovolemic shock—Rapidly administering fluids without compromising the pulmonary circulation. Fluids given too rapidly could cause pulmonary edema and congestive heart failure.**
   - **Anaphylactic shock—Maintaining an adequate airway and monitoring client response to the antigen.**
   - **Septic shock—Identifying the microorganism causing the septicemia, initiating antibiotic therapy, and lowering the body temperature in the warm phase.**
   - **Neurogenic shock—Preventing further spinal cord injury and maintaining adequate systemic arterial pressure.**
   - **Cardiogenic shock—Maintaining an adequate cardiac output while monitoring for cardiac arrhythmias, decreasing the workload on the heart, and revascularization of the heart.**

   Specific nursing responsibilities with the administration of crystalloid and colloid solutions include:

   - **Establishing baseline vital signs, lung sounds, heart sounds, central venous pressure, and pulmonary artery wedge pressures**
   - **Monitoring and recording vital signs every 15 minutes until stable**
   - **Monitoring and recording hourly urinary output**
   - **Monitoring for signs of congestive heart failure or pulmonary edema: dyspnea, cyanosis, cough, crackles, or wheezes**
   - **Monitoring for signs of dehydration: dry lips, dark-colored urine, and urinary output less than 30 cc per hour**

- Monitoring for signs of circulatory overload: jugular neck vein distention, increase in central venous pressure, and an increase in pulmonary artery wedge pressure
- Monitoring prothrombin, partial thromboplastin times, and platelet counts
- If administering dextran or plasma protein fraction, having epinephrine and antihistamines available for any signs of hypersensitivity, such as fever, chills, rash, headache, or wheezing

Specific nursing responsibilities with the administration of adrenergics (sympathomimetics) include:

- Using an IV route with continuous infusion pumps. Titrating the dose according to the client's response and the physician's orders and the agency's protocols
- Monitoring and recording vital signs and hemodynamic paramaters before administering the medication and every 15 minutes after until stable and thereafter according to the agency protocols
- Monitoring and recording hourly urinary output to ensure an output of greater than 30 cc per hour
- Not mixing sympathomimetics with sodium bicarbonate or alkaline solutions
- Monitoring the IV insertion site for infiltration. Infiltration of vasoconstrictors can cause localized tissue ischemia and necrosis.

Specific nursing responsibilities with the administration of vasodilators include:

- Protecting these medications from light by wrapping the IV bag in the package that is provided
- Mixing with D_5W only and no other medications
- Infusing with an infusion pump and discarding any unused solution within 4 hours
- Monitoring and recording vital signs and mental status every 15 minutes until stable and according to agency protocol thereafter
- Monitoring, recording, and reporting to the physician adverse reactions to the medications, such as dizziness, tachycardia, arrhythmias, hypotension, and adventitious breath sounds. Should any of these symptoms occur, slowing the rate of infusion to a keep-open rate

Specific nursing responsibilities with the administration of blood and blood products include:

- All of the measures under crystalloid and colloid solutions
- Assessing for previous blood reactions
- Using blood administration tubing and initiating a saline solution administration to flush the tubing and filter
- Administering the blood immediately
- Checking and documenting that the name of the client, client's name brand, and the name on the blood bag are identical
- Ensuring that the number on the unit of blood is identical to the one on the requisition for the blood
- Checking compatibility of blood type and Rh factor
- Checking the expiration date on the blood

- Checking the unit of blood for bubbles or discoloration
- Taking and recording the vital signs prior to administering the blood
- Initiating an infusion rate of 2 ml per minute for the first 15 minutes
- Monitoing the client for hypersensitivity or hemolytic reactions and taking and recording vital signs per agency protocol
- After the first 15 minutes, if there are no adverse reactions, increasing the rate of administration to ensure that the unit of whole blood infuses within 3–4 hours
- Immediately stopping the infusion if an adverse reaction occurs
- Keeping the vein open with saline
- Taking and recording the vital signs
- Returning the blood and tubing to the lab
- Following agency protocols for collecting urine and blood specimens
- Continuing to monitor the client

2. Utilize the data in the preceding question to develop and prioritize a list of nursing diagnoses with three nursing interventions and one outcome criteria for each client.

Huang Mei Lan

Risk for Altered Tissue Perfusion related to progression of septic shock as evidenced by decreased cardiac output, increased metabolic rate, hypotension, and massive vasodilation.

Outcome: Demonstrate increased perfusion as evidenced by peripheral pulses present, vital signs within normal range, and balanced I & O

Interventions:

- Monitor vital signs, hemodynamics, and heart and lung sounds
- Administer antipyretics as prescribed
- Review lab work

Richard Tanner

Decreased Cardiac Output related to decreased myocardial contractility

Outcome: Demonstrate hemodynamic stability

Interventions: Review lab work, determine baseline vital signs and hemodynamic parameters; position with head of bed in semi-Fowler's position.

Jane House

Fluid Volume Deficit related to hemorrhage

Outcome: Improve fluid volume to a functional level

Interventions: Administer fluids as ordered; maintain adequate IV access for fluid resuscitation; monitor vital signs and hemodynamic parameters.

Timothy Murphy

Risk for Ineffective Breathing Pattern related to cervical fracture and bucking the ventilator

Outcome: Establish an effective respiratory pattern

Interventions: **edicate with sedatives and muscle relaxants as ordered; assist with establishing a patent airway and respirations through endotracheal intubation and mechanical ventilation; reduce the client's fear and anxiety by answering monitor alarms promptly.**

Steve Cron

Impaired Gas Exchange **related to obstructed airway**

Outcome: **Demonstrate improved ventilation and adequate oxygenation**

Interventions: **Note respiratory rate, depth, cyanosis, adventitious breath sounds, and use of accessory muscles; evaluate pulse oximetry to determine oxygenation; provide supplemental oxygen at the lowest concentration indicated by the laboratory results.**

Reflective Writing

Suppose you are the emergency room nurse in charge of the care for Jane House. Jane's parents arrive in the emergency department insisting they need to see their daughter while you are implementing care for her shock. They are in control but upset. What would you do? Why?

Having determined that they are in control, the nurse should ask them if they would like to be with their daughter in the ER. The nurse should briefly describe what the parents would encounter in the ER, accompany one or both parents into the ER, and stay with them to provide physical and emotional support. Encouraging verbal and physical interaction, as is possible, between Jane and her parents is crucial.

This is a critical time for both Jane and her parents. All three can find comfort and support with one another. Jane's parents will not have to wonder if everything was done or what happened behind the closed doors. Jane won't have to worry about where her parents are or what they know. Should Jane die in the ER, the moment at the time of death is a very precious spiritual and emotional time. Separation from their daughter at that time could cause difficulties in their grieving process.

References

Hudak, C., Gallo, B., & Morton, P. (1998). *Critical care nursing: A holistic approach,* 7th ed. Philadelphia: Lippincott.

LeMone, P. & Burke, K. (2000). *Medical surgical nursing: Critical thinking in client care,* 2nd ed. Menlo Park, Calif.: Addison-Wesley.

Doenger, M. & Moorhouse, M. F. (1998). *Nurse's pocket guide: Diagnoses, interventions, and rationales,* 6th ed. Philadelphia: F. A. David Company.

Vanderbeek, J. (2000). Till death do us part. *American Journal of Nursing,* 100(2), 44.

CASE # 17 CLARK AUSTIN

Learning Objectives

1. Discuss nursing implications for medications and treatments prescribed for clients with pneumonia.
2. Provide problem-focused effective teaching to clients with pneumonia and their family members.
3. Use the nursing process to assess, plan, implement, and evaluate patient's needs and care for clients with pneumonia.

4. Discuss immediate and later complications regarding respiratory status following surgery.
5. Understand different diagnostic tests and related nursing care commonly used to evaluate respiratory conditions.

Clark Austin is a 75-year-old retired engineer who lives with his wife Ann. He is admitted to your hospital with acute cholecysitis. He has undergone a cholecystectomy and has been transferred to your floor the second day postop. He has a nasogastric (NG) tube to continuous low wall suction, a Foley catheter in place, one peripheral IV, a large abdominal dressing, and a history of emphysema. In addition, he is on O_2 2L/min per NC and receives a continuous pulse oximetry monitoring. His orders include: $D_5{}^1/_2$NS with 20mEq KCl/L at 125cc/hr, Morphine 5mg IV q2hr prn, turn, cough, and deep breathe q2h, incentive spirometer q2h while awake.

Focus Questions

1. What is pulse oximetry? What is the normal range? What are the nursing considerations when using pulse oximetry on a patient?

   - **A pulse oximeter is a noninvasive device that measures oxygen saturation (O_2 saturation), which means the percentage of oxygenated hemoglobin in arterial blood. It is often used to detect hypoxemia before clinical signs and symptoms develop. It is a less expensive, noninvasive method of monitoring arterial oxygen saturation without the risks associated with arterial blood gas measurement or continuous arterial catheters.**
   - **The normal oxygen saturation is 95% to 100%. An O_2 sat below 70% is life threatening.**
   - **When a pulse oximeter is in use, nurses need to make sure that the sensor is appropriate to the client's size, set safety alarms, check the site on a regular basis, record the application of the pulse oximeter, type and size, and record nursing assessments. Nurses also need to be aware that certain factors will affect the accuracy of readings, such as severe anemia, nail polish, and carbon monoxide poisoning.**

2. What are the immediate and the later complications regarding respiratory status for a patient such as Mr. Austin undergoing abdominal surgery?

Immediate respiratory complications:

- **Airway obstruction, hypoxia, aspiration, and laryngospasm. All these are to be assessed at post-anesthesia care unit (PACU), and measures to prevent and treat these complications need to be in place.**

Later complications regarding respiratory system:

- **Respiratory infection due to aspiration and/or nosocomial microorganism infections: it often occurs in persons with preexisting diseases (e.g., COPD, diabetes, malignancy, and CAD) or impaired host defenses (e.g., recent surgery, invasive devices, and indwelling catheters).**
- **Pulmonary embolism: a clot occludes a pulmonary vessel and alters the pulmonary circulation. Dyspnea is the most common patient complaint. Other symptoms include chest pain, anxiety, diaphoresis, tachypnea, tachycardia, and rales in the affected lung.**
- **Atelectasis: an incomplete expansion or a collapse of lung tissue. It may involve all or part of the lung and it usually occurs within hours to a few days after surgery.**

3. Identify nursing interventions to promote Mr. Austin's pulmonary functions and decrease his risk for pulmonary infections?

- **Teach the patient about the asking for pain medication as soon as he experiences pain and correct any potential misconceptions about pain management. Effective pain control is crucial so patient can perform turn, cough, and deep breath as ordered.**
- **Demonstrate correct cough and deep breathing techniques. Cough and deep breathing help to promote expectoration of secretions and lung expansion.**
- **Explain and demonstrate the correct use of the incentive spirometer. Incentive spiromoter promotes lung expansion and provides feedback for Mr. Austin as to whether he is taking in enough air or not to expand his lungs.**
- **Encourage early ambulation and assist him to ambulate safely.**
- **Give enough fluid to thin secretions. Usually give at least 3 liters per day as long as the patient can tolerate that amount.**

This morning, when you enter his room, Mr. Austin appears quite anxious and coughs a lot. He complains of shortness of breath and pain in his chest and his incision site. He states: "I feel hot, and I am extremely tired."

Focus Question

1. Identify and prioritize your nursing activities at this time.
   - **Assess respiratory effort, such as method of breathing, use of accessory muscles, etc.**
   - **Auscultate lung sounds**
   - **Check his IV rate and site (possibly the IV is running too fast and causing fluid overload)**
   - **Position him in a high Fowler's position or orthopneic position to facilitate breathing**
   - **Complete check of vital signs, especially temperature and heart rate**
   - **Note perfusion**
   - **Determine the intensity of pain**
   - **Call the physician with your findings**

Your assessment reveals the following: His respiration is labored and shallow with the use of accessory muscles of the neck and abdomen. VS: 142/80, P 120, R 26, T 103.4° F. O_2 sat 88% on O_2 at 2L/min per NC. There are scattered crackles thoughout the right lung fields and LUL, rhonchi over large airways, and breath sounds are diminished from fourth intercostal space to the base on the left side. His IV is running at the prescribed rate and there are no signs of infection of the IV site. His pain level is at 5 on a scale of 1–10. The physician prescribes the following orders after you called him or her immediately after your assessment: continue IV of $D_5{}^1/_2$NS with 20mEq KCL/L at 125 cc/hr; STAT blood culture and sensitivity (C& S) sputum C & S; STAT chest x-ray (CXR) and ECG; Ampicillin/Sulbactam (Unasyn) 1.5g IVPB q6h; and Acetaminophen 650mg po for temp over 102°F.

Focus Questions

1. Based on your assessment findings, what do you think is going on with Mr. Austin? State your rationale.

- **He is experiencing tachycardia and tachypnea. His blood pressure is slightly elevated. All these may be due to incisional pain, fever, or hypoxemia (SaO_2 88% is below normal).**
- **Temperature is elevated. Slight elevation of temperature is expected immediately following surgery. However, 103.4°F is too high to indicate a normal postop reaction. Probably there is a new infection responsible for this temperature elevation.**

2. Before starting Unasyn, what nursing assessment and interventions should you perform and why?
   - **Pain medication needs to be given to the patient to alleviate the discomfort. Patient cannot tolerate and function normally at a pain level of 5. This needs to be dealt with immediately to promote patient's well-being.**
   - **Blood cultures need to be drawn before giving the antibiotic. Otherwise, antibiotic might interfere with the growth of microorganisms, causing an inaccurate result.**
   - **Always check allergies before starting an antibiotic, especially Penicillin. Penicillin is one of the most common drugs that cause allergic reactions, especially anaphylactic reactions.**
   - **Obtain sputum sample as early as possible, such as in the morning or after postural drainage. If unable to obtain, Mr. Austin may be suctioned.**
3. Why does the physician order a culture and sensitivity test? How are the results being used?
   - **A culture is a growth of an organism on a nutrient media to identify the microorganisms. Any body fluids, drainage, or tissue sample can be cultured for microorganism identification. In conjunction with the culture, after a microbe is isolated, its susceptibility to specific antibiotics is tested and determined. Microorganisms are then classified according to their reaction to a number of antibiotics as resistant, sensitive, or intermediately sensitive. Therefore, the C&S results are used to choose a more suitable antibiotic to fight the microorganism. Frequently, before the C&S results are available, a broad-spectrum antibiotic is prescribed first to initiate the therapy.**

The CXR reveals LLL pneumonia, and the results of the blood culture reveal that Mr. Austin has an infection caused by methicillin-resistant staphylococcus aureus (MRSA) and he is sensitive to Vancomycin. The physician changed the antibiotics to Vancomycin 1g IVPB q12h. He/she also orders peak and trough level of Vancomycin with third dose.

Focus Questions

1. What are the factors that might predispose Mr. Austin to pneumonia?

   Pneumonia is more likely to result when defense mechanisms become incompetent or are overwhelmed by the virulence or quantity of infectious agents.

   For Mr. Austin, the risk factors to developing pneumonia could be grouped into three categories:

   (a) preexisting conditions: emphysema and age

   (b) compromised defense system: recent surgery, Foley catheter in place, IV lines, and large wound

   (c) environmental factors: living at a hospital also increase the chance to develop pneumonia.

2. Mrs. Austin is extremely anxious about starting a new medication and asks you why the doctor changed the medication. Discuss the rational for changing the medication. In addition, what kind of patient education are you going to perform?

   - **The change of medication is based on the result of culture and sensitivity, so the antibiotics will function more effectively to eradicate the responsible microorganisms, in this case, S. Aureus.**

   - **Information, such as the need to adhere to drug regimen and not to interrupt the dosage of this new drug, Vancomycin, needs to be provided to the patient and his wife. In addition, they need to promptly report any signs of side effects, especially ringing in ears, since the drug may cause damage to the auditory branch of eighth cranial nerve and could result in deafness.**

   - **Give them information regarding MRSA. Make sure Mrs. Austin and other visitors wash their hands before leaving Mr. Austin's room to prevent cross-contamination.**

3. Explain the order for the peak and trough level. How is this going to be obtained and used?

   - **Peak and trough level are often ordered when a patient is on Vancomycin because of its nephrotoxicity and ototoxicity. It is used to adjust drug dosage and/or frequency to achieve an effective therapeutic level while minimizing the chance of drug toxicity.**

   - **Peak level measures the highest plasma drug level of circulating medication. It helps to monitor for possible toxic levels. It is usually drawn 30 minutes after the medication is totally administered.**

   - **Trough level measures the lowest plasma drug level of circulating medication. Usually, for vancomycin, it is drawn 30 minutes before administration of the next dose of medication, and it indicates whether the therapeutic level has been maintained.**

4. Identify at least three top priority nursing diagnoses that apply to Mr. Austin at the present time.

   - **Ineffective airway clearance related to decreased energy, pain, and inflammation**
   - **Knowledge deficit related to unfamiliarity with information**
   - **Ineffective breathing pattern related to pleural chest pain**
   - **Pain related to pleural inflammation and recent surgery**
   - **Activity intolerance related to hypoxemia**

 Mr. Austin recovers from his pneumonia and is preparing for discharge.

Focus Question

1. What discharge teaching should you give to him and his wife regarding the prevention of another pulmonary infection?

   - **Teach the importance of getting immunization with pneumococcal vaccine (one-time injection only) because of his history of emphysema and his age.**
   - **Teach the importance of getting a yearly influenza vaccine.**
   - **Avoiding exposure to people with colds/flu.**
   - **Drinking plenty of fluids (at least 2 liters per day) to thin pulmonary secretions and facilitate expectoration.**

- **Good hand-washing technique and proper handling and disposing of secretions.**
- **Teach the patient the importance of having good oral care to clear mouth of pathogens to help prevent pneumonia.**

Reflective Writing

More and more people with pneumonia are being discharged early to home or are being entirely treated at home. What roles can nurses play to promote those patients' recovery and well-being?

This case has presented an elderly person with hospital-acquired pneumonia. For those people who are either discharged early to home or those whose pneumonia are treated at home, nurses play an important role in disease treatment and health promotion. Good assessment and education are essential to the patient's successful recovery. Normally, persons discharged from the hospital after being admitted still require about 4 weeks before they feel completely well. The older the person, the longer the period of recovery. First, nurses act as patient advocates. They need to carefully assess patient's condition and living arrangements and work together with social worker case manager to make sure that there is someone in the home at least part of each day to assist with ADL. Nurses need to make sure that the patients will be monitored closely by their health care provider and to arrange assistance in going to follow-up appointments. Second, nurses are also educators. They need to teach the patient about medication, diet and nutrition, hydration, sleep and rest, gradually increasing activities, and measures to prevent future infections.

References

Phipps, W. J., Sands, J. K., & Marek, J. F. (Eds.). (1999). *Medical-surgical nursing: Concepts and clinical practice*, 6th ed. St. Louis: Mosby.

Caclianno, C. (1996). Nosocomial pneumonia: Repelling a deadly invader. *Nursing*, 26(5), 34–39.

CASE #18 MR. ALVAREZ

Learning Objectives

1. Identify the normal signs and symptoms of a client with cataracts.
2. Discuss preop care teaching necessary for a client undergoing cataract surgery.
3. Discuss postop teaching following cataract surgery.
4. Discuss physical findings and rationale for a detached retina.
5. Explore ways to communicate with others assertively.

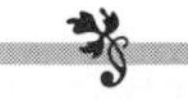

Mr. Alvarez is a 77-year-old retired graphic artist. He has been married for 52 years to his wife, Maria. They live alone as all eight children are grown and gone from home. He is being seen today for his yearly routine eye exam. He states he needs new glasses because his eyesight is hazy.

Focus Question

1. What additional assessment data should the nurse collect?

   Interview: How has his eyesight changed over the past year? Does anything make it worse or anything make it better? Does he have any pain in his eyes or any headache? Does changed eyesight affect his day-to-day activities? What medications does he take?

   Physical exam: Vital signs, Snellen chart, and inspection of his eye.

Physical exam shows vital signs to be T—98 P—80 R—20 BP 130/76. Inspection reveals an opaque right lens with the right pupil being grayish-white in appearance. The left eye appears normal. Snellen chart in right eye = 20/150, left eye = 20/50. Mr. Alvarez states he takes Hydrochlorothiazide 50mg every day for high blood pressure with a glass of orange juice. He states he is afraid to drive anymore and that the glare from headlights blinds him. He denies any headaches or eye pain and states his vision remains hazy no matter what he tries. His eyesight has gotten to the point that he is unable to read or engage in his artistic hobbies. His physician diagnoses a right eye cataract and recommends surgery.

Focus Questions

1. What preoperative teaching should be done?

   Explain the procedure to Mr. Alvarez and his wife including type of anesthesia, length of surgery, sounds and smells of the operating and recovery rooms, postoperative monitoring and eye patching procedures, and expected postoperative outcomes. Give Mr. Alvarez ample opportunity to ask questions and express his concerns. Offer reassurance and answer his questions. Make sure Mr. Alvarez does not have an upper respiratory infection for you do not want him coughing after surgery, which will increase intraocular pressure.

2. Since this is an out-patient surgery, what postoperative instructions will be given prior to discharge?

   Teach patient and his wife ***eye drop instillation*** **procedure; have them return demonstrate procedure. Procedure includes pulling the lower lid down to expose the conjunctival sac. Have patient look up and away and squeeze the prescribed number of drops into the sac. Release lid and have him blink to distribute medication. If medication is absorbed systemically, gently press thumb on inner canthus for 1–2 minutes while patient closes eyes. To apply the eye patch, close the eye but do not squeeze shut and apply gauze pad and shield. Apply tape over the shield to keep in place. Give written instructions and visual illustrations of eye drop instillation and patching procedures to patient and his wife.**

   Activity restrictions: **Watch TV for only brief periods of time. Engage only in sedentary activities such as listening to music, audiotapes, and audiobooks. No driving, writing or art work for 2 weeks. No straining, lifting, or bending at the waist.**

   Reduce risk of eye injury: **Wash hands before touching eye. Do not squeeze eye shut or rub eye. Pat tears under the eye gently. Wear eye patch/shield at night. Wear dark glasses for glare. Keep the affected eye dry when showering or washing hair. Abstain from sexual intercourse until allowed to resume by physician. Have traffic areas well lit, especially at night. Clear walking paths for easy passage.** ***Recognizing and reporting abnormal symptoms:*** **Nausea/vomiting, eye pain, decreased vision or change in vision, signs of infection such as redness, pain, edema, and increased non-clear drainage.**

Mr. Alvarez is sent home following an uneventful cataract removal and lens implant of the right eye. His wife brings him to the emergency room two days postop, and Mr. Alvarez states his eyesight has changed and he feels like he is "looking through a veil, seeing flashing lights and floaters in his right eye." He denies any eye pain. In examining his peripheral vision, you find no peripheral vision present in his right eye. His left eye is normal.

Focus Questions

1. What do you expect is happening to Mr. Alvarez and why? Are these normal findings following cataract surgery?

These are not normal findings, and you suspect a detached retina since this is a possible complication following cataract surgery. A detached retina is painless because the retina has no sensory nerves. The "flashing lights" are caused by vitreous traction on the retina and the "floaters" are minute hemorrhages at the point of separation.

2. What do you expect will be the intervention for Mr. Alvarez?

   He will have both eyes patched to prevent eye movement that will worsen the detachment, and he will be admitted immediately for a retinal detachment repair.

3. What additional teaching is needed postoperatively?

   Ice compresses to decrease the edema. Expect mild discomfort after this surgery.

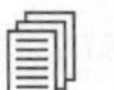

Reflective Writing

You are caring for Mr. Alvarez on the surgical unit after his surgery for retinal detachment. You also have six other clients, one of whom is actively hemorrhaging. You ask a colleague to help you by hanging an IV for Mr. Alvarez so you can manage your hemorrhaging client. She responds, "Sorry, I'm busy, too. You'll have to deal with it!" You note that she has been talking with her husband on the phone for the last 20 minutes. How can you respond in an assertive manner?

- **To be assertive, a person stands up for his or her rights in a way that others are not violated.**
- **Use "I" statements—this is what I feel, think, and want.**
- **Avoid "you" statements.**
- **Timing is important. Because of the emergency you are experiencing, you may not be able to respond to her inappropriate response to you immediately. However, do not ignore it. Discuss it with her later.**
- **In approaching her later, you might say, "Yesterday when my client was hemorrhaging I needed your help. I'd like to talk to you about this."**
- **You need to explain to her what your feelings are and what you'd like to see happen in the future: "I felt not supported and I'd like to feel I could count on you next time."**
- **Remain calm, do not raise your voice, use eye contact, stand up straight, and don't whine.**

References

Bastable, S. B. (1997). *Nurse as educator: Principles of teaching and learning*. Boston: Jones and Bartlett.
Diseases. (1993). Springhouse, PA: Springhouse Corporation.
Kearney, K. M. (1997). Retinal detachment. *American Journal of Nursing*, 97(8), 50.
Nursing procedures. (1996). Springhouse, PA: Springhouse Corporation.
Sheldon, N. E. Burton, S. (1994). *Assertiveness skills.* Burr Ridge, Ill.: Business One Irwin/Mirror Press.

chapter **5**

Annotated Miscellaneous Cases

CASE #1 AUNT LUCY

Learning Objectives

1. Assess for fall risk factors in later life.
2. Summarize environmental modifications promoting safety of the environment.
3. Formulate nursing diagnoses and goals based on assessment data.
4. Identify the manifestations of different types of urinary incontinence.
5. Describe nursing interventions to control and manage urinary incontinence.
6. Adapt teaching tools and strategies to needs of older adults.
7. Identify factors influencing the quality of nursing care she/he provides to older adults.

Your 75-year-old Aunt Lucy lives alone in an apartment in a continuing care retirement community. You have always been very close, almost like her child, since she never married and had no children of her own. She has fallen three times in the past several months. The rest of your family is encouraging her to move into a more secure environment. She doesn't want to move, although she is concerned about her recent falls. She and your family ask you for advice.

Focus Questions

1. Given the information provided, what would be your priority nursing diagnosis and goal?

   High risk for injury r/t a history of falls; Aunt Lucy will ambulate safely and avoid falling in the next week.

2. What additional questions would you need to ask to determine your aunt's fall risk factors?

   Falls in people over 75 usually are the result of a combination of medication and disease related factors; falls in those younger than 75 more typically are caused by interactions between environmental hazards, age-related changes, and gait-balance changes. Students should formulate questions related to the following: musculoskeletal performance, pain in joints, balance, use of medications creating risk for falls, other medical conditions associated with falls or osteoporosis, history of fractures, dietary intake of calcium and vitamin D, amount and types of exercise, alcohol intake, depression, cognitive status

3. What environmental factors might you modify to increase the safety of your aunt's apartment?

Areas for assessment and potential modification would include:

- **Assistive Devices—available? Being used safely and properly?**
- **Bathroom—Grab bars? Rubber mat or tub seat? Appropriate toilet seat height or elevated toilet seat?**
- **Bedroom—Bed height appropriate? Mattress provides firm support for sitting on the edge? Pathway between bedroom and bathroom clear? Any method for turning on a light before getting out of bed? Bedside commode?**
- **Furniture—Chairs have arm rests and right height and depth? Tables stable? Furniture placed away from walking path?**
- **Illumination—lighting adequate but nonglare? Nightlights? Easy to reach light switches?**
- **Kitchen—Frequently used objects easily accessible? Nonslip mats in front of sink?**
- **Stairways—lighting adequate? Light switches at both top and bottom of stairway? Even steps with nonskid treads? Securely fastened handrails and colored tape to mark edges of stairs?**
- **Overall Safety—Sturdy shoes with nonskid soles? Door thresholds nonhazardous? Doorways wide enough for assistive devices? Use of stools etc. to get to out-of-reach objects and to change light bulbs? Telephones accessible? Cordless portable phone and/or emergency call system?**

As you talk to your aunt, she hesitantly admits that for several years she has had difficulty with "leaking," especially when she coughs, sneezes, or exercises. She states that she gets up to urinate about four to five times a night because she is afraid of "wetting the bed," and each time she has fallen she was on her way to the bathroom at night. Aunt Lucy also tells you that she has limited her fluid intake to four glasses per day and that she never drinks anything after five P.M. Lastly, Aunt Lucy says, "You know, I haven't left the house for longer than two hours at a time for about a year. I'm so afraid of having an accident."

Focus Questions

1. What assessment questions would you ask to determine your Aunt Lucy's incontinence risk factors?

Students should formulate questions related to the following categories:

- **Medications—Anticholinergic agents, calcium channel blockers, sedative-hypnotic agents, adrenergics, adrenergic blockers**
- **Cognitive Impairments**
- **Functional Impairments**
- **Myths and Misunderstandings**
- **Pathologic Conditions—Urinary tract infection, constipation**

2. Illustrate age-related changes in urinary elimination with a diagram. Include this with the case.

Students' diagrams should include changes in the kidneys, urinary muscles, renal tubules, and cerebral cortex

3. What type(s) of urinary incontinence does Aunt Lucy have? Support your answer.

   Stress incontinence—this type of incontinence is associated with the sudden leakage of urine in relation to activities that increase abdominal pressure. With the current data it is difficult to rule out all other types of UI.

4. Write a nursing diagnosis, a goal, and three interventions for Aunt Lucy.

   - **High risk for injury r/t a history of falls secondary to altered urinary elimination**
   - **Goal: Client will not suffer any injury**
   - **Interventions:**

   a. **Teach Aunt Lucy about normal age-related changes and risk factors contributing to incontinence.**

   b. **Teach Aunt Lucy about the importance of adequate fluid intake and mechanisms by which inadequate fluid intakes may contribute to incontinence.**

   c. **Discuss importance of comprehensive evaluation, emphasizing that incontinence is not a normal part of aging.**

You want to teach Aunt Lucy about falls and incontinence. Aunt Lucy says, "Honey, I'm too old. Besides, there's nothing to learn. It is just part of getting old."

Focus Questions

1. How would you respond? Why?

   Students' responses should reflect empathy for Aunt Lucy's feelings while also addressing the perceptions of falls and incontinence as a normal part of aging. Students should identify the importance of not discounting Aunt Lucy's feelings. "It sounds like you might be feeling a little hopeless or discouraged about things being different because of your age. Could we talk about that a little bit?"

2. How would you modify your teaching to address common age-related changes in hearing, vision, and cognitive function?

   - **Hearing**

     Minimize use of high frequency consonants—c, ch, f, s, sh, z

     Reduce or eliminate background noise

     Reduce the speed of speech

     Combine visual and audio cues

     Emphasize correct diction and enunciation

     Face the learner

   - **Vision**

     Make sure glasses are clean and in place

     Use nonreflective materials and surfaces

     Eliminate irrelevant information and decoration

Cluster information within the narrowest cone of vision

Combine type with graphic symbols when possible

Use print materials with large (14–16 point) type

Use high contrast to help discrimination

Avoid or limit use of blue, green, violet

Use soft white light to decrease glare

- **Cognitive Function**

  Teach in a familiar environment

  Relate information to past experiences

  Make information personally relevant

  Use analogies and examples

  Allow learner to set the pace

  Emphasize problem solving and application

  Provide advance organizers and organizing aids

Reflective Writing

In the second paragraph, Aunt Lucy mentions that she drinks 4 glasses of fluids per day and never drinks after 5 P.M. Did you consider assessing for alcohol use? Why/why not? What factors might have contributed to your consideration or omission of alcohol as a potential issue?

Most students do not associate alcoholism with the elderly. However, alcohol use could be a problem for Aunt Lucy. Her fall and incontinence should have triggered this possibility for students. Often older people do not volunteer information on their alcohol consumption, as they do not see it as relevant to their health. The nurse should ask specific questions regarding alcohol consumption: "Many older people enjoy a cocktail in the evening or a beer while watching television. What alcohol do you drink and when?" This will allow the client to divulge this information in a socially acceptable format.

References

Eliopoulos, C. (1997). *Gerontological nursing* (4th ed.). Philadelphia: J. B. Lippincott.

Miller, C. A. (1995). *Nursing care of older adults: Theory and practice* (2nd ed.). Philadelphia: J. B. Lippincott.

CASE #2 EVA HOMESON

Learning Objectives

1. Discuss ethical and legal aspects of the Patient Self-Determination Act.
2. Analyze responsibilities of health care providers for clients with a Living Will.
3. Explore the concepts of loss and grief in severe illness.
4. Apply concepts from the ANA Code for Nurses and International Council of Nurses Code for Nurses.

Eva Homeson is a 44-year-old single woman. She has a BA in Psychology, is a Roman Catholic, and is employed as a crisis intervention counselor at the Women's Center. She has smoked 3 packs of cigarettes per day for the past 10 years. Eva is admitted for left upper lobectomy for large cell cancer. The contact person is her mother, Janice Slocum, who lives 30 minutes from Eva. Eva does not have a living will but was given the information for one with hospital admission forms. Chart data includes the following: Tumor was 5 cm. in size, nonadherent to bone, in the left upper lobe, and a small nodule was also found in the right anterior neck. The mass and adjacent tissue was removed and a tracheostomy was created to provide a patent airway because of anticipated excessive postop neck edema. At the time of the nurse's visit, Eva is 3 days postop and receiving ventilatory support via the tracheostomy. She is alert, oriented, follows simple instructions, writes notes to communicate, and is assisting the ventilator 100%. The ventilator settings are: 0_2, 30% rate 10, Tital volume 750cc, Sigh 6/hour. She has an upper and lower chest tube on the left side. The lower chest tube is draining maroon-red bloody fluid, 900cc total output. R 18/min., BP 140/72, Pulse 98 regular, Temperature 99°F oral, Oxygen Saturation 85%. Eva relates to the nurse that she is comfortable with her life accomplishment. "I have no children or husband depending on me. I do not want to be a burden to my mother or the community. I could not live in a nursing home. I am very independent and must be able to return to my prior lifestyle or life is meaningless. This is not quality living. If my heart stops, I do not want all that 911 stuff like on TV." Eva's mother cries every time she visits. Janice also states that she needs her daughter and could not stand by and watch her die. Janice states that she plans to have Eva move in with her so that she can care for her. During the physician's visit, Eva requested to be made a No Code. The physician listened and reassured her that he understood Eva's request. The physician did not write the No Code nor inform Eva of this decision.

Focus Questions

1. What are the legal and ethical issues in this case? Be sure to consider the Self-Determination Act, the State Nurse Practice Act, the International Council of Nurses Code for Nurses, the American Association of Nurses Code for Nurses, and principles of ethical decision making.

   - **Legal Issues**

     Eva does not have an Advanced Directive and is requesting the No Code status.

     The physician did not write a No Code order as requested by Eva.

     Eva's legal rights within the Self-Determination Act were obstructed.

     Eva assumed that the physician would write the order for the No Code.

     The role of the nurse is to be a client advocate.

   - **Ethical Issues**

     The physician breached the moral principle of open honest communication with Eva.

     By not writing the No Code order, the Principles-based theory and Relationship-based theory of moral frameworks were breached.

     Eva is expressing autonomy, but she may be making an emotional, impulsive, uninformed decision for the No Code.

     Eva's significant other, Janice, does not want the No Code.

     Based on principles of nonmaleficence, beneficence, justice, fidelity, and veracity, the nurse should inform the client and advocate for Eva with the physician.

     Principles of client advocacy in the International Council of Nurses Code for Nurses and the American Nurses Association Code for Nurses support the nurse intervening for Eva.

2. What should the RN do? Justify your decisions.

   Based on the codes for nurses and, ethical principles, the nurse needs to be a client advocate. As a client advocate, the RN should explore Eva's understanding of her illness, the No Code, and the Advanced Directive. The RN needs to clarify Eva's decision, the motivating factors, and her comprehension of the expected outcomes. The RN needs to discuss with the physician Eva's request for No Code as indicated in the above conversation and understand the guiding principles for the physician's decision. The RN should inform Eva that the physician did not immediately write the No Code order. Based on the clinical situation and the answers to the above action plan, the nurse may need to pursue the nursing chain of command policy for the agency and involve the agency's ethics committee.

3. What additional assessment data are needed?

   Eva's understanding of her illness, No Code protocol, and Advanced Directive.

   Eva's decision, the motivating factors, and her comprehension of the expected outcomes. Assessment of all functional health patterns.

4. Can the nurse tell Eva and Janice about the physician's decision not to write the No Code?

   As client advocate the nurse should inform Eva that the No Code was not written. The nurse cannot assume or imply anything from physician's action. For client confidentiality the nurse should not inform Janice unless directed by Eva.

5. How can the nurse effectively communicate with and assess Eva?

   Explore various methods of nonverbal communication since Eva is on the ventilator. Some options are pencil and paper, computer, letter board, and picture book. Depending on Eva's energy level, muscular-skeletal strength, and literacy, communication may need to take place over several short blocks of time.

6. What losses is Eva experiencing at this time? What type of grief response could she be expressing?

   - **Losses**

     Effective communication, oral communication

     Mobility

     Oral intake

     Role in the workforce

     Self-concept

     Unrestricted movement of arms, torso, and face due to IVs, ventilator tubing, and chest tubes

     Freedom of pain and discomfort

     Social interaction

     Control or usual privacy for elimination function

   - **Grief**

     Shock and disbelief

     Anger

     Depression

Two hours after physician's visit, the nurse notices that there is no tiding in either of the chest tubes. The output in the lower chest tube collector is now full with a total of 2,000cc red fluid. Eva's R is 24/min., oxygen saturation 80%, BP 138/80, pulse 106 regular. Eva indicates that she feels short of breath (SOB). Eva suddenly has a seizure, becomes unconscious, and is pulseless. Cardiac monitor shows sinus tachycardia.

Focus Questions

1. Should the nurse start CPR?

   Yes. Based on the data in this case study, the legal aspects of the Self-Determination Act, and most state laws, the nurse must start CPR. A written order by the attending physician for a No Code must be present on the unit before the nurse can legally not initiate CPR.

2. If the physician had written a No Code order, what are the responsibilities of nurses and the health care agency?

   - **Communication such that all care providers are aware of the order.**
   - **Client continues to receive comfort measures, respect, hygiene care, skin care, fall precautions, and psychosocial care.**
   - **Based on the client's living will, she may continue to receive hydration and nutrition and medications.**
   - **In the event of pulselessness or apnea, no intervention should be done.**
   - **Some agencies require review and renewal of a No Code order on periodic basis.**
   - **Some agencies require specific documents and documentation.**

Reflective Writing

Suppose Eva requests you, as her nurse, to witness an Advanced Directive and Organ Donation Consent to donate organs and tissues. Her mother, Janice, tells you to ignore Eva's request, claiming it is against her (Janice's) religious beliefs and that Eva is mentally incompetent at this time. You believe that Eva is mentally competent. How do you feel about this, and what should you do?

- **This case facilitates students to explore their spirituality, values, and beliefs. This may be very difficult for some students and cause significant personal conflict.**
- **There are several legal issues in this situation. For most agencies the RN may sign the documents as witness to the client's signature only. Some agencies may prohibit the nurse from signing one or both of these documents.**
- **This is Eva's life and decision. Janice may be attempting to exert some control over the situation and is expressing her religious beliefs. The nurse can assist Janice to recognize this conflict as well as Janice's anticipated loss and grief. It may benefit both Janice and Eva if they dialogue about Janice's concerns and resistance to these decisions.**
- **The nurse needs to assess Eva's understanding of the Advanced Directive and Organ Donation decisions to ensure Eva is making an informed decision.**
- **The nurse also needs to assess Eva's mental competency and document specific data.**

References

Kozier, B. Erb, G., Berman, A., & Burke, K. (2000). *Fundamentals of nursing: Concepts, process, and practice.* 6th ed. Upper Saddle River, N.J.: Prentice Hall.

LeMone, P. & Burke, K. (1996). *Medical surgical nursing: Critical thinking in client care.* Menlo Park, Calif.: Addison-Wesley.

CASE #3 AMBULATORY CLINIC

Learning Objectives

1. Identify students' own attitudes and beliefs about clients who come from different socio-economic backgrounds.
2. Describe how a client's treatment in the health care setting is impacted by the nurse's attitude and beliefs about their client's socio-economic background.
3. Identify approaches that can be used when colleagues have disparaging views toward a client's socio-economic background.
4. Develop a personal plan to increase sensitivity to client's socio-economic background in providing nursing care.

***Attention Instructor: An optional activity prior to introducing the case: Have the students break into two groups and do the following exercise.**

Half of the group is asked to write down everything they have ever heard, felt, thought, or believed about the rich. The other half of the group is asked to write down everything they have ever heard, felt, thought, or believed about the poor. Each student then writes their responses on a blackboard, so that all the students can see them. After all the words describing each group are listed on the board, students are asked to individually put a check beside the words they feel are true based on their own experiences. With this data revealed, the teacher can ask the following kinds of questions to help students realize that their beliefs come from their experiences and the views held by people around them.

- **Have any of you ever felt unfairly treated because of your socio-economic situation? How did it make you feel?**
- **Have you ever felt uncomfortable around someone who is from a different socio-economic background? Either they were more affluent or less affluent than you were. How did you feel? What kinds of comments did you or others around you make at that time?**
- **What beliefs, values, and prejudices did you recognize in the comments?**
- **How would those beliefs, values, and prejudices influence or impact on the care a nurse would give to someone from a different socio-economic status than her or his own?**

You are a nurse working in an ambulatory outpatient surgical clinic of a large city hospital. The vascular surgery clinic is being held, and 25 patients are scheduled to be seen today. The vascular surgery clinic starts at 8:30 A.M., and then at 1 P.M. the neurosurgery clinic will be held in the same area. There are three nurses (you, Helen the charge nurse, and Ted), two physicians (Howard Smith and Grace Meyer), and one aide (Harriet) managing the clinic. Helen the charge nurse says at the beginning of the shift, "Now we really need to get done on time today.

We have an inservice with Dr. Stan Brown who is going to talk to us about a new surgical technique. You all know how great a speaker Stan is. We will order lunch to be delivered in the conference room at noon."

The clinic starts and you, the other nurses, and the aide bring the patients to the rooms, do initial assessments, and follow through with discharge teaching instructions as the patients finish with the doctors. You notice that Helen is quick to work with patients that are easy to bring into the rooms and are clean and well dressed. Because of their vascular problems, many patients come to the clinic in wheelchairs, but Helen usually avoids those patients. Between patients, while the nurses have a quiet moment, you hear Helen complaining to Ted that she doesn't understand why some of these patients miss their appointments and don't come for two or three weeks. "By then their dressings are filthy. Don't they know they are making the ulcers worse? They just don't care, I guess." At 11:45 A.M. Helen says, "Ok, lets get finished up as soon as we can. Both doctors are on their last patient. Who wants to set up the conference room? We have to get finished with lunch by 1 P.M. because we have a huge neurosurgery clinic this afternoon."

Focus Questions

1. Based on the above data, what are the primary values that Helen holds?

   Suggested answers would include, but are not be limited to:

   efficiency

   being on time

   being responsible for own care

   being compliant to health care recommendations

   wants to spend time with people she identifies with, i.e., physicians and colleagues, not "poor patients," values cleanliness

2. How do Helen's values regarding time, patient compliance, and patient's socio-economic status influence her nursing care?

   Helen is unable to see beyond her own values to see the world from the patients' perspective. She implies that people who don't come for care are doing it on purpose. She tends to avoid and also to blame the patient when they do not behave the way she thinks they should.

3. What else would you like to know about Helen?

   What kind of socio-economic background did she come from? Where did she learn her values? What does she believe the nurse's role should be in caring for the poor? Has she always believed the way she does or did something happen along the way to make her change her mind?

4. Compare and contrast how Helen talks to her staff about patients and physicians.

   She talks in polite and admiring terms about the physician who is going to talk at noon versus the disparaging way she talked about some clients. She talks down to other staff and doesn't come across as having any insight or interest in why clients behave the way they do.

At 11:50 A.M., Mr. Elias Jones, a 68-year-old man comes to the clinic with his great-grandson. He is using a cane and is obviously limping. He is wearing house slippers that have been cut open to allow room for his severely swollen feet. His right foot poking out from his pants has a very dirty, old dressing wrapped around it. Mr. Jones in a soft-spoken voice says that he has an appointment this morning to see the doctor. Helen approaches him and says, "You're too late. We stopped seeing patients at 11:30. You will have to make another appointment and come back next week. Anyway your appointment was for 9:00 A.M. this morning." Mr. Jones says, "I had to wait for my grandson to help me take the bus, and he didn't get there until 10:30 A.M." You have just finished up with Dr. Smith's last patient and overhear the above conversation.

Focus Questions

1. What are the implications of not having Mr. Jones see the physician today?

   There is a great possibility that his wound is already not doing well. A further delay in seeing the physician would cause the wound to get worse with greater consequences to Mr. Jones' over-all health. There is also no guarantee that Mr. Jones could easily come back for another appointment. There is always the potential for serious complications of gangrene, septicemia, and other life-threatening conditions developing if he is not cared for. When a patient is refused care, he is unlikely to want to come back again, and this could be detrimental to his health.

2. How do you think the patient felt to be told that he would have to make another appointment?

   He might feel very humiliated, angry, discouraged, depressed, hopeless, and powerless.

3. What is the most professional way for you to react to this situation?

   Intercede for Mr. Jones by asking the physician, Dr. Smith, if he would be willing to see the client. Tell the physician the circumstances and the reason you are concerned that Mr. Jones receive care today. Offer to assist the physician and to do the discharge care so that other staff are free to go to lunch.

4. What difference did Mr. Jones' perceived socio-economic status play in this situation?

   It caused him to have to rely on a bus to come to the clinic. Most likely Helen drove to the hospital that day and had ready access to transportation and is not aware of how difficult it is to rely on the bus. Mr. Jones was viewed in an impersonal way, and because his bandage was dirty, he may have been viewed as noncompliant and therefore not worth helping.

5. What, if anything, would you say to Helen?

   Approach Helen using "I" statements and describe your beliefs and feelings related to Mr. Jones' need. Learn more about Mr. Jones' situation, and if it seemed helpful, share the details with Helen. Try to be an advocate without putting down Helen's need. Try to find out why she feels so strongly about this.

Reflective Writing

Develop a personal plan to increase sensitivity to client's socio-economic background when providing nursing care by answering the following statements and questions:

1. Identify your own beliefs, opinions, and biases related to working with clients from a different socio-economic status.
2. What is the hardest part about caring for someone that is less affluent or more affluent than you are?

3. What biases, beliefs, attitudes, and opinions could prevent the nurse from giving the most professional care?
4. Describe how your personal beliefs about socio-economic status influence your nursing care.

The answers to the questions are very individual to each student. The questions are posed to encourage the students to consider how their values and beliefs might impact the care of a person who is from a different socio-economic background than the students'. Nurses need to understand their own beliefs and values in order to recognize their own biases and then make sure they do not impose them on their clients. Without this understanding nurses cannot show respect to clients who are from different backgrounds. The nurse especially needs to learn to be an advocate for the poor. Many clients who a nurse cares for will have complex problems that have been impacted by their poverty. This writing will help students examine their own feelings and beliefs and hopefully help them become more sensitive to the poor clients they will care for.

References

Andrews, M. & Boyle, J. (1995) *Trancultural concepts in nursing care,* 2nd ed. Philadelphia: J.B. Lippincott Co.

Gropper, R. (1996) *Culture and the clinical encounter: An intercultural sensitizer for the health professions.* Yarmouth, Maine: Intercultural Press.

CASE #4 MRS. WHITE

Learning Objectives

1. Delineate age-related changes that affect sleep and rest patterns.
2. Examine psychosocial, environmental, attitudinal, and physiologic risk factors that influence sleep and rest in older adults.
3. Discuss consequences of altered sleep patterns in later life.
4. Describe effective strategies for minimizing negative effects of sleep pattern changes.

Mrs. White is a 70-year-old Caucasian woman who lives alone in an apartment in a senior housing complex. Her medical diagnoses include glaucoma, depression, and congestive heart failure. Her health is declining, and she acknowledges that she sometimes forgets to take her medications. When you are interviewing her about her experiences of health and aging, she remarks that her sleeping is disturbed. She says that she is anxious and irritable because she doesn't "get my eight hours."

Focus Questions

1. What additional information from Mrs. White would lead you to determine that she was experiencing age-related changes in sleep?

The initial questions are designed to enhance students' awareness of salient assessment data as well as myths regarding sleep and the elderly, which may affect both the direction of their assessment and the information volunteered by elderly clients. These questions also provide a springboard for the discussion of differences between commonly occurring health problems in the elderly population and senescence. Limitations of

research on aging changes may also be discussed at this time. Age-related changes in sleep often include:

a. increasing time in bed including a greater number of daytime naps

b. decreasing proportion of time in actual sleep

c. longer time required to fall asleep (prolonged sleep latency)

d. increased number of awakenings during night (one-fifth of night may be spent in periods of wakefulness).

These sleep patterns are related to changes in the sleep cycle:

a. Throughout adulthood, duration of Stage I sleep increases gradually (5% of younger adult's sleep to 7–12% of older adult's sleep); this accounts for longer periods of drowsiness without actual sleep; during the night older adults have frequent shifts in and out of Stage I sleep.

b. Stage II does not change significantly.

c. There appears to be a greater degree of variability in Stage III in older adults as compared to younger adults.

d. Stage IV decreases to the point where it is virtually absent in older adults, especially men.

It is important to point out that there is controversy as to whether sleep pattern changes are true age-related changes or are attributable to disease states (physical discomfort, periodic leg movement syndrome, lower auditory threshold level).

2. What are some common myths about sleep in later life? How might a belief in these myths affect health?

   a. It is commonly believed that total sleep time changes drastically in later life. In reality, total daily sleep durations tend to be the same for healthy older and younger adults, although as indicated previously, changes do occur in quality and continuity of sleep.

   b. It is a myth that if total sleep time changes drastically, then older people usually need naps. Excessive daytime sleeping, especially when it replaces physical activity, often contributes to sleep disturbances.

   c. Health care professionals and clients often think that older people sleep the same as younger people and that "sleeping pills" constitute an effective long-term treatment for insomnia. This belief, along with the accompanying conclusion that arousals during the night are unhealthy, lead to the diagnosis of insomnia and treatment with sedative-hypnotic medications.

   d. The rigid belief in the necessity of always getting 8 hours of sleep per night also leads to false definitions of insomnia and the concomitant pharmacological treatment.

   e. A belief in the myth of the effectiveness of an alcohol "nightcap" also may contribute to sleep disturbance.

3. What psychosocial, environmental, and physiological (disease) factors might be affecting Mrs. White's sleep?

   a. As indicated in the initial paragraph, Mrs. White has also been diagnosed with depression. If students do not identify the possible relationships between depression and sleep disturbance, this should be pointed out. People who are depressed also typically take longer to fall asleep, have less deep sleep and more light sleep,

and awaken more frequently during the night and early in the morning. Possible daytime boredom—if she is depressed, does she withdraw from activities? stay in bed during the day from boredom, lack of motivation, or lack of concentration?

b. In terms of environmental factors, possible influences may include the length of time she has lived alone, any fears at night, noise level of the environment, and additional comfort factors, such as temperature.

c. Students are informed that Mrs. White has also been diagnosed with congestive heart failure. Studies of coronary patients found significant relationship between severity of condition and extent of sleep disturbances. Coronary artery disease and angina may be exacerbated during sleep, especially during REM sleep stages.

d. Other conditions that may be exacerbated include hypertension, duodenal ulcers, and COPD.

e. Sleep apnea, the involuntary cessation of airflow for 10 seconds or longer, is associated with advanced age and should also be considered as a potential factor in sleep disturbance. Other factors associated with sleep apnea include obesity, dementia, depression, snoring, hypothyroidism, and use of nicotine, alcohol, and medications that depress the respiratory center. More than 5–8 of these per hour are considered pathological. Although one-third of adults 60 and over experience this, the majority however report satisfactory sleep; consequently, the association with sleep disorders is unclear.

f. Lastly, the assessment should include questions to ascertain whether Mrs. White is experiencing periodic leg movements in sleep (PLMS), brief muscle contractions of intervals of about 30 seconds that may cause leg jerks and brief arousal. These may occur several times nightly and may last for an hour or more. The prevalence of this in later life is similar to apnea, and as with sleep apnea, there are associations between this and diminished sleep time, but not with subjective sleep complaints.

When you ask her about management of her health problems and use of medications, Mrs. White brings out all her pill bottles for you to look at. The labels on the pill bottles indicate that the following medications have been prescribed for Mrs. White:
Multivitamin forte every day
Lasix 20 mg. 2 bid (twice a day)
Lanoxicaps 0.1 mg., qd (every day) except Monday and Thursday
Ecotrin qd (every day)
Transderm-Nitro 0.2 mg/hr. qd (every day)
Zoloft 50 mg qd (every day)
Cardizem 60 mg tid (three times a day)
Timoptic 0.25% bid (twice a day)
You notice that the Zoloft (antidepressant) bottle is full. When you ask her about this, Mrs. White states that the Zoloft was giving her severe headaches, which you know is a side effect of this medication. She indicates that because of this she stopped taking it after one week.

Focus Question

1. Given this new information, what do you think could be happening? What additional information would you want to support your hypothesis?

   These questions are designed to stimulate critical thinking regarding polypharmacy in the elderly population, as well as the impact of cognitive-perceptual factors on medication misuse in the older population. Depending on the prior emphasis on pharmacology in the curriculum, students might be provided with pharmacology books or nursing drug handbooks to assist them in addressing the questions.

a. In the discussion, students should be asking the following questions: What are some adverse medication effects of these drugs? When were her medications last reviewed? Have there been any other health changes that may indicate a need for elimination and/or reduction of drugs (scenario states health is declining)? Are there methods you might use to enhance her ability to take medications? Are sensory deficits contributing to difficulties in taking medications? Other ways to enhance adherence? Could any of the medications be affecting her abilities? For example, depending on the time of administration, Lasix may cause awakening for nocturia.

b. If students have not already begun to question the reasons for Mrs. White's "declining health" and her forgetting to take medications, this data should be pointed out to them.

c. Although Mrs. White stated that she had stopped taking the Zoloft because of headaches, as indicated headaches may also be a side effect of Lanoxin. Lanoxicaps are to be used cautiously in the elderly; possible side effects include headache, hallucinations, confusion, nausea, vomiting.

d. Studies indicate about 59% of older adults in a community dwelling make medication errors in self-administration with overdosage and omission being the most common errors. Over 3 million elderly people exhibit confusion/delirium; an estimated 30% of confusion and/or delirium is drug-induced.

Depending on the curriculum, age-related changes may also be discussed:

1. *Absorption*—rate at which a drug leaves its site of administration
   (a) Age-related changes in gastric emptying and altered intestinal motility influence rate of absorption of oral medications
2. *Distribution*
   (a) Decline in cardiac output, (b)decrease in total body water: water-soluble drugs such as cimetidine (Tagamet), digoxin, (Lanoxin), and ethanol will be reflected in a higher than usual blood level in the elderly, (c) increased body fat: lipid soluble drugs may be stored in fatty tissue, extending and elevating drug effect, (d) decrease in lean body mass, (e) decrease in albumin levels: drugs bind with albumin; diminished albumin leads to more free active drug circulating and contributes to overdose and toxicity; highly protein bound drugs include aspirin, Coumadin, Motrin, Dilantin, Naproxen, Orinase, Thorazine, Haldol, Mellaril, Procardia, Diuril, Lasix, Valium
3. *Metabolism*—physical and chemical reactions that drugs undergo
   (a) Changes in liver function extend half-life (time required for plasma concentration of a drug to be reduced by half) of a drug
4. *Elimination*—Majority of drugs eliminated by the kidneys
   (a) Age-related changes that lead to decreased renal function are responsible for reduction in excretion of many drugs in the elderly; reduction in excretion ability leads to higher serum levels of many drugs over a prolonged period of time; dehydration will prolong and elevate blood levels of drugs

General principles related to adverse drug reactions

1. The signs and symptoms of an adverse reaction to a given drug may differ in older persons.
2. A prolonged time may be required for an adverse reaction to become apparent in older adults.

3. **An adverse reaction to a drug may be demonstrated even after the drug has been discontinued.**
4. **Adverse reactions to a drug that has been used over a long period of time without problems can develop suddenly.**

Risk factors for polypharmacy

Inclusion of several medications in drug regime

Debilitated or frail state

Malnourishment or dehydration

Multiple illnesses

An illness that interferes with cardiac, renal, or hepatic functioning

Cognitive impairment

History of adverse medication effects

Recent change in health or functional status

Negative functional consequences of polypharmacy

Increased probability of adverse effects

Unpredictable therapeutic effect

Mental changes and other functional impairments

Mrs. White's daughter stops by the apartment while you are there. She says to you, "Did my mother tell you she and her neighbor trade pills? She's been taking her neighbor's sleeping pills for six weeks. She forgets that, though."

Focus Questions

1. What could be the effect of the "sleeping pills"?
   a. **Most hypnotics interfere with REM sleep; Benzodiazepines can also cause awakening secondary to apnea**
   b. **Tolerance usually develops within several days**
   c. **Adverse effects likely to occur, especially if dose increased due to tolerance**
   d. **Paradoxical effects—nightmares and agitation**
   e. **Very long half-lifes, interfering with nightime sleep by causing daytime drowsiness**

   As stated before, over 3 million elderly people exhibit confusion/delirium; an estimated 30% of confusion and/or delirium is drug-induced.
2. What would you say and do?
   a. **Students might ask if Mrs. White's daughter knows the exact medication being used**
   b. **Further assessment of Mrs. White's cognition and depression, including possibility of intentional omission of medications as well as existential issues of meaning and hope**
   c. **Further assessment of side effects of medications experienced by Mrs. White**
   d. **Further assessment of Mrs. White's method of medication administration**

Reflective Writing

Suppose that Mrs. White's daughter informed you that her mother had been coming home at 2:00 or 3:00 A.M., and asks you for your advice on what to do about her mother. What would your first reaction be? What assumptions would be challenged by this information?

This prompt is used to further challenge students to identify assumptions, underlying beliefs, and implications for practice. Students may question assumptions regarding Mrs. White's cognitive status and her ability to live independently, expressing concerns about her safety. Students also discuss concerns regarding Mrs. White's ability to provide accurate assessment data. Issues regarding confidentiality are sometimes discussed, as well as the role of family members in provision of health care to the elderly client. The following information is then shared with students:

Postscript:

As you conduct your nursing assessment, you ask Mrs. White what gives her life meaning. Mrs. White confides that she is in love and often stays at her gentleman friend's house, but she has not shared this information with her daughter. She states that she needs and enjoys the companionship and sexual satisfaction provided through this relationship, but she is fearful that her daughter will be embarrassed by her actions and will question her judgment. Mrs. White, in fact, states that she has not been taking her friend's sleeping pills, but told her daughter she had been. She indicated to her daughter that because of the sleeping pills she sleeps so soundly that she does not hear her phone late at night when her daughter calls to check on her. Students typically do not identify sexuality and sexual behavior as a possible issue in this case. The postscript provides an opportunity to discuss reasons for this, as well as possible factors contributing to Mrs. White's hesitance in volunteering this information to her daughter or the nurse. This case can then be used as an introduction to the next class or unit on sexuality and aging.

Reference

Miller, C. A. (1995). *Nursing care of older adults: Theory and practice* (2nd ed.). Philadelphia: J. B. Lippincott.

CASE #5 PAULA POWELL

Learning Objectives

1. Problem-solve issues related to managing nursing staff consisting of experienced and novice nurses.
2. Discuss advantages and disadvantages of various approaches to solving problems encountered by a dysfunctional team of nurses working on a unit.
3. Explore team building exercises.

Paula Powell, 38 years old, is the nurse manager for an inpatient medical-surgical unit. During the past three months, there have been several new hires among the nursing staff. The evening shift now consists of one new graduate, two experienced nurses who are new to the facility, and three nurses who have several years experience on the unit. The newly hired nurses have satisfactorily completed their probationary periods. Paula has scheduled time to be on the evening shift to discuss the new hospital policy about paid days off. She meets with the staff, answering questions and clarifying the policy. Toward the end of the meeting, Paula senses that there is an undercurrent of edginess.

Focus Questions

1. What possible explanations could exist for Paula's feeling?

   There may be additional questions or concerns about the policy changes that staff members are uncomfortable in asking. There may be a patient situation that is affecting the responses. Inner turmoil among the staff members may exist. A conflict situation with staff from another unit or a physician may be occurring.

2. What possible actions could she take at this time?

   There are four possible actions: open the discussion to any topic that a staff member wants to address; end the meeting and delay her departure to allow for anyone to approach her privately; ignore the emotional climate in the belief that it is best for the staff to work out their own problems; and acknowledge the emotional tone and ask for a discussion of the issues.

3. What are the pros and cons of each identified action?

   - *Invite open discussion:* **Pros—Makes the staff aware that she is interested in their issues, regardless of the topic. Provides an opportunity for staff to address their concerns with a facilitator present. Cons—Paula does not know what their issues may be and she may be unprepared to facilitate such topics. There may not be sufficient time to address their concerns.**

   - *End the meeting and delay her departure:* **Pros—She would have opportunity to do fact-finding about the issue(s) affecting the staff. Staff members may feel more comfortable approaching Paula individually rather than speaking in front of the group. Paula can gather information without being responsible for assisting the group to formulate decisions. Cons—Paula may not have the time to meet with each staff member individually. Paula must hear from all staff members to develop a full picture of the perceptions of the issue(s).**

   - *Ignore the emotional climate:* **Pros—This affords the staff the opportunity to solve their own problems. This avoids making a large problem from a relatively small problem. Cons—The staff may develop the impression that Paula is not concerned about their problems. Paula will not be in touch with the thoughts and feelings of her staff members.**

   - *Acknowledge the emotional tone and ask for the issue(s):* **Pros—This approach makes the staff aware that their distress is noticeable and that Paula is interested. This provides for an open discussion focused on the emotional climate. Cons—The issues may be personal and not appropriate for discussion by the group. The time available for this discussion may not be sufficient today.**

4. What should Paula do?

   The instructor asks students for their preferred action and facilitates students to explore the rationales for their choices and possible reasons for making other selections.

At the conclusion of the meeting, Paula stays on the unit to complete some paperwork. The new graduate asks to speak privately with her. He shares with Paula his concerns about the cold, and sometimes critical, treatment he has recently received from the more experienced nurses. As Paula listens to his story, she is concerned that there is more to the situation than just a simple personality difference.

Focus Questions

1. What possible actions exist for Paula at this time?

   The following actions are available: talk individually to each staff member and gather additional information; discuss strategies for the new graduate to use in working with the more experienced nurses; and encourage the new graduate to allow more time for the relationships to develop.

2. What are the advantages and disadvantages of each action?

   - *Talk individually with each staff member:* **Advantages—Paula would gain information about each person's perception of the situation. Just expressing her concern to each person may bring about a change in behavior. No one is put in the position of having to reveal information with anyone else listening. Disadvantages—This approach is time-consuming for Paula. The staff may look to Paula in the future to solve their problems.**
   - *Discuss strategies for the new graduate to use in working with the more experienced nurses:* **Advantages—Equipping the new graduate with additional skills will encourage professional growth by allowing him to solve this problem himself. Addressing his concerns facilitates a sense of trust between Paula and the graduate. Disadvantages—This approach does not address any negative behaviors that may be occurring on the part of the more experienced nurses. Impacting their behavior is important to the success of future new graduates who come to work on this unit.**
   - *Encourage the new graduate to give the relationships more time:* **Advantages—Encourages the new graduate to persevere in forming relationships with the more experienced nurses. Disadvantages—The new graduate may feel that Paula is not interested in how well he is doing. He may be reluctant to speak with Paula about unit issues in the future.**

3. What action should she take?

   The instructor should facilitate discussion about the choices and assist students to select the behavior(s) they deem appropriate. The best response may be a combination of discussing the issue with each nurse and discussing strategies for the new graduate to use in working with the more experienced nurses.

After gathering information about the issues and meeting again with the graduate nurse, Paula decides that the underlying concern is that this group has not come together as a team. They are operating as small cliques, with the new graduate on the outside.

Focus Questions

1. What approaches are possible at this time?

   Paula may decide to schedule another unit meeting and address her concerns to the whole group at one time. She may discuss her concerns with each staff member individually. She may request assistance from human resources in planning several team-building sessions with this staff.

2. What advantages and disadvantages exist for each approach?

   - *Schedule a unit meeting and address her concerns to all:* **Advantages—Everyone will have the opportunity to discuss the issues and formulate responses to the concerns. As a result of the open discussion, staff members may feel a greater sense of obligation to develop workable solutions. Disadvantages—Staff members may become**

defensive and resist suggestions for improving the emotional climate of the unit. Blaming one particular staff member may result from the open discussion.

- *Discuss the concerns individually with all staff members:* **Advantages—All staff members can respond to suggestions without any fear of reprisal from other staff members. Staff members who have been exhibiting less than professional behavior can be confronted in private. Disadvantages—The opportunity to blame others is more possible in the private sessions. As time is required to speak individually with all staff members, it takes longer for everyone to arrive at the same end point.**
- *Request assistance from human resources in planning some team-building sessions:* **Advantages—The main purpose here is to achieve a higher functioning unit. Team-building activities will assist the staff members in learning how to work productively together. No one is singled out as causing the problem; everyone is responsible for the solution. Disadvantages—Sessions will have to be short and to the point to avoid disrupting the unit activities.**

3. Explore various team-building activities and report on one you think would be effective in this situation.

   The instructor should direct students to resources that provide team-building exercises.

Reflective Writing

What actions by Paula could have possibly prevented this entire problem or was there anything she could have done? If you were the new graduate in this scenario, how would you see the situation? If you were one of the experienced nurses, how might you see the situation?

Perhaps a preceptor for the new graduate would have provided him with some security as he made the transition to the evening shift. Paula could offer her new graduates the opportunity to meet with her periodically just to talk about how their work is progressing. Paula may not have been able to prevent this situation from occurring. The new graduate likely experienced frustration and lowered self-esteem from his treatment. He may have experienced thoughts about moving to another position or leaving nursing altogether. The experienced nurses may not have considered the potential impact of their behaviors to be negative. They may be wondering what all the fuss is about. Changing their behaviors will undoubtedly create frustration for them.

References

Huber, D. (1996). *Leadership and nursing care management.* Philadelphia: W. B. Saunders.

Marquis, B. L. & Huston, C. J. (2000). *Leadership roles and management functions in nursing: Theory & application* (3rd ed.). Philadelphia: Lippincott.

CASE #6 THE BANCEK FAMILY

Learning Objectives

1. Apply the nursing process to families with a chronic illness.
2. Demonstrate assessment strategies to use with families.
3. Plan appropriate interventions based on family nursing diagnoses.
4. Apply principles of family nursing.

Mr. Bancek is a 59-year-old Caucasian male who was diagnosed 7 years ago with Alzheimers disease. He is cared for in the family home by his wife and children with the help of a home care nurse several days a week. He is unable to care for himself and while ambulatory reguires assistance with all ADL. Prior to his illness, he was a factory worker at an automotive plant. He and his wife have 9 children, ages 13 to 28. The three youngest still live in the home, and the others live in the community. There are three grandchildren. The entire extended family attends the same church. They have lived in their home for 30 years.

Focus Questions

1. Using the Friedman Family Assessment Model, identify data you would need to collect from this family.

    - **Identifying data—religion, leisure activities**
    - **Developmental stage and family history—history of family origin, present developmental stage, extent of family developmental task fulfillment**
    - **Environmental data—support systems, home characteristics, neighborhood, family association with community**
    - **Family structure—(1) communication patterns between members, (2) power structure—decision making process, power base, finances, (3) role structure—formal, informal, (4) family values—what is important**
    - **Family functions—(1) affective—need-response patterns, closeness, connectedness, (2) socialization—child rearing practices, value of children, (3) health care function—definition of health and illness, dietary practices, sleep and rest habits, activity and leisure, knowledge level related to chronic illness, values and beliefs about health and health care, health history**
    - **Family Stress and Coping—(1) stressors—short and long term, (2) coping mechanisms—what strategies have been used in past; how do different family members cope**

    In this case, the nurse would want to assess how the family is coping with Mr. Bancek's illness. All the above data needs to be collected in order to assess strengths, challenges, and where the nurse needs to focus his/her intervention. This family needs to function effectively, even though there is a chronic illness present. The most important information would include the family's perception of their problem, if they have one.

2. What assessment strategies might be used to elicit the data needed in question 1?

    Interview with all family members to ascertain each one's perception of the use of formal instruments such as the family Apgar or FILE, which measures family stress. Remember that in this case we are focusing on the family as the client, not specific family members.

3. If a family genogram is constructed, what might it look like? What is the purpose of this assessment strategy?

    This a pictoral representation of the family that maps relationships of members of both the nuclear and the extended family. It helps the nurse to see patterns of health and to generate possible hypotheses about what is happening within the family. It delineates information about age, gender, birth, divorce, marriage, illness/health status, death, race, social class, ethnicity, religion, occupation, and place of residence. From the given information, a skeleton genogram could be constructed showing the marriage of Mr. and Mrs. Bancek, their nine children, and their grandchildren. It should include Mr. Bancek's occupation and chronic illness. Obtaining additional information would be required to complete the strategy.

You are to be the new home care nurse. You have met with the family to discuss arrangements. Mrs. Bancek was a homemaker until her husband's illness. She had to return to work full time 4 years ago to meet the family's financial needs. All of the family members want to help with Mr. Bancek's care and are very supportive. The Bancek's oldest daughter shares most of the care giving with her mother.

Focus Questions

1. What family nursing diagnoses might be identified for this family?
   - **altered family process, caregiver strain**
   - **family coping, potential for growth**
   - **parenting, altered**
2. Prioritize a plan of care for the Bancek family.

   Plans could focus on having the family as a group using problem solving to identify possible solutions and arrangements as to how to share in Mr. Bancek's care. All family members have some strain, but particularly the mother, the oldest daughter, and the children still at home. The nurse needs to help the family use strategies that have worked for them before in making decisions. The nurse might help them identify community resources.
3. Identify family strengths.
   - **Close knit family—all members want to help**
   - **Religion**
   - **Stable family—lived in same place 30 years**

Mrs. Bancek shares with you that she tried to get a placement for Mr. Bancek in an adult day-care setting; however, he did not meet enough of the criteria. She shares that when the case worker asked him who Mrs. Bancek was, Mr. Bancek replied, "Mother." Mrs. Bancek cries and becomes quiet. Her oldest daughter cares for her father two days a week. When asked if this is a burden, she says, "No, my mother has it the hardest. It's like she doesn't have a husband or anyone to talk to. Her husband is dead, but he isn't."

Focus Question

1. How should you, as the home care nurse, respond to Mrs. Bancek and her daughter?

   The best strategy is to listen and show empathy to the family. (Instructor may wish to have students role-play the interaction. Debriefing of how each felt during the interaction could help students see the situations from different perspectives.)

Reflective Writing

Write about the role of **support** for the family nursing: where does support come from and what forms can it take?

This will provide the students a way to look globally at their role in working with families. Support can come from within the family unit, as well as from multiple sources in the community (church, extended family, health care team). Support can take many forms such as emotional, tangible, and informational. Students should mention all of these ideas in exploring the role of support for families.

References

Friedman, M. (1998). *Family nursing : Research, theory, and practice.* (4th ed.). Stamford, Conn.: Appleton & Lang.
Hanson, S. & Boyd, S. (eds). (1996). *Family health care nursing: Theory, practice, and research.* Philadelphia: F. A. Davis Co.

CASE #7 DELTA COUNTY HEALTH DEPARTMENT

Learning Objectives

1. Identify parameters that need to be assessed when concerns arise about an identified aggregate in the community.
2. Describe methods that can be utilized to assess an identified aggregate's health status.
3. Analyze data to arrive at a nursing diagnosis (conclusion) about an identified aggregate.

The Delta County Health Department (DCHD) is a large official tax-supported agency located in a major urban center, serving the geographical area of Delta County. It has a team of about 50 staff members who make home visits. These staff members include community health nurses, registered nurses, licensed practical nurses, social workers, occupational and physical therapists, homemakers, and certified home health aides. In weekly team meetings over the past several months, various members have voiced concern about the social isolation that they believe they are seeing among their elderly clients. There is limited public transportation, and thus, unless clients drive or have family members who do, there are few alternatives for leaving home. There is voiced concern that depression and confusion are resulting. After discussion by the team, there is consensus that the concern should be investigated thoroughly and objectively to ascertain whether or not the isolation should be a priority problem with resources budgeted to address it. A date and time for a meeting is set.

Focus Questions

1. Identify objective data that are currently available about the population 65 years and older in Delta County. What can these data tell the team?

   Census data, morbidity and mortality data, numbers of visits made by DCHD staff, and numbers isolated at home as assessed by DCHD staff. When they are compared in terms of percentages with data from another county or with state data, a decision can be facilitated as to whether there are "large" numbers of people over 65, married, isolated, etc. These data are relatively easy to collate and are usually readily available.

2. Identify parameters about the people under study, not part of census data, who should be investigated. Develop one question to be asked about each parameter.

   Along with demographics, investigate religion, roles of community members, and history of the community, values, customs, and norms. For example, if clients could easily leave home, where would they like to go? If clients go to church, are there people there who help them get around? How often do the clients want to leave and cannot?

3. Identify parameters about the environment and the health care delivery system that should be investigated. Develop one question to be asked about each parameter.

   - **The health care delivery system: kinds and types available in the area served by DCHD.**

- **The environment: the social environment including transportation sources, industry, types of communication, recreation, technology, politics, religion; biological environment including food supply.**
- **Sample question: What is the primary source of news for elderly clients in Delta County? Where do they buy their food on a regular basis?**

In the second weekly team meeting, the leader asks the group to think about *how* the data identified at the last meeting can be collected. Keep in mind that time and money is limited.

Focus Questions

1. A basic principle is that the identified aggregate (clients 65 and older) should help identify the problem and possible solutions. Discuss methods for obtaining input from the aggregate and the advantages and disadvantages of each. Which of the questions identified at the last meeting should be asked of them?

   Focus groups, mailed surveys, interviews with individual clients, talks with clubs, church and synagogue groups, phone interviews. It may be difficult for the elderly to get to group gatherings, so individual clients can be interviewed at home. Natural gatherings such as clubs can be identified to collect this information.

2. What key community informants should be interviewed? What questions identified at the first meeting should be asked of them?

   Clergy, directors of housing projects, politicians, city planners, professionals in other health care organizations, senior citizen groups. This group of people will help to solve identified problems so they also need to know the extent of the problem, if there is one. These informants can address the questions identified in paragraph 1.

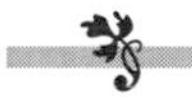

Over the course of the past two months, data have been gathered from many people. Statistical data have been collected. Following are some of the results: the number of people over 65 in Delta County are declining as "baby boomers" move in to gentrify the county which is historically rich. The county is ethnically diverse, and there does not appear to be social and political cohesion among the numerous subcultures. There is limited public transportation, and city planners have no plans to enlarge the system since "we have no demands for it from most of the county's population." Of the 25 clients interviewed, 8 said that lack of transportation was a very serious problem for them. No morbidity or mortality could be objectively linked to the transportation issue.

Focus Question

1. The problem of social isolation and lack of transportation has been investigated. Decide what conclusion(s) should be reached from the data gathered. Is social isolation among elderly clients served by DCHD a priority problem?

   Because resources are limited, problems addressed must be those that are a priority. Data do not support the statement that isolation and lack of transportation are a priority problem for people 65 and older in Delta County. It might be interesting to discuss why there seemed to be a problem: Is it human nature to have biases, even for health professionals? Perhaps some team members felt very strongly about their concern for their clients and voiced this strongly and frequently? It is for these reasons and others that concerns must be objectively investigated to ascertain their validity and depth. Because this is a problem for some people, perhaps there can be brainstorming to develop some solutions for those concerned.

Reflective Writing

Though there are not many people who suffer from isolation, some really do. How do you as a health professional deal with the ethical dilemma of knowing that you cannot help everyone, even those with severe problems?

There is no right answer—as is the case with ethical dilemmas. It is important for nurses to have self-understanding about their own beliefs and actions when they face such dilemmas. Just as some nurses find euthanasia an acceptable alternative, others find it abhorrent. The critical factor is coming to terms with one's own beliefs and having an understanding of why that belief is held. Further, it is important for community health organizations to have ethics committees that are part of the standards of accreditation. No one person should have to make difficult decisions alone, and there are experts in the field of ethics who can assist organizations with these situations. Further, community organizations need to discuss and come to terms with what they are capable of doing or not doing, and make this known to their employees and to the general public. Nurses need support during the times they are dealing with difficult situations. Without this, burnout is a given. Burnout or leaving the profession results from continual feelings of inadequacy. The community setting can be a "setup" for burnout because there are so many needs and often too little money.

Reference

Clemen-Stone, S., McGuire, S. L., & Gerber Eigsti, D. (1998). *Comprehensive community health nursing. Family, aggregate, and community practice.* St. Louis: Mosby Year Book.

CASE #8 BILL GROOMS

Learning Objectives

1. Identify abnormal vital signs (T, P, R, BP)
2. Identify factors that affect body temperature, pulse, and respirations.
3. Discuss possible rationales for altered vital signs (T, P, R, BP)
4. Identify sites where pulse may be taken.
5. Discuss common errors in blood pressure assessment.

Bill Grooms is a 48-year-old white male. He is in the recovery room postinguinal hernia repair under a general anesthetic. Vital sign are: Temp—99°F, BP—120/80, P—80, R—18.

Focus Questions

1. Are Bill's vital signs within normal limits? List normal adult vital signs.

Bill's Vitals		**Normal for adult**
Temperature:	**99°**	**Range: 98–98.6°F**
Pulse:	**80**	**Range: 60–100**
Respiration:	**18**	**Range: 12–20**
BP:	**120/80**	**Range: 90/60–140/80**

There is a slight increase in temperature.

2. What factors might affect body temperature?
   - **Environmental temperature (i.e., hot room, cold weather)**
   - **Stress (it causes increase production of epinephrine and nonepinephrine, which increases heat production)**
   - **Hormones (especially with women at time of ovulation—increase temperature)**
   - **Exercise (increases temperature)**
   - **Circadian rhythms (temperature highest between 8:00 P.M. and midnight; lowest between 4:00–6:00 A.M.**
   - **Age (older adults and infant most susceptible to changes)**
   - **Infection (causes temperature elevation)**
3. What are some varied sites that the nurse might take the client's pulse? What sites are most commonly used?
   - **Temporal**
   - **Carotid**
   - **Apical—commonly used**
   - **Brachial**
   - **Radial—commonly used**
   - **Femerol**
   - **Popliteal**
   - **Posterior Tibial**
   - **Pedal**
4. What factors might influence respiratory rate?

Increase	Decrease
Exercise	**Cold environment**
Stress	**Increased intracranial pressure**
Hot environment	**Medications (narcotics and analgesics)**
Increased altitude	

Two hours postoperative, Bill complains of abdominal pain. Vital signs: Temp 99.2°F, BP 90/60, P—120, R—24.

Focus Questions

1. What could Bill's vital signs indicate? What nursing interventions are indicated?
   - **Hemorrhage—decrease in blood volume results in *decreased blood pressure—increase in pulse* due to blood loss, as the heart tries to compensate for the lost blood volume—*increased respirations,* as respirations follow pulse rate**
   - **Nurse needs to check for blood loss (check dressing, turn client to see if blood is running down side to back)**

- **Monitor for further vital sign changes**
- **Administer fluids (po or IV) to raise blood volume**
- **Elevated temperature could be due to dehydration from being NPO and surgery**

2. What clinical signs indicating fever might the nurse assess with Bill?
   - **Chills at onset**
   - **Warm skin**
   - **Thirst**
   - **Aching muscles, fatigue**
   - **Glassy-eyed appearance**
   - **Drowsiness**
   - **Herpetic lesions of the mouth**
3. If his fever persists and increases for a few days, what might the nurse suspect is happening and what might be done?
   - **Indicates possible infection (if over 100.4°F for more than 4–8 hours after the first day postoperatively)**
   - **Nurse needs to:**

     —check dressing for purulent drainage

     —force fluids

     —give antipyretics as ordered

     —keep bed dry

     —give tepid sponge bath

     —help with oral care

     —I & O

     —monitor white blood cells (WBC)

     —monitor VS

     —assess for sites of possible infection such as lungs for congestion, urine for urinary tract infection, etc.

Bill does well and is to be discharged. However, when the physician checks the chart, he notices that Bill's blood pressure is charted to be both high (190/100) low (90/50) and average (120/80) depending upon which nurse or aide had taken it. Since BP is an indicator of the client's condition, he asked the head nurse to investigate this variation. The physician checked his pressure three times within an hour period and found it to be stable and normal at each reading.

Focus Questions

1. What are some common errors in blood pressure assessment that result in erroneously high or low readings?

High Readings	Low Readings
—too small or narrow cuff	**—too wide or big cuff**
—unsupported arm	**—repeat procedure too soon (low diastolic)**
—client not at rest prior to measurement	**—deflate cuff too quickly (low systolic)**
—repeat procedure too soon (high systolic)	**—arm above heart level**
—cuff too loose or wrinkled	
—deflate cuff too quickly (high diastolic)	
—deflate cuff too slowly (high diastolic)	
—assess during pain, smoking, eating	

2. How might the head nurse educate her staff regarding proper BP techniques?
   - **Seminar to reeducate (if abnormal repeat and assess, why up or down?)**
   - **Devise a game to assess knowledge of common errors in procedure (Jeopardy, Trivial Pursuit, etc.)**
   - **Demonstration/return demonstration**

Reflective Writing

If you were a nurse on a busy postoperative unit and a nurse's aide has been repeatedly not getting accurate vital signs, how would you approach her? Would your response differ if (a) she was not even taking vital signs, just charting what seemed normal *or* (b) she was incompetent in taking vital signs and charted what she thought was accurate?

In either instance, the nurse must talk with the aide or report her to the head nurse/supervisor so someone can stop her behavior, as well as document her behaviors. The approach needs to be to first assess her competence and then address her "not doing" her job, if that is the case. If she is unable to take accurate vital signs, she must be retrained and checked until she is competent. If she is simply not doing her job, she must be counseled regarding the importance of vital signs in postoperative clients and the possible consequences if changes are not documented. The aide needs constant supervision until you are certain she is competent. If this fails, she may need to be terminated.

Reference

Kozier, B., Erb, G., Berman, A., & Burke, K. (2000) *Fundamentals of nursing: Concepts, process, practice.* Upper Saddle River, N.J.: Prentice Hall.

CASE #9 MANDY AND AMY, STUDENT NURSES

Learning Objectives

1. Identify breech of ethics and legality.
2. Discuss appropriate behaviors of nurses dealing with private and confidential information.
3. Reflect on ways to respond ethically to situations involving sharing of confidential information.

Mandy and Amy are student nurses working in the postpartum unit. Mandy's client, Jill, is a newly married new mother to a baby boy. Jill is excited and tells Mandy how wonderful her husband Jim is. She tells her how Jim has stood by her and how loyal he has been throughout their courtship and marriage. Amy's client, Ashley, is a 16-year-old adolescent with a newborn daughter. She, too, cannot quit telling Amy how wonderful her boyfriend is and how they are going to be married soon. While Mandy and Amy are charting, a man approaches the nurses' station and asks what rooms Jill George and Ashley Cole are in? Mandy gives him the information. She notices he has two bouquets of flowers. "Can you keep these flowers here till I finish visiting Jill?" he asks Mandy as he hands her one bouquet.

Focus Questions

1. What conclusions might you come to regarding this man?
   - **Maybe the man is the father to both babies. (The "Jim" they both talk about.)**
   - **Maybe one woman is his wife and one is his cousin or friend (but why did he want Mandy to keep the second bouquet?)**
   - **Maybe he is the father of neither baby and is a relative or a friend to both.**
2. How should Mandy respond to the man?
   - **"Yes, of course, I'll keep them right here for you." His intentions are none of Mandy's business, despite what her assumptions might be.**

The man leaves the nurses' station and heads to Jill's room. Later he returns to the station and retrieves the second bouquet of flowers. He then heads to Ashley's room. Mandy and Amy discuss this scenario at the nurses' station and decide that he is the father of both babies. They proceed to tell the other nurses and students on the unit about this "jerk" and debate how they will let Jill and Ashley know about their so-called loyal and loving husband and boyfriend.

Focus Question

1. Have Mandy and Amy done anything ethically and/or legally wrong? If so, what?

   Yes, they have assumed something about the man that may or may not be true. They have no right to tell other staff who are not involved. In fact, neither of them should tell anyone about this. By discussing this, they have breeched confidentiality and may be spreading untrue rumors about him, which could result in their being sued for slander should they be overheard.

Upon leaving Ashley's room, the man returns to the nurses' station. Mandy and Amy are still in the station. "Excuse me, I'm Pastor Jim from the Holycrest Baptist Church. May I leave my card for you? Two of my church members are here, and if they feel the need to talk with me, I'd be glad to come back. Feel free to call me or encourage them to do so."

Focus Question

1. What should Mandy and Amy do now? Is there a way to "right" the rumors they spread to the staff?

   They must immediately remedy the falsehoods they assumed about Jim. They need to acknowledge their wrong-doing and use it as a learning experience for staff and other students. We cannot *assume* things based on our own perceptions, nor can we spread private information about clients, families, etc., to others (even if the information is

true). They might call a meeting for all staff to discuss this issue to ensure the rumor goes no further.

Reflective Writing

As a nurse, you will encounter many situations where you will be faced with knowing private and confidential information about another person or a family. What are your responsibilities as a professional nurse? How will you deal with keeping this information to yourself, especially if you feel it is information that needs to be shared with the client, the family, or the physician?

Nurses need to respect one's privacy and confidential information. It must not be shared with anyone who does not have to be aware of it in order to provide adequate care to the client. Often nurses feel conflicted in their loyalties and obligations to patients, families, and other staff members. The nursing code of ethics says a nurse's first loyalty is to the client. Sometimes telling a client the truth can do more harm than good for the client. Nurses need to analyze the consequences of their actions before acting so as to assure the best for their clients.

(Faculty might want to discuss ethical decision-making models such as Thompson & Thompson (1985), Cassello and Redman (1989), Chally and Loriz (1998), or other models.)

References

Cassells, J. & Redman, B. (1989). Preparing students to be moral agents in clinical nursing practice. *Nursing Clinics of North America*, 24 (2), 463–473.

Chally, P. & Loriz, L. Ethics in the trenches: Decision making in practice. *American Journal of Nursing* 98(6), 17–20

Kozier, B., Erb, G, Berman, A., & Burke, K. (2000). *Fundamentals of nursing: Concepts, process, and practice.* Upper Saddle River, NJ: Prentice Hall.

Thompson, J. & Thompson, H. (1985). *Bioethical decision making for nurses.* Norwalk, Conn.: Appleton-Century Craft.

CASE #10 RITA JENKINS, SCHOOL NURSE

Learning Objectives

1. Discuss nursing interventions to identify, treat, and prevent head lice in the school setting.
2. Discuss hepatitis A, its symptoms, the way it is spread, and how a school nurse can intervene to prevent its spread and educate staff.
3. Identify information pertinent for teachers to know about caring for a child with seizures.

Rita is the school nurse for a rural school district that has two elementary schools, one junior high school, and one high school. She spends one day per week at each of the schools and uses the fifth day as one to "catch up." Today she is at one of the elementary schools where head lice is becoming more and more prevalent. She is scheduled to do "head checks" in all of the classrooms.

Focus Questions

1. What procedure should she use to check children?
   - **Inspect scalp using a magnifying glass/lamp**
   - **Go through the entire head using applicator sticks or a fine-toothed comb (use new applicators or comb for each student)**

- **Look for lice and nits, noting location**
- **Look for head irritation due to itching and/or secondary infections**

2. If lice or nits are found, what should she do?
   - **Children should be sent home and are not allowed to return until they are nit free.**
3. How might she educate students and families about identifying, preventing, and treating lice?

   Use of written information as well as verbal teaching on:
   - **Methods of disinfection of clothing and bedding (washing, drying, ironing, storage in plastic bag)**
   - **Treatment of myths (cutting hair won't decrease risk; use of disinfecting spray won't kill lice and eggs)**
   - **Treatment of hair (topical shampoo, i.e., Nix, Rid, R&C, Ovide), in compliance with manufacturer's instructions for application. Follow treatment with another one in 7–10 days to kill eggs. Use comb to remove lice and nits.**
   - **Prevention—children should not share hats, combs, etc. Families need to prevent reinfestation by treating furniture, carpets, bed sheets, automobile upholstery, etc.**
   - **Follow-up posttreatment with recheck at school**
   - **Classroom teachers need to be taught prevention strategies (no sharing of head gear, pillows, etc., separate coat hooks, keep hats in coat sleeves or pockets).**

The next day Rita is working at the other elementary school when Mrs. Borden, a teacher for multi-handicapped children, approaches her to discuss a child in her class who has been diagnosed with hepatitis A. Even though the child is no longer at school, Mrs. Borden is afraid that she and the other children might be at risk, and she wants Rita to help and to give her advice and information on the disease.

Focus Questions

1. What should Rita tell Mrs. Borden about hepatitis A?
   - **Formerly known as infectious hepatitis**
   - **Caused by the hepatitis A virus (HAV)**
   - **Commonly reported in older children and young adults**
   - **Fatality rate is 0.6%—rapid recovery occurs with most cases**
   - **Makes up 50% of the reported cases of all hepatitis**
   - **Transmission by person to person through oral ingestion of fecal contaminants**
   - **Often transmitted because of poor personal hygiene**
   - **May be due to food handlers who have contaminated food with feces (don't wash hands after toileting)**
   - **Symptoms—fever 100–102°F, nausea and vomiting, malaise, anorexia, jaundice within 1–5 days of flu symptoms; as jaundice progresses may have dark urine and clay-colored stools**
   - **Diagnosis with blood test (look for IgM anti-HAV)**

2. What interventions should occur since hepatitis A has been diagnosed in the school?
   - **Teachers and staff need to be taught about the spread of hepatitis A by the fecal-oral route, especially those who work with special needs children who may require diapering or have fecal incontinence.**
   - **In-service for all school staff on importance of frequent hand washing and how to care for children with fecal incontinence (gloves, disposal, hand washing, etc.). Also teach about disinfecting toys or materials that children may put into their mouths.**
   - **All classrooms (children) need to be instructed on hand washing by the school nurse or by their teacher (who has been taught by the nurse).**
   - **Children deemed at risk should be identified, and their parents should receive information on the spread of hepatitis A and the potential for fecal-oral transmission. They also need to be encouraged to discuss prophylaxis with immune globulen (IG) with their physician.**
   - **Hepatitis A must be reported to the health department.**

Rita is scheduled to give an in-service to the high school teachers on how to care for an epileptic child experiencing a seizure. This request for the in-service occurred as a result of one of the teachers witnessing a girl having a grand mal tonic-clonic seizure in the cafeteria because of her epilepsy.

Focus Question

1. What topics should Rita cover in her in-service?

   a. **Definition of epilepsy**
   - **Chronic disorder of the brain resulting in recurrent seizures**

   b. **Definition of seizures**
   - **Uncontrollable episodes of excessive electrical discharges in the brain resulting in either tonic-clonic movements where the person stiffens and jerks or absence episodes where there is staring or blinking (often confused with day-dreaming)**

   c. **What to assess regarding seizure as it occurs**
   - **Describe what you see**
   - **Time lapse—how long did it last?**
   - **Events that preceded it**
   - **Was there an aura?**
   - **What body parts moved/behavior?**
   - **Levels of consciousness**

   d. **Medication/Treatments**
   - **Anticonvulsant medications (Phenobarbital, Tegretol, Dilantin)**
   - **Valium for status epilepticus or severe recurrent seizures (given rectally)**
   - **Oxygen administration**
   - **Surgery in extreme cases**

e. **Classroom modifications for safety**
   - **Adequate room—move furniture**
   - **Avoidance of contact sports**
   - **If child has an aura, teach him/her to get into open area prior to seizure to prevent injury**

f. **Safety during seizure including preventing aspiration**
   - **Stay with child**
   - **Loosen restrictive clothing**
   - **Protect head**
   - **Move furniture away**
   - **Keep child as safe as possible**
   - **Don't restrict movement**
   - **Put on side if possible**
   - **Clear secretions from mouth**
   - **Don't use tongue blade**
   - **Check respirations after seizure ends**

g. **Support Peers—fear may occur for other children**
   - **Remove other children if possible**
   - **Explain epilepsy—give information**

h. **Emergency procedures in case of Status Epilepticus**
   - **Call 911**
   - **Give Valium if ordered (rectally)**
   - **Provide safe environment**

Reflective Writing

Discuss the responsibilities and challenges of school nursing. What personal and professional characteristics must the school nurse demonstrate in order to work in this area of nursing?

- **Record keeping (immunizations, screening, health rx)**
- **Community focus**
- **Care for individuals, families, and groups of children**
- **Health promotion/prevention important aspects**
- **Teaching is a major responsibility—children, teachers, and staff**
- **Give routine medications**
- **First Aid**
- **Screenings (eye, hearing, scoliosis, etc.)**
- **Flexible**
- **Knowledgeable**
- **Able to work without supervision**

- **Like kids**
- **Like to teach**

References

Epilepsy Foundation of America, 4351 Garden City Dr., Landover, MD 20785
Wong, D. (1999). *Whaley and Wong's nursing care of infants and children.* 6th ed. St. Louis: Mosby.

CASE #11 ELSA HUNGER

Learning Outcomes

1. Distinguish between spirituality and religion.
2. Describe components of a spiritual assessment.
3. Recognize the difference between a spiritual and a psychological nursing diagnosis.
4. Identify nursing interventions for spiritual needs.
5. Examine personal beliefs about spirituality.

Elsa Hunger, a 72-year-old female of Italian Polish heritage, is being seen by the home health nurse twice a week for chronic obstructive pulmonary disease, shortness of breath, and complaint of burning with urination. She is being monitored on several respiratory medications and an antidepressant. She had been using an antibiotic for a urinary tract infection but is not on it presently. She uses oxygen continuously and has been known to increase the rate herself, even though she has been told the danger of this practice to her condition. She had smoked for over fifty years but stopped three months ago. She has four grown children all living nearby; however, she is estranged from three of the children, frequently making angry statements about them. Her youngest son Peter, age 32, comes to see her weekly. She tells the nurse that although he is her youngest and her favorite, she is also angry with him because he is an alcoholic, is always asking her for money, and is unable to keep a job. A home health aide comes three times per week to assist her in activities of daily living. She used to attend mass weekly but has not been able to go for the last six months. Her priest comes weekly to give her communion. She cries frequently and calls the home health nurse often with miscellaneous complaints. When the nurse planned to decrease the number of visits per week, Elsa started complaining of burning with urination. A catheterized specimen was negative. Frequently on arriving at the home, the nurse finds Elsa with a rapid respiratory rate of 40, which immediately slows to normal when the nurse sits down with her. Today she is talking about a friend who had called her and told her about a problem at the church that she is upset about. During the visit Elsa complains that "nobody cares that I am alive, not my family, not my friends, not God."

Focus Questions

1. Define the difference between spirituality and religion.

   This should include a general discussion about what are spirituality and religion. The students' ideas on how they are alike or different could evolve. The differences between spirituality and religion can be defined as seen in the Sumner (1998) article: Spirituality is a broad concept of a basic human phenomenon that helps create mean-

ing and gives purpose to life. Moberg describes it with vertical and horizontal aspects. Well-being in relation to God is the vertical aspect, while the horizontal aspect relates to one's sense of the purpose of life, hardiness, serenity, peace, connection, and hope. The vertical concerns our eternal being; the horizontal, our earthly existence. Sumner defines religion as both a concept and a social system that supports group expression and devotional activity. It is a formal medium for expressing belief in God or gods. Religion is a part of spirituality, but it is not necessarily related.

2. Identify components of a spiritual assessment. What assessment data should the nurse obtain from Elsa?

Components of a spiritual assessment of Elsa should include:

I. Observations:

A. Nonverbal behavior

1. Observe affect. Does the client's affect or attitude convey loneliness, depression, anger, agitation, or anxiety?

2. Observe behavior. Does the client pray during the day? Does the client rely on religious reading material or other literature for solace?

B. Look for symbols of worship

1. Look for visual cues on patient's person and in home regarding spiritual religion orientation, such as spiritual books, i.e., Bible, Torah, Koran, or others. Symbols of religion, i.e., cross, Star of David, medals, pins, plaques, rosary, statues, etc.

C. Interpersonal relationships:

1. Does the client have visitors or is she or he alone a lot?

2. Are the visitors supportive or do they leave the client feeling upset?

3. Does the client have visitors or friends from church?

II. Listening—Carson (1989)

A. Does the client seem to complain out of proportion to his illness?

B. Does the client complain of sleeping difficulties?

C. Does the client ask for unusually high doses of sedation or pain medication?

D. Does the client talk about prayer, faith, hope, or anything of a religious nature?

E. Does the client refer to God in any way?

F. Does the client talk about church functions that are a part of his life?

G. Does the client express concern over the meaning and direction of life?

H. Does the client express concern over the impact of the illness on the meaning of life?

III. Interviewing: Areas to be covered in a spirituality interview of Elsa should address the following from Stoll (1979):

A. Concept of God:

1. Is religion or God important to you? If so, can you describe how?

2. Do you use prayer in your life?

3. **Do you believe God or a deity is involved in your personal life? If so, how?**
4. **What is your God or deity like?**

B. **Sources of Strength and Hope:**

1. **Who are your support people?**
2. **Who is the most important person in your life?**
3. **Are people available to you when you are in need?**
4. **Who or what provides you with strength and hope?**

C. **Religious Practices:**

1. **Is your religious faith helpful to you?**
2. **Are there any religious practices that are meaningful to you?**
3. **Has your illness affected your religious practices?**
4. **Are there any religious books or symbols that are helpful to you?**

3. Distinguish and prioritize Elsa's spiritual and psychosocial nursing diagnoses.

From Sumner (1998) students should synthesize the knowledge related to signs of spiritual concerns, signs of spiritual distress, and signs of spiritual despair, and then apply to Elsa:

I. **Signs of Spiritual Concerns could include:**

A. **Discouragement**
B. **Mild anxiety**
C. **Expressions of anticipatory grief**
D. **Inability to participate in usual spiritual practice**
E. **Expressions of concern about relationship with God or higher power**
F. **Inability to obtain foods required by beliefs**

II. **Signs of Spiritual Distress could include:**

A. **Crying**
B. **Expressions of guilt**
C. **Disturbances in sleep patterns**
D. **Disrupted spiritual trust**
E. **Feeling remote from God or higher power**
F. **Moderate to severe anxiety**
G. **Anger toward staff, family, God, or higher power**
H. **Challenged belief or value system**
I. **Loss of meaning and purpose in life**

III. **Spiritual Despair:**

A. **Loss of hope**
B. **Death wish**

C. **Severe depression**

D. **Flat affect**

E. **Refusal to participate in treatment regimen**

Elsa's issues could be organized in the following way, distinguishing the psychosocial from the spiritual

Spiritual Concerns

- **discouragement**
- **mild anxiety**
- **not able to participate in church activities with others**
- **statement that God doesn't care**

Spiritual Distress Symptoms

- **feeling remote from God**
- **anxiety**
- **anger toward family and God**
- **loss of meaning in life**

Emotional Issues

- **social isolation**
- **loss of ability to get out**
- **loss of ability to care for self**
- **change of role**
- **change of self-esteem**
- **powerlessness toward own situation, son's alcoholism, relationship with other children**
- **abandonment**
- **anger with family, friends**

Although some of these symptoms and concerns may overlap, it is important to try to distinguish the root causes. If the person is feeling disconnected from God, that is a severe loss and needs to be addressed. A client's relationship with his or her God can bring a great source of hope, and nurses should encourage this.

4. Identify appropriate spiritual caring interventions.

Based on her answers to the interview questions about her concept of God, her sources of strength and hope, and her desired religious practices, encourage her with specific comments or suggestions that would reinforce those responses that are hopeful. Reminding her of God's care and love for her and God's presence with her all the time can be an encouragement. If Elsa responds that her favorite spiritual practices are reading scripture or other devotional material or praying, the nurse can participate with the client if he/she is comfortable doing so. The nurse should feel free to offer to participate in spiritual practices but should always obtain the client's permission before engaging in these practices. Other caring behaviors include the nurse's continued pres-

ence and therapeutic communication techniques of reflections and restatement. Clarification or silence can also be helpful. Share your concerns with her priest and ask him or other lay church members to come regularly. Find out if there is a parish nurse who could visit.

A month later the nurse learns that Elsa's son Peter was killed in a drinking-related accident. The nurse plans a visit. At the visit she finds Elsa very upset. The nurse learns Elsa was able to attend the funeral because her son John took her, but she hasn't heard from John since then. She tells the nurse that her daughter-in-law made all the funeral arrangements on her own, and although they had a visitation, Peter was cremated. Elsa was very disturbed by this and said that the church doesn't allow it. She was also very upset that her daughter-in-law had Peter "laid out with his baseball cap on." Her daughter-in-law told her, "I wanted him to have it on since he loved baseball so much." Elsa cried quietly while talking about this, then said, "There isn't any reason for me to be here now." She said one of her daughters did call her after the funeral, but Elsa doesn't care if the daughter visits her or not. Her medical condition remains unchanged.

Focus Questions

1. Identify the components of the grief process that Elsa is experiencing. How do these relate to her spiritual needs?

   Based on the new data, Elsa seems to be experiencing anger and resignation in the grief process. The death of a child, even though an adult, is significant. Spiritual concerns connected with the death include (a) implied fear of lack of a final spiritual security for her son because he was cremated, (b) discomfort with the daughter-in-law's choices, (c) sense of powerless to change circumstances, (d) hopelessness, (e) fear of the change in the family structure and the resulting impact in all areas of Elsa's life.

2. Identify how her spiritual nursing diagnosis may change based on this new data.

   Elsa has probably moved from Spiritual Distress to Spiritual Despair because she does not want to see family, she has a death wish, and she is suffering from severe depression and hopelessness, which are all symptoms of her despair.

3. Identify appropriate nursing interventions that could be offered based on this new data.

   Continue with previous spiritual interventions. Additional new interventions include contacting the priest for follow-up, connecting Elsa with a grief support group, and sharing scripture passages that gives comfort because of messages of eternal life.

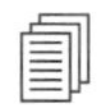

Reflective Writing

List your own beliefs, opinions, and biases related to spiritual care.

Describe how your personal definitions of religion and spirituality influence your nursing care.

What additional learning do you need in order to become competent in assessing spiritual needs and in providing spiritual care?

The answers to the questions are very individual to the student. The questions are posed to encourage the student to consider how their values and beliefs might impact the care of a person needing spiritual support. Nurses need to understand their own beliefs and values in order to recognize their own biases. Without this understanding nurses cannot show respect to clients regarding their beliefs and values. It should

always be the nurse's goal to provide spiritual care that meets the client's needs and not impose the nurse's beliefs on the client. (From the various readings, students will increase their knowledge regarding spiritual care, yet they may still feel uncomfortable in this role. This writing will help them express their fears and anxieties in helping the client with spiritual distress.)

References

Barnum, B. (1996). *Spirituality in nursing from traditional to new age.* New York: Springer Publishing Company.

Carson, V. (1989). *Spiritual dimensions of nursing practice.* Philadelphia: W. B. Saunders Company.

Dossey, B. (1998). Holistic modalities and healing moments, *American Journal of Nursing* 98, (6), 44–47.

Dossey, B. & Dossey, L. (1998). Body-mind-spirit: Attending to holistic care, *American Journal of Nursing,* 98, (8), 35–38.

Fish, S. & Shelly, J. (1983). *Spiritual care: The nurse's role,* 2nd ed. Madison, Wis.: Intervarsity Press.

Jost, K. (1995). Psychosocial care: Document it. *American Journal of Nursing 95,*(7), 46–49.

Mason, C. (1995). Prayer as a nursing intervention. *Journal of Christian Nursing,* 2(1), 4.

Shelly, J., John, S., & others, (1983). *Spiritual Dimensions of Mental Health,* Madison, Wis.: Intervarsity Press.

Stoll, R., ed. (1990). *Concepts in nursing: A christian perspective.* Madison, Wis.: Intervaristy Press.

Stoll, R. (1979). Guidelines for a spiritual assessment. *American Journal of Nursing 79;* 1574–1577.

Sumner, C. (1998). Recognizing and responding to spiritual distress. *American Journal of Nursing, 98,*(1), 26–31.